THE YOGI DIET

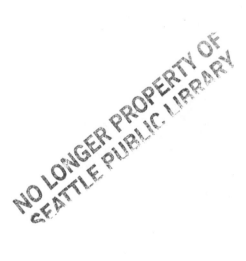

THE YOGI DIET

Spirituality and the
Question of Vegetarianism

James Morgante

PERMISSIONS GRANTED

Scriptural quotations: from the New Revised Standard Version Bible, copyright © 1989, Division of Christian Education of the National Council of the Churches of Christ in the USA. All rights reserved.

Text material: from Sri Aurobindo's *The Message of the Gita*, permission by Sri Aurobindo Ashram Trust, http://www.sriaurobindoashram.org/; from Gary Gran, permission by Gary Gran, ayurvedalessons.com and evanstonschoolofyoga.com; from *Sri Aurobindo and the Mother on Food*, permission by Vijay of The Sri Aurobindo Society, http://www.aurosociety.org/; from the works of Ellen G. White, permission by Ellen G. White Estate, Inc., http://www.whiteestate.org/; from George Ohsawa's *Zen Macrobiotics*, permission by the George Ohsawa Macrobiotic Foundation, www.OhsawaMacrobiotics.com; from Michio Kushi's *The Book of Macrobiotics*, permission by Alex Jack, http://www.amberwaves.org/; from Rudolf Steiner's lectures in *Nutrition and Stimulants, Lectures and Extracts*, permission by the Bio-Dynamic Farming and Gardening Association, Inc., https://www.biodynamics.com/; from the *Jivaka Sutta* [sic], permission by Bhikku Bhante Samāhita, "What the Buddha said in plain English!" http://whatbuddha-said.net/; from the work of Weston Price, permission by the Price-Pottenger Nutrition Foundation, http://ppnf.org/.

Illustrations: Macrobiotic pyramid and pie chart by permission of Alex Jack; Orthomolecular Health illustration by permission of the International Schizophrenia Foundation, http://www.orthomed.org/, http://www.helpyourselfcommunity.org/; *Mediterranean Diet Pyramid* illustrations by permission of Oldways Preservation and Exchange Trust, http://oldwayspt.org/; *Power Plate* illustration by permission of the Physicians Committee for Responsible Medicine, http://www.pcrm.org/; *Healing Foods Pyramid* illustration by permission of the Regents of the University of Michigan; low-carbohydrate pyramid by permission of Steve Aycock.

To Lady Wisdom, in all her multitudinous forms,
who wishes health for all her children;
and to all health seekers
who in seeking health seek Lady Wisdom

Contents

ILLUSTRATIONS

TABLES

FOREWORD

I am not a conspiracy theorist. But from the strange mélange of claims and counterclaims that cross each other every day, I could easily conclude that there is a pervasive conspiracy to delude and confuse the American public about diet.

Of course, you don't need to posit a conspiracy. In all probability, the confusion simply arises from the clamor of countless different voices, each of them proclaiming the supreme truth of its message and denigrating all the others.

Some of this din comes from the flocks of researchers promoting their own highly disparate findings. Often these findings are first hailed as breakthroughs and then disclaimed as errors. To take one example: One study in the 1990s found a correlation between tomato consumption and reduced risk of prostate cancer. But a 2007 news item from WebMD tells us, "The news that tomatoes could prevent prostate cancer sounded too good to be true, and apparently it was. . . . Subsequent studies have been either contradictory or inconclusive."[1]

Not so fast. Maybe tomatoes work after all. A BBC news item from 2014 asserts that "men who consume more than ten portions of tomatoes each week reduce their risk by about 20 percent, according to a UK study."[2]

To take another example, in recent times, we have witnessed supposedly authoritative opinion seesaw back and forth about the relative merits (and risks) of protein and carbohydrates. In one decade, it's fine to have a steak, as long as you don't have a baked potato with it; in the next decade, it's the other way around.

I'm reminded of my grandmother, who subscribed to J. I. Rodale's *Prevention* magazine in the 1960s. She gave it up because, she said,

"One month they tell you that milk is good for you, and the next month they tell you it isn't."

Even if you grant the validity of these findings, many of them raise the issue of sheer feasibility: what would I have to do in order to eat those ten portions of tomatoes a week? Perhaps I ought to forget about tomatoes and turn to broccoli. Three or four years ago my doctor told me that, according to the best research, if you ate two bushels of broccoli a day, you would never get any kind of cancer. (He was not actually recommending that I try this.)

The matter becomes still more perplexing when you add in the connection between diet and spiritual illumination. Spiritual teachers seem constantly to be pointing us toward foods that will allegedly put us on the fast track to enlightenment. Then there are the countless vegans and vegetarians who contend that by eating meat, you are simultaneously poisoning yourself and committing an atrocity.

For all these reasons, James Morgante's book *The Yogi Diet* is particularly welcome. In many ways, it is unique: it sets out a wide range of claims about diet (focusing on spiritual contexts) and tries to sort through them both humbly and objectively. Anyone who is interested in diet and spirituality should read this book. I do not know of any others that even attempt to be as fair and even handed.

To my mind, one of the most important statements in this book comes from Sri Aurobindo: "Food . . . is a question of hygiene, and prohibitions laid down in ancient religions had more a hygienic than a spiritual motive." For example, he adds, "Tamasic food [from the Sanskrit *tamas*, "darkness"] . . . is what is stale or rotten with the virtue gone out of it."

Hygiene, I believe, has been far more pervasive a factor in diet than it may seem. Take one thing explored here: the Greek philosopher Pythagoras's curious prohibition against eating beans. The wildest explanations have been given for this taboo. Here is the biographer Diogenes Laertius, citing Aristotle: Pythagoras forbade the eating of beans "either because they resemble some part of the human body, or because they are like the gates of hell (for they are the only plants without parts); or because they dry up other plants, or because they are representatives of universal nature, or because they are used in elections in oligarchical governments."[3]

In short, by the time of Aristotle, two hundred years after Pythagoras, it was impossible to tell why Pythagoras had forbidden beans.

In my book *Forbidden Faith: The Secret History of Gnosticism,* I wrote, citing the belief that Pythagoras studied in Egypt:

> The simplest explanation [for this prohibition] appears in Herodotus: "The Egyptians sow no beans in their country; if any grow, they will not eat them either raw or cooked; the priests cannot endure even to see them, considering beans an unclean kind of pulse." If indeed Pythagoras studied in Egypt, he might have picked up this food taboo, much as an American today who studies spirituality in India or Japan may become a vegetarian.[4]

This idea made (and makes) sense to me, but the theory has another twist. After my book was published, a woman wrote to me and pointed out that the only beans known in the Old World were fava beans (also known as broad beans), and fava beans can cause medical conditions such as oxidative stress and hemolytic anemia.[5]

We are back to hygiene. Pythagoras may have picked up this food taboo from the Egyptians, but it may have been instituted in the first place because fava beans can make some people sick. Since the exact mechanism of the cause was unknown, it seemed safer to prohibit beans entirely.

Another item that struck me was in Morgante's concise and intelligent account of the traditional Hindu diet based on the three *gunas,* or "principles," each of which describes a type of temperament and has foods related to it. One, *tamas,* is "darkness." We have already seen how tamasic food is "stale and rotten with the virtue gone out of it." As Morgante quotes on page 9 of this book, the Bhagavad Gita tells us also that "the tamasic temperament . . . even accepts like the animals the remnants half eaten by others" (Bhagavad Gita 17:7–10).

But who would accept food left over by others? Only a very poor person. This casts a new light on the Hindu dietary scheme. The first guna, *sattva,* is equated with harmony and knowledge, while the second, *rajas,* refers, in Morgante's words, to "energy, motion, passion, struggle, and effort." It is then easy to see how the gunas relate to the four castes: Brahmins, the priests and teachers, would be most likely to eat sattwic food, promoting clarity and serenity; Kshatriyas, the warrior caste, would favor stimulating rajasic food; while the lower castes would be drawn toward the tamasic, which might include items left over from higher-caste meals.

This schema fits in perfectly with the traditional Hindu perspective. The three gunas are universal; they exist everywhere. They are expressed in the system of castes (portrayed in Hindu texts, such as the Laws of Manu, as an organic part of the universe), in the temperaments, and in the foods that are best suited for those temperaments. While few today would care to see a return of the caste system, it does reflect a unified and organic view of the universe.

What constitutes the most desirable sattvic food? If readers today were asked to guess, many would no doubt think of dishes like those served in, say, a hippie restaurant from 1972. Not quite. As Morgante shows, the lists usually include such present-day dietary malefactors as butter and sugar.

In the mid-1970s I chanced to have dinner at a Hare Krishna community in Boston's Back Bay. The dinner was free, but I did not think the food was very good. I remember that it was extraordinarily sweet and sugary, and rather unsubstantial. Was this a low-grade diet that the crafty cult leaders were inflicting to keep their minions subjugated, or were they simply following the traditional sattvic yogi diet?

Another fascinating point in this book has to do with traditional diets. Morgante discusses the work of the early twentieth-century dentist Weston A. Price, who did a comparative study of dental caries. Surveying people around the world, he found a wild variance in caries between those who followed "traditional diets" and those who followed "modern diets." Among Seminole Indians, for example, of those who followed the traditional diet, only 4 percent had caries, while the percentage of those who followed a modern diet was 40 percent. But viewed globally, as Morgante writes, "No single diet . . . was the 'key' to robust health." In fact, the diets of healthy groups had little in common. "Some were high in protein and fat and based almost entirely on animal foods or fish; others contained various mixtures of plant and animal foods. But all these diets produced healthy teeth . . . and excellent health" (page 95).

Price had his own theories about this phenomenon, but I might note the one thing that these diets all had in common was that they were *traditional*. That is, people in those areas had been eating these foods for centuries if not millennia. Could it be that the most important factor in a healthy diet, for any given population, is simply long habituation? Humans adapt to different environments in all sorts of ways; why should they not also adapt to local food? In that case, Seminole Indians might see higher rates of caries, not only if they followed modern diets, but if they followed other traditional diets as well.

This has disturbing implications for Americans. Like the Athenians, who "spent their time in nothing else, but either to tell, or to hear some new thing" (Acts 17:21), we are constantly in search of novelty—in diet above all things. For us it would be hard to say what a traditional diet would consist of, since American diets change radically, often over the course of a generation or two.

Here is a snapshot from the past—the diet of an ordinary family in Muncie, Indiana, around 1890, as described by a housewife: "steak, roasts, macaroni, Irish potatoes, sweet potatoes, turnips, cole slaw, fried apples, and stewed tomatoes, with Indian pudding, rice, cake or pie for dessert." This was the diet in the winter. In this season, "we never thought of having fresh fruit or green vegetables and could not have got them if we had." As a result, most people suffered from "spring sickness," remedied by sarsaparilla and "salads of all sorts" as soon as they became available. In any case, meat was served universally, and many people did not believe that a meal was complete without it.

By the 1920s, this picture had changed somewhat, and it was increasingly possible to get fresh fruit and vegetables throughout the winter. There was also a trend toward more use of commercial canned foods.[6]

I am not suggesting this diet as a norm or a benchmark; it is simply a glimpse of what typical Americans ate over a century ago. Obviously many changes have taken place since then, including, as

Morgante points out, a move away from meat. The trend is accelerated by the constant stream of new health foods, whose value is, almost always, at best unproven—and by the strange metamorphosis of these health foods into junk foods. Yogurt starts as a beneficial fermented milk and ends as soft ice cream; Dr. Kellogg's wholesome cornflakes morph into Count Chocula. A recent *New York Times* article claims that today's granola is more of a dessert than a genuine breakfast food.[7] Even Coca-Cola started as a health tonic.

One of the central themes in Morgante's book is vegetarianism, which is so widespread today that we tend to forget that it is by no means universal—certainly not as a matter of preference. A traditional Chinese peasant might have eaten little or no meat, but it was very likely not a matter of choice. Rather, it is the omnivorous diet that is universal. Vegetarianism is possibly an innovation of the Indian subcontinent. The great religions of India—Hinduism, Buddhism, and Jainism—all espouse it to certain degrees, and it is most prevalent where the influence of those religions is the strongest. On page 113, Morgante writes:

> A survey of the major traditions reveals a remarkably mixed picture. In the Far East, Hinduism supports vegetarianism, yet with qualifications; Buddhism's two major traditions—the Hinayana and Mahayana—are largely at odds, one opposing and the other supporting vegetarianism; Jainism requires vegetarianism; Sikhism rejects it. Among the Abrahamic traditions of the Near East (Judaism, Christianity, and Islam), vegetarianism plays no outwardly significant role.

I personally suspect that the doctrine of *ahimsa* ("harmlessness"), as entailing a prohibition of meat, was the innovation of Mahavira, the founder of Jainism in the sixth century, and spread to Hinduism and Buddhism thereafter. In regard to Buddhism, Morgante writes: "Daisetz Suzuki . . . says that advocacy for vegetarianism was a later response to criticism. . . . Followers of Jainism, in particular, criticized Buddhists for the seemingly inconsistent way of applying ahimsa" (page 124). As Morgante also notes, the earliest Buddhist texts show no sign of advocating vegetarianism. In Hinduism, vegetarian strictures were enjoined upon the Brahmin caste chiefly.

Vegetarianism has been known in the West since antiquity. Pythagoras, in the sixth century BCE, was the best-known exponent of the practice, and even up to the nineteenth century vegetarianism was sometimes called "the Pythagorean diet." Where did Pythagoras get his aversion to meat? It is tempting to think that in some way it goes back to India, because other elements of Pythagoras's teaching, including reincarnation and number mysticism, share features of Indian thought. But there is no direct evidence for a connection, so the idea must remain speculative.[8]

The Pythagorean magus of Tyana, who lived in the first century CE, was said to be a vegetarian, following the example of his master. Apollonius's biographer, Philostratus, has him saying, "My abstention from animal food comes from [Pythagoras's] wisdom."[9] Although Philostratus's biography dates over a century after Apollonius's lifetime, the claim that he was a vegetarian was probably true.

The rise of vegetarianism in the modern West, which has taken place largely since the nineteenth century, is best seen as the result of Eastern influence through such mediums as H. P. Blavatsky's Theosophy. (The Theosophical Society was founded in 1875.) Although Blavatsky was not a vegetarian herself, early Theosophists were encouraged to follow a vegetarian diet; and Blavatsky's successor, Annie Besant, preached it energetically as one of her many causes. Later in the twentieth century, this practice spread along with Hindu and Buddhist movements in general.

Until recently, then, vegetarianism was regarded as an import vaguely connected with Eastern religion. The picture changed in 1975, with the publication of *Animal Liberation* by the Australian philosopher Peter Singer. Singer preached vegetarianism on grounds based on utilitarian philosophy, classically formulated by Jeremy Bentham and John Stuart Mill. Utilitarianism argues that moral judgments should be based (only or at any rate principally) on their consequences—promoting pleasure and preventing pain. Since animals are capable of feeling pain, it is mere "speciesism" (Singer's term) to restrict these criteria to the human race alone and make animals suffer by killing and eating them. Vegetarian, and later, vegan ideals were further advanced by the perception that large-scale animal husbandry causes a great deal of environmental damage.

Certainly these arguments have helped promote the move toward a more plant-based diet that Morgante discusses.

I myself have always been unsympathetic to vegetarianism and veganism, not as personal choices, but as proselytizing religions. From the perspective of spirituality, in the end I must rely on my own knowledge and experience. And my experience is this: I have been privileged to know a number of people over the years who seemed to me spiritually advanced. Practically none of these people were vegetarians, and none of them regarded it as a serious issue.

On the other hand, many vegans and vegetarians display an arrogant self-righteousness. I find this off-putting, of course, but I am also led to the conclusion that proselytizing in this way is a sign of limited spiritual development, a certain type of ego inflation that manifests in ideologies of all kinds. When you think about it, it is enormously presumptuous to tell the world what it ought to eat, when it is quite clear that individual (and collective) needs vary tremendously.

The arguments cited in favor of abstaining from meat do not always carry as far as one might think. Take the question of the cruelty of the meat industry: only a fool would pretend that it does not exist. But what would stop it? Boycotting meat altogether? Or pressing the industry to hew to high standards of humaneness? The industry is not likely to pay much attention to the people who are trying to put it out of business.

I could go further. Consider the population of horses and mules in the United States. This peaked at 25 million in 1920. By 1940, it had fallen to around 14 million. Although there were several reasons for this drop, the principal one was the mechanization of the American farm. By 1945 tractors had replaced draft animals on most US farms. Horses and mules were not needed nearly as much, and so fewer of them were bred. The US horse population was estimated at 9 million in 2005.[10]

Undoubtedly there are fewer horses mistreated than there were a hundred years ago. But then there are many fewer horses.

Similarly, if the meat industry were to be eliminated, fewer farm animals would be mistreated, but there would also be many fewer than there are now. Which leads to this Dostoevskian question: is it better to exist as an exploited farm animal, or not to exist at all?

I am not so much attempting to refute anti-meat arguments as to show that the issue is by no means as clear as one might pretend. And while I respect the dietary choices of vegans and vegetarians, I would like for many of them to show a similar respect for the choices of others.

One thing that particularly impresses me about *The Yogi Diet* is the modesty of its conclusions. In the end Morgante, speaking from his own experience, simply recommends a breakfast of whole grains. This is a refreshing contrast to most books on this subject, which proclaim the superiority of their dietary claims with the assurance of revealed scripture.

We are left asking what the best diet is for oneself. In the first place, I think it is useful to remember that this very question is a luxury that most people in the history of the world—and many people in the world today—could not afford to ask. For them, it is not an issue of what picks they should make out of a cornucopia of abundance, but whether they will be able to get enough food at all.

In the second place, if we go back to diet and the spiritual path, I think we come down to one central fact: The spiritual path is, at its core, a process of growth in self-knowledge. If you do not follow the old Delphic dictum "Know thyself," you are probably not on anything that genuinely resembles a path, whatever you think. And self-knowledge takes place at many levels. At the level we are talking about here, it has to do with the best diet you can follow for yourself. Some may need meat; some should avoid it. Some should eat plenty of grains; some should stay away from them. You have the right, and, I would add, the obligation to look into this question for yourself. But I don't believe you have the right to dictate the answer for others.

–RICHARD SMOLEY, Winfield, Illinois, October 2016

RICHARD SMOLEY is the author of books including *How God Became God: What Scholars Are Really Saying about God and the Bible; The Deal: A Guide to Radical and Complete Forgiveness; Supernatural: Writings on an Unknown History; The Dice Game of Shiva: How Consciousness Creates the Universe; Conscious Love: Insights from Mystical Christianity; Forbidden Faith: The Secret History of Gnosticism; The Essential Nostradamus; Inner Christianity: A Guide to the Esoteric Tradition;* and *Hidden Wisdom: A Guide to the Western Inner Traditions* (with Jay Kinney). He is editor of *Quest: Journal of the Theosophical Society in America.* His website is innerchristianity.com.

ACKNOWLEDGMENTS

Acknowledgements are due to the following persons: to my parents for providing the funding that allowed my taking a sabbatical year to complete the manuscript; to all cited authors and references for helpful inspiration and information; to friend, colleague, and editor Connie Eichenlaub for reviewing the original manuscript and making helpful suggestions; to my cousin John LaSpina for convincing me that the use of a pseudonym was a bad idea and insulting to my deceased father; to his wife, Barbara Sardarov, for help with myriad activities, including finding the missing page number to a reference in the box in the basement; to Lee Tillman, proprietor of the Admiral Junction Mailing Center, for facilitating the printing, mailing, and billing of proposals via email; to book agent Sheree Bykofsky for the critique that led to a helpful edit and for getting at least a look from several publishers; to editor Paul Dinas for pointing away from the wrong direction toward the right one; to friend and reader Kenneth Ingham, PhD, for insisting on the chapter-become-an-appendix becoming a chapter again (thereby restoring the original eight-chapter octave principle); to friends and readers Michael Martin, PhD, and Tim Marzen, PhD, for providing reviews that were helpful to a proposal; to the former editors of Quest Books, Sharron Dorr and Richard Smoley (before Quest decided to cease publishing operations)—to Richard for finding value in the original manuscript, to both for the many suggestions that led to fruitful additions and changes, and to Sharron for helping to prepare the manuscript for self-publication; to Marianne Arin for financial support with editing costs; to all acquaintances, relatives, and friends for interest, enthusiasm, support, and assurances of buying a copy (I hope you also read it and derive benefit from it); and lastly, once again, to everyone for an effort that was truly collaborative in ways I could not imagine.

INTRODUCTION

This book is entitled *The Yogi Diet* because the spiritual dietary teachings it explores begin with the tradition of ancient India and eventually end there, while it also considers the teachings of other diverse traditions and points of view.

The word *yoga*, from the Sanskrit root *yuj*, "to yoke," means "union" in the sense of union with the Divine. In ancient India, the practice of yoga was woven into the fabric of society itself and concerned everyone, especially in life's later stages. In this sense, *The Yogi Diet* is about a diet not just for yogis, but for everyone— everyone, that is, who acknowledges a spiritual dimension to life and seeks to cultivate it.

The Yogi Diet aims to foster the development of wisdom, or sound judgment, about vegetarianism and the role it should play in one's life, if at all. Its viewpoint is first and foremost spiritual, which is to say that spiritual teachings about spiritual dietary effects are highlighted, but the ultimate concern is holistic health, or the health of body, mind, and spirit, and so other points of view are also considered, including the views of contemporary nutritional paradigms.

The book's method is more descriptive than prescriptive, meaning that sometimes conflicting or even contradictory information is presented side by side. Conflict between opposing points of view in this sense is methodological, and intuiting what is right for oneself is necessary to resolve it. Nutrition, like politics and religion, is a controversial subject, requiring individual discernment.

Besides vegetarianism, the book's other major theme is the new carbohydrate foods of the agricultural revolution such as grains that are essential to a vegetarian diet but have come under increased

scrutiny and even criticism through the low-carbohydrate movement. Here, too, conflicting views require resolution and intuition.

The first five chapters focus on vegetarianism in the context of
holistic health and spiritual views and find that good reasons exist
both for and against vegetarianism, and so caution and discernment are necessary. The final three chapters focus on carbohydrates
and grains, providing the information for a final answer—the biblical ideal of a vegan diet in the book of Genesis (chapter 1) can
only be realized in the distant future when human evolutionary
development will have climaxed and animal foods are no longer
necessary. Until then, the role and form of vegetarianism in anyone's life necessarily becomes an individual question.

Chapter 1 introduces the Bhagavad Gita's teaching as the archetype for spiritual dietary instruction. The Gita does not name
specific foods, but instead talks about dietary effects, essentially
recommending a holistic diet nourishing body, mind, and spirit
together. Yet the question arises as to whether meat can be included in such a diet, which seems to be the case, at least for yogis of
the high Tibetan plateau where meat is eaten for warmth. A final
answer is left open pending additional information.

Chapter 2 focuses on spiritual dietary effects and the religious
and spiritual teachings that discuss them. Many, but not all, such
teachings advocate vegetarianism, and what emerges are advantages and disadvantages to both vegetal and animal foods.

Chapter 3 takes up dietary psychological effects as indicated by
orthomolecular medicine and the work of Weston Price, suggesting
the importance of whole foods and grains in particular, but also parental diet (for healthy embryo structures) and the soil (for nutrient
content) as well.

Chapter 4 focuses on physical dietary effects in the view of modern nutritional paradigms. The trend toward vegetal foods is contrast-
ed with the animal-foods emphasis of low-carbohydrate paradigms.
At the heart of the debate are the carbohydrate and fat hypotheses
of disease. A potential resolution points to the confounding health
effect of mixing fats and carbohydrates—either alone can be healthy
to the extent that the other is limited. A lingering question, however,
is whether some form of animal food is necessary for physical health.

Chapter 5 addresses religious and spiritual views on the question of vegetarianism specifically by surveying the major traditions of the East and West. The result is ambiguity and an unequivocal "yes" and "no" response. The consequence is the call for ethical sources of animal foods, as exemplified by those traditions with religious slaughtering practices.

Chapter 6 takes up carbohydrates and grains, discussing their historical and cultural importance and their critique from a low-carbohydrate point of view.

Chapter 7 takes up the three major dietary types (low carbohydrate, low fat, and low calorie) and contrasts advantages and disadvantages from a spiritual point of view.

Chapter 8 takes up the critique of carbohydrates and points to the transformations that are necessary, for foods and for human beings, to make carbohydrates fully nourishing. This transformational perspective includes human evolutionary development, the culmination of which finally allows veganism to become possible in a healthy way. The relationship between veganism and human evolutionary development is the final criterion offered for attaining sound judgment about vegetarianism.

THE YOGI DIET began as my master's thesis in a holistic psychology program some thirty-five years ago ("Nutrition, Consciousness, Spiritual Teachings, and Scientific Models"). My attempt to relate spiritual teachings about dietary consciousness effects to scientific models was not fully satisfying. It was only after completing the thesis that I encountered Rudolf Steiner's indications (reviewed in chapter 2), which seemed to offer greater insight. I included Steiner in a postscript and hoped to take up the subject again in the future.

This impulse received new impetus years later through my fleeting contact with the low-carbohydrate movement and then a chance conversation with a health professional, undoubtedly of the low-carbohydrate persuasion, who disparaged grains and religious myths characterizing them as "gifts of the gods." To him, this idea was yet another example of religion's deleterious cultural effects. Knowing the importance of grains, not just in spiritual teachings but in the agricultural revolution and modern food paradigms as well, I decided that any reworking of the topic of spirituality and nutrition would also need to focus on grains.

Knowing the range of views among spiritual teachings on diet, when I finally took up the project again I already anticipated the "yes" and "no" response to vegetarianism that comes at the end of chapter 5. Yet knowing also the trend toward vegetal foods among modern paradigms, I expected a net "plus" to accrue to vegetal foods and a net "minus" to animal foods, tipping the scales.

This developmental plan ran along smoothly until my full encounter with the low-carbohydrate movement in chapter 6. I anticipated that the movement would reveal itself as regressive because of its emphasis on animal foods. To my surprise, however, I found myself impressed with the evidence in favor of animal foods and against the agricultural revolution and carbohydrates like grains. I also began to penetrate more deeply the conflict between the carbohydrate and fat hypotheses of disease that accounts to some extent for the biases for or against animal or vegetal foods. Reflecting on the ambivalence of spiritual teachings toward vegetarianism, which also included positive assessments of meat, I concluded that the low-carbohydrate movement was not regressive at all but instead provided an important brake to hastily embracing vegetal foods, vegetarianism, and especially veganism.

Resultantly, the book's shape and contents changed. Chapter 4 grew to include the case for animal foods, the low-carbohydrate movement as an alternative health paradigm, and an attempt to reconcile the carbohydrate and fat hypotheses. Weston Price's influence led to questioning whether animal food in some form was necessary to physical health, and chapter 3 grew to include his research into the relationship between diet and mental functioning. Chapter 6 grew to include the Paleo dietary revival and the arguments against carbohydrates and the agricultural revolution. Chapter 7, which originally intended to emphasize the value of low-fat/high-carbohydrate diets, grew to include their negative side, the positive side of low-carbohydrate diets, and the value of mixed diets. Chapter 8, which was not in the original plan at all, became necessary to deal with the critique of carbohydrates and finally to resolve the enigma of a biblical injunction in favor of carbohydrates. The epilogue was also added to reemphasize important points about animal foods and the framework in which vegetarianism must be considered.

In short, much changed regarding the book's contents, but more importantly regarding my own thinking. As a result, I want to express a deep debt of gratitude to the low-carbohydrate movement for stimulation culminating in a more balanced and deeper presentation.

The low-carbohydrate movement's significance was one unforeseen development. Others also came to light: the importance of the Blood-Type Diet and the many issues relating to blood types (see chapters 4, 7, and 8); the relationship of creation mythology and sacrificial rituals to meat eating and the communion meal of Jesus as the culmination of this mythology and these rituals (see chapter 5 and appendix A); the importance and troubled history of the vegetarian undercurrent in the Abrahamic traditions of Judaism, Christianity, and Islam (see chapter 5); and the significance of grain cultivation and the application to the biblical tradition's enigmatical vegan command (see chapters 6 and 8).

In the face of all these surprising developments, I can only acknowledge having held the ship's wheel during the journey of research and writing, but not having determined the course or final destination. In a paradoxical but real way, I have been this book's "reader" as well as writer. Perhaps that always has been and always will be the experience of authors everywhere. In any case, the process has been personally enlightening in many ways.

THE YOGI DIET has three intended audiences: religious believers and spiritual seekers; low-carbohydrate proponents; and vegetarians, especially vegans.

To the religious and spiritually inclined, the book's message is that diet has health significance beyond that of the body embracing the spirit and spiritual development. The consequence is not simplistic advocacy for vegetarianism because it has advantages and disadvantages. Fully understanding both benefits and detriments and applying them to one's life is what is essential.

The message to low-carbohydrate proponents is likewise that diet has spiritual significance, but with an emphasis on the potential detriments of animal foods. The consequence is not a rejection of animal foods, but understanding the health consequences of excess and balancing both sides of the animal/vegetal equation.

The message to vegetarians and especially vegans is the potentially negative effects of vegetal diets and the benefits of animal foods. Such seemingly surprising or even offensive assertions are well-articulated parts of the cultural tradition and worthy of attention. Balance is the key for everyone, and the perspective of an evolutionary journey may help to temper impatience about fully realizing the ideal in the present.

1

DIET AND THE BHAGAVAD GITA

We begin the exploration of spirituality and diet with Hinduism, reputed to be the world's oldest living religious tradition,[1] and the Bhagavad Gita, one of Hinduism's most revered spiritual texts. The Gita, also known as the Holy, Celestial, or Divine Song, is an episode within the great epic poem the Mahabharata and contains the spiritual instruction given to the warrior Arjuna on the eve of a great battle by Lord Krishna, an incarnation of the Divine.

In the story, Arjuna's resolve to fight is wavering due to uncertainty about the righteousness of participating in a battle against his own kinsmen. Krishna encourages him to fight by explaining how this battle fits within the divine plan and also uses the opportunity to provide Arjuna with the orientation that will lead him past all life's difficulties toward the final goal of salvation.

Part of that orientation involves diet, and what Krishna tells Arjuna about diet is related to three primal qualities, or modes of energy, that exist in nature and everything and are called *gunas*. Their names are *sattva* (or *sattwa*), *rajas*, and *tamas*. Because the gunas are a key to understanding the Gita's dietary teaching, it is important to review their significance:

> Sattwa is by the purity of its quality a cause of light and illumination, and by virtue of that purity produces no disease or morbidity or suffering in the nature . . .

> Rajas . . . has for its essence attraction of liking and longing; it is a child of the attachment of the soul to the desire of objects; . . .

> But Tamas . . . born of ignorance, is the deluder of all embodied beings. . . .

7

> Sattwa attaches to happiness, rajas to action . . . ; tamas covers
> up knowledge and attaches to negligence of error and inaction.
>
> (Bhagavad Gita 14:6–9)[2]

Another guna commentary relates sattva to equilibrium, harmony, balance, sympathy, virtue, and knowledge; rajas to energy, motion, passion, struggle, and effort; and tamas to inertia, inconscience, ignorance, incapacity, darkness, and obscurity.[3]

When the gunas manifest in different things of the world, one or the other may dominate. When they manifest in humans, however, the interaction between them is dynamic and ever-changing:

> Now sattva leads, having overpowered rajas and tamas . . . now rajas, having overpowered sattva and tamas; and now tamas, having overpowered sattva and rajas.
>
> When into all the doors in the body there comes a flooding of light, a light of understanding, perception and knowledge, one should understand that there has been a great increase and uprising of the sattwa guna in the nature.
>
> Greed, seeking impulsions, initiative of actions; unrest, desire—all this mounts in us when rajas increases.
>
> Nescience, inertia, negligence and delusion—these are born when tamas predominates.
>
> (Bhagavad Gita 14:10–13)[4]

The spiritual path outlined by the Gita involves the pursuit of "free spiritual consciousness," and on this quest, the gunas must be transcended because all of them bind the spirit to nature: sattva binds through attachment to knowledge and happiness; rajas through attachment to works; and tamas to negligence, indolence, and sleep (Bhagavad Gita 14:6–8.)[5] Yet sattva is the "mediator between the higher and lower nature" and should be strengthened first because its power is useful for transcending the restraints of the others. Once those have been transcended, sattva's own restraints are then easier to shed.[6]

A final point is that the gunas represent *tendencies* towards qualities, but not the qualities themselves: "Sattva guna is the tendency towards purity but is not purity itself. Similarly rajas guna is that force which tends to create action but is not action itself."[7]

What this means is that guna tendency does not always determine the manifested quality, which remains changeable. We will see some examples with foods.

The above understanding of the gunas prepares us now to better understand the Gita's teaching on diet:

> The food...which is dear to each [human] is of triple character. ...Hear...the distinction of these.
>
> The sattvic temperament . . . turns naturally to things that increase the life, increase the inner and outer strength, nourish at once the mental, vital and physical force and increase the pleasure and satisfaction and happy condition of mind and life and body, all that is succulent and soft and firm and satisfying.
>
> The rajasic temperament prefers naturally food that is violently sour, pungent, hot, acrid, rough and strong and burning, the aliments that increase ill-health and the distempers of the mind and body.
>
> The tamasic temperament takes a perverse pleasure in cold, impure, stale, rotten, or tasteless food or even accepts like the animals the remnants half-eaten by others.
>
> (Bhagavad Gita 17:7–10)[8]

We see, hopefully not with too much disappointment, that the Gita is adept at throwing curves. While we expect or would like particular foods to be associated with the various gunas, they are associated instead with human temperaments. Some food characteristics (succulent, sour, and stale) are named, but the Gita's focus is on health effects. This is the reason for preferring the sattvic temperament's choice.

As for those health effects, we see that the Gita's conception is holistic, or all-inclusive. The choice of the sattvic temperament nourishes inner and outer strength; the mental, vital, and physical forces; and mind, life, and body together. Of the three forces that are named, the vital is undoubtedly unfamiliar. It embraces the realm of desires, impulses, and passions.[9] This holistic conception of dietary effects on various human dimensions is a recurring theme among spiritual teachings that we will see again in the chapter ahead.

In sum, the Bhagavad Gita's dietary teaching relates the gunas to human temperaments and to food choices made by those temperaments, but not to specific foods. A few descriptive characteristics and the health effects that result are named, but foods themselves are not named. The question, of course, that remains concerns any application to individual foods. In turning to interpretations, we see that commentators do relate the gunas to specific foods. Yet opinions vary, and other important considerations also come into play.

INTERPRETING THE GITA'S DIETARY TEACHING

Jayadayol Goyandka, before commenting on the Gita's teaching, refers to a passage from the Chhandogya Upanishad (7.26.2).[10] Further research led me to find the passage as follows:

> Now is described the discipline for inner purification by which Self-Knowledge is attained:
>
> When the food is pure, the mind becomes pure.
> When the mind is pure the memory becomes firm.
> When the memory is firm all ties are loosened.[11]

Goyandka cites this passage because purity is a sattva-related theme and then matches the gunas with individual foods:

- Sattva: Milk, clarified butter, vegetables, fruits, sugar, wheat, barley, rice, and other grains

- Rajas: Tamarind, lemon, overly hot foods, chilies, parched grains, mustard seeds; foods that cause discomforts like a burning sensation or watering of the eyes

- Tamas: Meat and eggs (because they involve the destruction of life); liquor, drugs, and tobacco; foods that lack succulence due to overcooking, spoiling, or being out of season; foods that smell offensively like garlic and onion, and those that are "foul" due to fermentation or chemical processing[12]

Although Goyandka designates grains as sattvic, he adds that parching makes them rajasic and overcooking, tamasic. Here we see that the guna tendency is not fixed, but malleable and subject to change. (A similar indication notes that sattvic foods can become rajasic or tamasic through the addition of excess salt, spice, or sugar.)[13]

Swami Prabhupada, another commentator, matches the gunas with foods in the following way:

- Sattva: Dairy, sugar, rice, wheat, and fruits and vegetables because they are pure by nature, increase life's duration, and aid physical and mental health

- Rajas: Foods that are overly bitter, salty, or hot, producing mucus and leading to misery and disease

- Tamas: Meat, which is "untouchable" because it involves unnecessary killing; liquor (also untouchable); foods that are spoiled or have been cooked more than three hours prior to eating (unless blessed!)[14]

In these designations, we see a close similarity to those of Goyandka above.

Dr. Rudolph Ballentine, however, emphasizes a more dynamic understanding of the relationship between the gunas and foods. With respect, for example, to meat (designated as tamasic by both Goyandka and Prabhupada), he differentiates between tamasic and rajasic,[15] which a more dynamic understanding allows.

Tamasic foods create heaviness and lethargy and add substance to the body, but they do not increase "energy, vitality and consciousness." Producing restlessness and irritability, they can lead to cruel and thoughtless actions. Processed and chemically treated foods acting as irritants are tamasic, as are alcohol and meat tainted with toxins that result from cellular degeneration.

Yet although decayed meat would be considered tamasic, Ballentine notes that the ancients considered fresh fish and wild game that were properly prepared—and meat, too—as rajasic. Such foods energize, yet in an unbalanced way, impelling toward activity. They promote aggressive, worldly behavior, qualities that were considered appropriate for soldiers, rulers, and politicians who played an active role in life. Spiced foods that stimulate the appetite and sensual pleasure and can lead to overeating are also rajasic, as are coffee, tea, and tobacco (Goyandka designates tobacco as tamasic).

Ballentine continues that the purpose of the guna system was not to judge food goodness or healthiness, but to clarify effects so that diet could be chosen according to need. Meat and wine were considered appropriate for rulers but forbidden to Brahmins (scholars, teachers, and spiritual seekers) due to overly stimulating effects. The sattvic foods appropriate to Brahmins promote "calm alertness" and a "state of quiet energy," nourishing both body and consciousness and adding steady inner vitality instead of weighing one down (tamasic) or pushing one beyond one's capacity (rajasic). Sattvic foods promote inner strength, not the muscular strength that comes from rajasic foods. Sattvic foods supreme are fresh fruit, grains, and raw, fresh milk. Sour or spoiled milk, however, becomes tamasic.

Despite the differences between Ballentine and previous commentators, there are also similarities. Like the others, he considers milk, grains, and fruit as sattvic. Yet his distinction between rajasic and tamasic meat and the notion of food appropriateness according to effect and need (meat and wine being appropriate for rulers) add new dimensions to the discussion.

Sri Aurobindo is a commentator who questions the concern with sattvic food at all, emphasizing instead hygienic and health effects. He also cautions about fixed associations between the gunas and foods:

> I think the importance of sattwic [sic] food from a spiritual point of view has been exaggerated. Food is rather a question of

hygiene, and many of the sanctions and prohibitions laid down in ancient religions had more a hygienic than a spiritual motive. The Gita's definitions seem to point in the same direction—tamasic food, it seems to say, is what is stale or rotten with the virtue gone out of it, rajasic food is that which is too acrid, pungent, etc., heats the blood and spoils the health, sattwic food is what is pleasing, healthy, etc. It may well be that different kinds of food nourish the action of the different gunas and so are directly helpful or harmful apart from their physical action. But that is as far as one can go confidently. What particular eatables are or are not sattwic is another question and more difficult to determine. Spiritually, I should say that the effect of food depends more on the occult atmosphere and influences that come with it than on anything in the food itself.[16]

Aurobindo's comments are important for several reasons. While not denying a relationship between the gunas and particular foods, he questions a simplistic identification, just as we have heard that the gunas represent tendencies, not fixed qualities, and that sattvic rice becomes rajasic or tamasic through cooking, and meat is either rajasic or tamasic depending on freshness. Moreover, Aurobindo stresses that health and hygienic effects are the most important considerations, which appear to be the Bhagavad Gita's own concerns. As for "occult atmosphere and influences," the compiler of Sri Aurobindo's remarks relates that these can include the consciousness of growers, cooks, and servers that is passed on to foods and perceptible to those who are sensitive, vibrations and energies in the environment, and even the manner of cooking.[17]

Commenting not on the Bhagavad Gita but on the sattvic diet, Gary Gran, a yoga teacher and Ayurvedic practitioner, stresses flexibility, noting that the yogic attitude toward animal foods depends on criteria like indulgence:

Yogis are advised not to indulge in flesh foods. It is said that the fear and anger of the animal being killed is transferred to the person eating the flesh. Fresh meat is considered rajasic, and old meat is considered tamasic. Another approach is to avoid the flesh of mammals, especially if one is using dairy products.

How can one eat the flesh of one's (symbolic) mother? This approach allows for some high-quality fish, poultry or eggs. Even then it is recommended to abstain from flesh foods a minimum of three days a week with at least two prolonged periods of abstention from all animal foods every year. Purists rely on dairy for supplemental protein as it is given freely and is considered non-harming.[18]

Gran also notes, like Ballentine, that in yoga and Ayurvedic practice, food effects are observed so that each individual can determine the makeup of a sattvic diet; moreover, that yogis in high-altitude Tibet sometimes eat meat for warmth because vegetarian diets tend to have a cooling effect.[19]

Gran's remarks also point to an emphasis on health effects and raise the additional questions of whether a sattvic diet can include meat and, if so, to what extent. These are questions to ask now while awaiting the input of further points of view.

In summarizing the Gita's teaching and the various commentaries, we can say the following:

- Foods may have inherent guna qualities, but these are malleable tendencies depending on variables like quality (in the case of meat) and preparation (in the case of rice).

- Dietary appropriateness depends on guna effect and social activity and role, but most importantly on health effects. The preferred sattvic choice imparts inner and outer strength while nourishing the mental, vital, and physical forces—life, body, and mind—together.

The Bhagavad Gita's dietary framework is holistic and focuses on health effects. In the chapters ahead, we will examine in more detail this idea of beneficial effects on the entire human being, beginning with other spiritual teachings that share a holistic perspective and whose special concern is effects on the spirit and spiritual development.

2

NOURISHING THE SPIRIT: RELIGIOUS AND SPIRITUAL TEACHINGS

A holistic point of view is a recent development in modern thinking. Only since the last half of the twentieth century has it become more common in fields such as sociology and science.[1] Philosophy and religion, in contrast, have viewed human nature holistically for millennia. The West speaks of body and soul (with the soul understood to contain a spiritual component), or body, soul, and spirit. The Bhagavad Gita similarly speaks of mental, vital, and physical forces (or mind, life, and body). In both systems, the various dimensions are understood to interconnect and interact dynamically.

Of Indian philosophy's three forces, the vital force (see chapter 1) encompasses the realm of desires, impulses, and passions. Vital activity is expressed in the mental realm through imaginations, dreams, and thoughts. Vital desires and passions, however, can overshadow the intelligence and will. Vital activity is expressed in the physical realm through habits, instincts, and the nervous system. The effect of the vital on the physical has the potential to benefit health, yet the mind can disturb its influence:

> It [the vital] gives health and strength to the body. It knows what is beneficial or what is injurious to the system. If left to itself, it would have been the safest guide in regard to health. But in civilized persons it is seldom left unimpaired; the activity of the mind has created great confusion.[2]

Sri Aurobindo also relates the vital to what Theosophy calls the "astral" realm, which similarly involves sensation and feeling.[3]

What follows are spiritual teachings that share a holistic perspective with dynamic interaction between various dimensions and that speak of dietary effects on the blood, body, consciousness, emotions, mind, nervous system, passions, soul, and spirit. One teaching speaks directly of vital effects, and two of astral effects that are synonymous with the vital. The ultimate concern, however, of all these teachings is the impact on the spirit and spiritual development.

THE MOSAIC DIETARY CODE

The Mosaic dietary code, found in the biblical books of Leviticus (11:1–47) and Deuteronomy (14:3–20), specifies the animals, fish, birds, and insects that are allowed or forbidden for consumption. The Mosaic code is similar to other ancient dietary codes, but while those apply to "priests and saints" specifically, the Jewish code applies to all of the people.[4]

Attempts to understand the reasons for distinguishing "clean" (allowed) creatures from "unclean" (forbidden) ones vary and include allegorical, hygienic, mystical, national, philosophical, and psychological explanations. Yet a significant feature of unclean animals and birds is their carnivorous and predatory nature.[5] The most illuminating explanations from a holistic perspective relate to effects on the body and soul.

Writing about bodily effects, the nineteenth-century German rabbi Samson Raphael Hirsch suggests the negative effects of meat compared with vegetal foods:

> The human body is the medium which connects the outside world with the mind of man. . . . Anything which gives the body too much independence or makes it too active in a carnal direction brings it nearer to the animal sphere, thereby robbing it of its primary function, to be the intermediary between the soul of man and the world outside. Bearing in mind this function of the body and also the fact that the physical structure of man is largely influenced by the kind of food he consumes, one might

come to the conclusion that the vegetable food is the most preferable, as plants are the most passive substance; and indeed we find that in Jewish law all vegetables are permitted for food without discrimination.[6]

Samuel ibn Seneh Zarza, a fourteenth-century Spanish philosopher, speaks of dietary effects on both body and soul. Forbidden foods "deprave the blood and make it susceptible to many diseases," thereby polluting body and soul.[7] Yet the fourteenth-century Spanish rabbi Isaac ben Moses Arama rejects adverse bodily effects while speaking more precisely about the soul effects:

> These foods defile and pollute the soul and blunt the intellectual powers, thus leading to confused opinions and a lust for perverse and brutish appetites which lead men to destruction, thus defeating the purpose of creation.[8]

Arama adds that a meat diet (i.e., of those creatures that are allowed) is appropriate for the less evolved, but the spiritually evolved "possessed of divine wisdom and removed from worldly desires" have always refrained because of a coarsening effect.[9] In a similar vein, the Cabalist view associates nonkosher animals with an impure spirit that is completely evil, but kosher animals with a spirit that mixes evil and good.[10]

Nachmanides (1194–1270) writes that the prohibition against predatory creatures protects against developing aggression and cold-bloodedness. Rabbi Joseph Albo (1380–1444) implicitly extends such an effect to a lesser extent to allowed creatures as well.[11] Echoing both Nachmanides and Albo, the renowned twentieth-century rabbi Abraham Isaac Kook notes that allowed creatures are more similar in nature to human beings and that consuming them does not have the same corrupting effect as does consuming predatory and forbidden creatures.[12]

An editorial footnote to Kook's text cites the pseudepigraphic "Letter of Aristeas," which asserts that the Mosaic code was allegorically intended: unclean carnivorous and predatory birds serve as a "sign" to practice justice and righteousness and to guard one's character from destruction. Philo of Alexandria similarly advances an allegorical understanding.[13]

The allegorical understanding certainly belongs to the interpretive debate and cannot be dismissed. Most of the authors cited above, however, suggest direct and immediate effects from consuming creatures on the human being. We shall see that this same theme recurs in the teachings that follow.

PYTHAGORAS AND THE PYTHAGOREANS

Pythagoras is a towering figure in Western antiquity. Born about 570 BCE on the Greek island of Samos, he reportedly traveled and studied throughout the ancient world, becoming initiated into the mysteries of numerous schools before developing his own unique blend of wisdom.

About 530 BCE, Pythagoras reportedly relocated to the Greek colony of Krotona in Southern Italy and started his own school, teaching various disciplines including dietetics, which he considered the most important part of medicine.[14]

No original writings of Pythagoras exist, and whether he wrote anything at all is uncertain. Teachings at that time were conveyed orally for deliberate reasons: People differed in the capacity to understand, and different degrees of teaching applied to different levels of understanding. Moreover, the dialogue of question and answer was considered the best way to promote philosophical enquiry. Despite a lack of original Pythagorean writings, however, the accounts of his teachings by biographers are considered reliable.[15]

Before turning to Pythagorean dietary teachings, it is important to mention some underlying principles that illuminate his thought and undoubtedly that of others as well.

The first is that philosophy as the pursuit of wisdom aims at "assimilation to God," which involves not only intellectual endeavor but a way of life, hence the "Pythagorean way of life" known in antiquity.[16] The second principle relates to harmony. Cultivating the harmony between body and soul was thought to lead to understanding divine harmony, and diet was a therapeutic means to harmonize the soul with qualities such as temperance, prudence, fortitude, and justice.[17] Expounding on temperance and the variations found among people, the Pythagorean biographer Iamblichus explains the relationship to diet:

> For each kind of food . . . becomes the cause of a certain peculiar disposition. [Quantity] is as important as quality; for sometimes a slight change in quantity produces a great change in quality, as with wine. First it makes men more cheerful, later it undermines morals and sanity. This difference is generally ignored in things in which the result is not so pronounced, although everything eaten is the cause of a certain peculiar disposition. Hence it requires great wisdom to know and perceive what quality and quantity of food to eat.[18]

We will hear very similar remarks later from a macrobiotic author.

Some final introductory remarks relate to symbolic meanings like those found in *The Pythagorean Symbols or Maxims*, which include dietary sayings. Iamblichus states that intended meanings are not always clear and require explanation; sayings may seem foolish, but when properly explicated, the wisdom becomes prophetic or even oracular.[19] Here again we hear about the importance of oral exposition, which safeguarded the life and truth of the tradition. As we shall see, teachings appear to have multiple layers of meaning not necessarily apparent and are subject to misinterpretation.

Dietary Interdictions: Animal Food, Beans, and Wine

The Pythagorean view about animal food is succinctly summarized by Iamblichus:

> The most contemplative of the philosophers, who had arrived at the summit of philosophic attainments, were forbidden . . . unjustifiable food, such as was animated, and [instructed] not to sacrifice animals to the Gods, nor by any means to injure animals, but to observe most solicitous justice towards them.

He himself lived after this manner, abstaining from animal food, and adoring altars undefiled with blood.[20]

Iamblichus continues that Pythagoras also forbade animal food to politicians—because how could they recommend acting justly to others if they themselves were guilty of giving in to "insatiable avidity"? He adds, "Eating of the flesh of certain animals was, however, permitted to those whose lives were not entirely purified, philosophic and sacred; but even for these was appointed a definite time of abstinence."[21] We see then that although Pythagoras himself abstained from animal food, abstention for others applied only to the most advanced. Flesh was prohibited to promote justice, engender a sense of kinship, and suppress unbridled desire.

Another passage asserts many reasons for prohibiting flesh, but chief among them is promoting peace: abhorring animal slaughter lessens the desire to kill and engage in war.[22] Other reasons include promoting temperance, avoiding greediness, and keeping alert the "genuine energies of the reasoning powers."[23] Another Pythagorean biographer, Diogenes Laertius, also notes the beneficial intellectual effect of a simple diet eschewing animal foods.[24]

Purity is another related theme. A pure and alert soul, as well as invariable bodily health, results from abstention.[25] Pythagoras also taught about the soul's immortality and asserted that purification through various means including diet leads to the memory of former lives.[26] Dietary purity also helps to cleanse the blood and equalize the breath, making both vigorous.[27] The avoidance of forbidden foods leads to the soul's cleanliness and to its redemption.[28] We heard similar ideas in chapter 1 (Jayadayol Goyandka quoting the Chhandogya Upanishad) and will hear them again.

Abstention from meat, however, was not absolute: It is reported that Pythagoras himself sometimes ate animal sacrifices;[29] yet he is said to have avoided bloodied altars and to have used bread, cakes, myrrh, and even an ox made out of flour for his own.[30] Occasional eating of animal sacrifices also extended to all Pythagoreans.[31] One commentary speaks of the injunction to avoid "too much flesh."[32]

Another aspect to abstention is the symbolic meaning. The maxim "Abstain from eating animals" is interpreted as "Have no conversation with unreasonable men."[33] Despite this additional dimension, it seems clear that Pythagoras taught the general avoidance of animal food because of the effects cited above on soul and body.

A final point about abstention relates to a jesting verse directed against Pythagoras:

> Pythagoras was so wise a man, that he
> Never ate meat himself, and called it sin.
> Yet gave he gave good joints of beef to others;
> So that I marvel at his principles;
> Who others wronged, by teaching them to do
> What he believed unholy for himself.[34]

Even though Pythagoras generally abstained from meat himself and expected the same from advanced students, he did not expect it of those less advanced. Such a differentiated practice appeared to some as hypocrisy. We are reminded of Iamblichus's caution about symbolic meanings: on the surface, they can be misleading. It seems clear that Pythagorean teachings were subject to misunderstanding by those not fully informed. As for applying different standards to different people, we shall see that this amounts to a general principle among spiritual dietary teachings.

Beans are a famous, or infamous, Pythagorean interdiction. As with meat, the reasons for prohibition are many. Iamblichus says that they included "physical, psychic, and sacred" ones.[35] Yet he also adds a symbolic dimension implying an approval of aristocracy (and a disapproval of democracy): beans are used to vote, while Pythagoreans appointed office holders.[36] Diogenes Laertius provides a more detailed summary of causes for interdiction, including negative effects on the stomach and dreams. The flatulence that beans cause relates to animal properties contained in beans. Avoidance promotes purity, hence the keepers of the temple mysteries prohibited them. Diogenes Laertius also notes symbolic reasons cited by Aristotle, such as the resemblance to genitals and their use in elections.[37] Other Pythagoreans mention symbolic and seemingly fantastic explanations for prohibiting beans. For example, when a piece of bean is buried, it grows into the shape of a vagina or an infant's head.[38] The association to genitals involves prohibiting anything that relates to "beginning, increase, source . . . end . . . [and] the first basis of all things."[39]

That such rationales against beans have been dismissed or even ridiculed is easy to understand. Yet Rudolf Steiner notes that beans are a source of protein and that protein digestion leads to creating mental images. Overconsumption, however, leads to an overabundance of images and becoming overwhelmed by them; and it is to prevent this, Steiner says, that Pythagoras advised refraining from beans.[40] Although one may well feel skeptical about the relationship between protein and mental images, linking beans with protein sheds light on the Pythagorean claim of a relationship to the "first basis of all things," as protein provides the building blocks of organic life. This astonishing and inadvertent insight into otherwise obscure remarks serves to underline Iamblichus's warning about symbolic meanings. Pythagoras was known for his spirituality and wisdom, and there appears to be more involved in his teachings such as those about beans than meets the eye.

The interdiction against wine is another consistent theme. Like animal food, wine is said to impede reason and is forbidden to the most contemplative philosophers. Yet it does appear on the daily program's supper menu, and Pythagoras is noted for never drinking wine "during the day."[41] As with animal food, it seems safe to conclude that a wine interdiction was not absolute but nevertheless practiced.

Animal foods, beans, and wine were not the only interdicted Pythagorean foods. Gurnards (a kind of fish) and various other sorts of fish, eggs, and animals that lay eggs were also discouraged.[42] As for what Pythagoras did eat, Porphyry writes:

> His breakfast was chiefly of honey; at dinner he used bread
> made of millet, barley or herbs, raw and boiled. . . . To quiet

hunger he made a mixture of poppy seed and sesame, the skin of a sea-onion, well washed until entirely drained of the outward juices, of the flowers of the daffodil, and the leaves of mallows, of paste of barley and chick peas, taking an equal weight of which, and chopping it small, with honey of Hymettus he made it into a mass. Against thirst he took the seed of cucumbers, and the best dried raisins, extracting the seeds, and coriander flowers, and the seeds of mallows, purslane, scraped cheese, wheat meal and cream, all of which he mixed up with wild honey.[43]

As for the effect, Porphyry continues:

This preserved his body in an unchanging condition, not at one time well, and at another time sick, nor at one time fat, and at another lean. Pythagoras' countenance showed the same constancy that was also in his soul. For he was neither more elated by pleasure, nor dejected by grief, and no one ever saw him either rejoicing or mourning.[44]

Constancy of body and soul, nurturing and maintaining their natural harmony, and striving to conform to divine harmony were the goals of Pythagorean dietetics. These were the reasons for the various interdictions, even if the prohibitions were not absolute. We will continue to see similar understandings in the teachings that follow.

THE LANKAVATARA SUTRA

The Lankavatara Sutra is a text from the Mahayana Buddhist tradition. Chapter 8 of the sutra discusses diet. In the teaching, the Buddha dialogues with a disciple who asks for clarification about eating meat so as to teach the *dharma* (the path of enlightenment) to others.

Buddha begins by appealing to compassion and the doctrine of evolution. Because all beings assume various forms of life during the course of evolution, have kinship with one other, and share the same nature, eating them would be unjust and uncompassionate:

In this long course of transmigration ... there is not one living being that ... has not been your mother, or father, or brother, or sister, or son, or daughter ... in various degrees of kinship; and when acquiring another form of life may live as a beast, as a domestic animal, as a bird, or as a womb-born, or as something standing in some relationship to you; [this being so] how can the [son of the Buddha engaged in the work of enlightenment and salvation,] who desires to approach all living beings as if they were himself and to practise the Buddha-truths, eat the flesh of any living being that is of the same nature as himself? ... So with Bodhisattvas whose nature is compassion, [the eating of] meat is to be avoided.[45]

The Buddha then talks about meat's negative effects on the body, contrasting that effect with the effects of proper food that "keeps away many evils":

In his eating he never knows what is meant by proper taste, digestion, and nourishment. His visceras are filled with worms and other impure creatures and harbour the cause of leprosy. He ceases to entertain any thoughts of aversion towards all diseases. ...

Now ... the food I have permitted [my disciples to take] is gratifying to all wise people but is avoided by the unwise; it is productive of many merits, it keeps away many evils; and it has been prescribed by the ancient Rishis. It comprises rice, barley, wheat, kidney beans, beans, lentils, etc., clarified butter, oil, honey, molasses, treacle, sugar cane, coarse sugar, etc.; food prepared with these is proper food.[46]

Subsequently, the Buddha repeats the prohibition against meat and specifies to whom this teaching applies—ascetics and yogis on the path to enlightenment who practice self-mastery, compassion, and love for all beings:

The interdiction not to eat any kind of meat is here given to all sons and daughters of good family, whether they are cemetery-ascetics or forest-ascetics, or Yogins who are practising the exercises, if they wish the Dharma and are on the way to the mastery of any vehicle, and being possessed of compassion, conceive the idea of regarding all beings as [to be loved as if they were] an only child, in order to accomplish the end of their discipline.[47]

Finally, the Buddha enumerates other foods to be avoided and then talks more specifically about the detrimental psychological and spiritual effects of meat:

So it is said:

5. Let the Yogin always refrain from meat, onions, various kinds of liquor, allium, and garlic. . . .

7. From eating [meat] arrogance is born, from arrogance erroneous imaginations issue, and from imagination is born greed; and for this reason, refrain from eating [meat].

8. From imagination, greed is born, and by greed the mind is stupefied; there is attachment to stupefaction, and there is no emancipation from birth [and death]. . . .

20. As greed is the hindrance to emancipation, so are meat-eating, liquor, etc., hindrances. . . .

24. Therefore, do not eat meat which will cause terror among people, because it hinders the truth of emancipation; [not to eat meat] this is the mark of the wise.[48]

As is apparent, meat is the special dietary concern of the Lankavatara Sutra for its effects on the body but more importantly on the mind and spiritual development. Other undesirable foods are mentioned as well—alcohol, onions, garlic, and allium—foods that are also discouraged by Bhagavad Gita commentators (onions, garlic, and allium as rajasic; alcohol as tamasic). The Lankavatara Sutra's recommended foods (grains, beans, butter, oil, honey, molasses, and coarse sugar) have the opposite effect of meat and are mostly foods Bhagavad Gita commentators cite as specifically sattvic foods.

SHINTO, MISOGI-HARAI, AND MONOIMI HO

Shinto is Japan's indigenous religion, and spiritual development in Shinto traditionally aims at soul pacification. Toward this end, purification exercises called *misogi-harai* preceded exercises dealing more intimately with inner transformation[49] (with the theme of purification, we hear the echo of Pythagorean teachings).

Misogi-harai applied to different dimensions of the human being. Exercises for the body included dietary change to help purify the body by gradually detoxifying bowels and blood. Initial rules stressed a vegetarian diet, food limitation, and abstention from alcohol, coffee, and tea. As cleansing began, more restrictive diets were implemented. Various schools observed different kinds of diet differently. Some allowed fish and dairy, but meat was prohibited.[50]

Purification was a concern because of the belief that uncleanliness opened the soul to the influence of evil spirits. Higher stages of purification were understood as a way to transcend human limitations and to open communication with the spiritual world.[51]

A modern-day Shinto sect whose doctrines grew out of the historical concern with purification is Shinshu Kyo, founded by Yoshimura Masamochi in 1880. Shinshu Kyo attempts to revive ancient Shinto practices and restore the old order, "when the Way of the Gods was completely interwoven with practical life and social ethics."[52]

According to Masamochi's teaching, knowing God depends on knowing one's spirit, which is not possible until body and mind have been purged of evil. Toward this end he advocated *monoimi ho,* or the "abstinence method" of purification, reviving ancient food taboos.[53]

One purpose is blood purification; others include strengthening the control of desires and changing the temperament to align it more closely with the Divine (once again, a Pythagorean theme).[54] Monoimi ho also stresses moderate eating, because too much food causes sluggish and idle behavior, and abstention from meat because it leads to anger and cruelty.[55] In fact, Shinto regarded meat as a cause of "pollution" until the Middle Ages.[56] Monoimi ho's teaching against meat is based on Shinto's "old order."

Masamochi's teachings, however, were also based on his own experience. Monoimi ho brought him improved health and alertness and beneficial changes in emotion and temperament.[57]

In this way, old Shinto and the modern-day Shinshu Kyo sect teach dietary purification as a prerequisite for inner transformation and spiritual attainment, and moderate eating and meat abstention are important parts of the process.

In Shinto we see once again the recurring holistic understanding of dietary effects, in a framework that particularly recalls Pythagorean teaching. Diet and especially eliminating meat are used to cleanse the body, control desires, benefit emotions and temperament, and heighten the mind's alertness and receptivity to the Divine.

ELLEN H. WHITE AND SEVENTH-DAY ADVENTIST TEACHINGS

Nutrition and health play such an important role in the Seventh-Day Adventist tradition that public nutrition classes are offered and missionary work includes instruction about diet and food preparation.[58] Ellen Harmon White, one of the church's founders, is responsible for this emphasis, having received in 1863 a vision that led to the dietary teachings which Adventists still follow today.[59]

Basics emphasize natural foods, in season whenever possible, and avoiding meat, refined foods, and substances like alcohol, drugs, and tobacco. A tribute to Ellen White's farsightedness notes that not until the twentieth century did science verify the hazards of the foods she recommended avoiding back in the nineteenth century.[60]

White indicates in her writings that God showed her a reform diet in order to lessen disease and suffering. The foods most healthful and nourishing for strength, endurance, and "vigor of intellect" are grains, fruits, nuts, and vegetables.[61] They provide all nutritional elements that are needed "free from the taint of flesh meat."[62] Health and strength is not what demands the use of meat, she says, but instead "a depraved appetite." Why such strong invective against meat? She replies:

> Its use excites the animal propensities to increased activity and strengthens the animal passions. When the animal propensities are increased, the intellectual and moral powers are decreased. The use of the flesh of animals tends to cause a grossness of the body, and benumbs the fine sensibilities of the mind.[63]

Citing the biblical prohibition on animal blood and fat, she continues that these accompaniments of meat cause additional trouble for the blood:

> Both the blood and the fat of animals are consumed as a luxury but the Lord gave special directions these should not be eaten [Leviticus 3:17]. Why? Because their use would make a diseased current of blood in the human system. The disregard for the Lord's special directions has brought a variety of difficulties and disease upon human beings. . . . If they introduce into their systems that which cannot make good flesh and blood, they must endure the results of their disregard of God's work.[64]

Like other spiritual writers, however, Ellen White prohibits other items besides meat: "We bear positive testimony against tobacco, spirituous liquors, snuff, tea, coffee, flesh-meats, butter, spices, rich cakes, mince pies, a large amount of salt, and all exciting substances used as articles of food."[65] Similarly, liquor, tea, coffee, and other exciting substances (onions, garlic, and allium) are all cited as rajasic and tamasic foods in Bhagavad Gita commentaries.

As we see, Ellen White's comments harmonize with those of others, especially about the effect of meat. It is worth noting that although she cites the prohibition against blood and fat in the Mosaic dietary code, the code did allow for meat consumption, albeit from "clean" creatures. In this sense, Ellen White's teaching and those of others against all meats are more extreme. Chapter 5 will say more about such differences. Most importantly, Ellen White also reveals a

holistic understanding of dietary effects. Her concern is effects not just on the body, but on the mind and spirit as well.

THEOSOPHICAL PERSPECTIVES: ANNIE BESANT AND C. W. LEADBEATER

The Theosophical Society was founded in 1875 with the goals of universal brotherhood and pursuing religious and spiritual truth. Annie Besant (1847–1933) and Charles Webster Leadbeater (1854–1934) were two prominent members of the early society. Besant was the second president until her death in 1933. Both she and Leadbeater were prolific authors and speakers whose topics included spirituality and diet.

Besant's lecture "Vegetarianism in the Light of Theosophy" takes up the effect of animal slaughter and meat consumption on the world of subtle astral forces and thereby on human and world evolution.[66]

In Besant's evolutionary perspective, the problem with eating meat is not kinship with animals through degrees of relationship over time (as in the Lankavatara Sutra), but progressive human development and the elevation of animals and the world. Humans, as part of an evolving chain of intelligences, should choose the path to higher and nobler life. Slaying animals for sensual gratification, or even misusing the powers of mind to create weapons of destruction, represents the antithesis to pursuing higher life.

Next to these considerations is the effect of slaughter on the astral world, a world that interpenetrates the physical world (the astral relates to the Bhagavad Gita's vital realm). Besant characterizes the astral world as an objective, perceptible reality involving thoughts, actions, and emotions:

> In that world you have the reflection and the imaging of what occurs on the material plane . . . thoughts also take image there, just as actions are there reflected, and this astral world lies between the material world and the world of thought. . . . It is this

which is so often felt by the "sensitive" . . . a subtle feeling that he may be unable to explain, something of the general characteristics of the atmosphere of that house, or hall, or city—whether . . . pure or foul . . . friendly or hostile; whether it exerts . . . a healthful or hindering influence.[67]

Besant then asks her listeners to imagine the astral reality of the slaughterhouse and the effect, not just on animals, but on humans and even the surrounding neighborhood:

Try to estimate . . . something of the passions and emotions which . . . are aroused . . . in the animals . . . being slain! Notice the terror . . . as they come within the scent of blood! See the misery, and the fright, and the horror with which they struggle to get away . . . as the life is suddenly wrenched out of the body, and the animal soul with its terror, with its horror, goes out into the astral world to remain there for a considerable time before it breaks up and perishes. And remember . . . that those react on the minds of men. . . . [68]

She adds that sensitives feel these atmospheric vibrations, recounting her own sense of oppression and depression upon entering the area of Chicago by train, which she attributes to the slaughtering houses there.

This astral effect of fear and terror reverberates upon humans even if they remain unaware, coarsening and degrading them by affecting their own subtle forces.

This continual throwing down of these magnetic influences of fear, of horror, and of anger, and passion, and revenge, works on the people . . . and tends to coarsen, tends to degrade, tends to pollute. It is not only the body that is soiled by the flesh of animals, it is the subtler forces of the man that also come within this area of pollution, and much, very much of the coarser side of city life, of the coarser side of the life of those who are concerned in the slaughtering, comes directly from this reflection from the astral world, and the whole of this terrible protest comes from the escaped lives of the slaughtered beasts.[69]

Next to this effect on everyone is the more specific effect on slaughterers—they become so coarsened that butchers are not allowed to serve as jurors on murder trials. This claim is corroborated by evidence today that affirms social recognition for the influences she describes.[70]

Like other authors, Besant also asserts that consuming meat has a coarsening effect on humans. It imparts something of the animal's nature, stimulating the lower human passions and retarding the reception of subtler impulses. The net effect is retarded human growth and animalization instead of spiritualization:

> Man ... makes his task either harder or easier ... according to the nature of the physical apparatus which that Soul is forced to use. ... And if in feeding the body he feeds ... with food which brings ... the passions of the lower animals and their lower nature; then, he is making a grosser and more animal body, more apt to respond to animal impulses, and less apt to respond to the higher impulses of the mind. ...
>
> And so the task ... is also rendered harder by this increase of the molecules that vibrate to the lower passions ... this animalizing of the human body, instead of the ensouling and spiritualising of it.[71]

Besant ends her lecture on vegetarianism by emphasizing once again an evolutionary understanding of life, cooperation with the Divine, and world ennoblement:

> You and I are either helping the world upward or pulling the world downward; with every day of our life we are either giving it a force for the upward climbing or we are clogs on that upward growth; and every true Soul desires to be a help and not a hindrance, to be a blessing and not a curse, to be amongst the raisers of the world and not amongst those who degrade it.[72]

Diet, in this respect, has far more significance than nourishing the body—it retards or hastens human and world evolution.

C. W. Leadbeater's lecture "Vegetarianism and Occultism" reiterates similar themes: human spiritual evolution is affected by the relationship with animals; slaughter causes astral pollution and especially degrades the slaughterer; and meat consumption imparts the degrading influence of animal passions, stifling spiritual development.[73]

Where Leadbeater differs, however, is in the detail given to health arguments for vegetarianism and the vociferousness of his judgment against slaughter and eating meat. The health arguments for vegetarianism (more nutriment, less disease, and greater strength) involve the enjoinder of striving for perfection. While Besant concedes that meat may increase strength (but still argues that slaughter is unjustified), Leadbeater denies any health advantage to meat eating. Its only rationale is "degraded and detestable lusts." Here he echoes Ellen White. We will hear, however, from other writers different assessments of the effects of meat and of the motivation for eating it.

Also noteworthy is Leadbeater's invocation of the dietary ideal expressed in Genesis 1:29:

> See, I have given you every plant yielding seed that is upon the
> face of all the earth, and every tree with seed in its fruit; you
> shall have them for food.

For Leadbeater, this is yet another argument for vegetarianism and against slaughter, and he also notes that the biblical Fall goes hand in hand with death and meat consumption. The relationship among these various elements—the biblical command in Genesis, the Fall, death, and meat eating—is important to the spiritual dietary puzzle we are trying to piece together. Chapter 5 will take these elements up in detail.

To sum up, Annie Besant and C. W. Leadbeater are two strong voices arguing that animal slaughter and meat consumption have no place in human and world evolution. They articulate more clearly than others heard so far the degrading effects on the environment and human beings through the paradigm of astral influences and effects. The net effect is negative—the atmosphere polluted, animal qualities absorbed, the lower passions stirred, and spiritualization hindered. In their view, animal slaughter and meat consumption are regrettable, and in this they are in harmony with previous teachings.

MAZDAZNAN PHILOSOPHY: OTOMAN ZAR-ADUSHT HA'NISH

Otoman Zar-Adusht Ha'Nish (1844–1936) was a modern interpreter of the Mazdaznan philosophy that traces its roots to the Zoroastrian tradition. He taught the "Mazdaznan Science of Daily Life," whose five fundamental principles include dietetics along with breath culture, personal diagnosis, eugenics, and gland therapy.[74]

Like other authors, Ha'Nish outlines characteristics of foods that affect human beings and shares the concern of expressing humanity's higher nature and unfolding "the attributes, talents and endowments . . . of body, mind, soul and spirit."[75] Yet he cautions that dietary principles only have value in conjunction with practicing the other Mazdaznan principles. As for dietary principles, he notes that foods ripening in the sun have a positive effect on consciousness and intelligence, in contrast to potatoes that ripen underground.[76] Peanuts are related to potatoes, and so too much consumption of them is also cautioned against.[77]

Ha'Nish also joins other authors in the concern about meat. He claims that substances in the juices stimulate the heart and other organic functions (i.e., rajasic effects) and arouse the animal nature. The effect of the intelligences in animal tissues on the human mind and spiritual nature are alleged to be even worse:

> These intelligences continue their work . . . by their allurements and the gradually increasing negative attitude, they [cause] the subjection of one's higher intelligence, until at last the unbalanced intelligences of brute nature appeal to the mind holding one enchained to the lowest conditions of existence. The sense of justice is lost and one no longer lives the life of a being, noble and sublime, but merely exists as a phenomenon of the brute reflecting through the human form.[78]

The total effect is physical, mental, and spiritual retardation.[79] We have heard this notion about absorbing animal qualities before, and we will hear it again from others, each with their own explanations.

As for recommended foods, Ha'Nish emphasizes wheat: "We find that the best guide for man as to the ingredients required by the human system is found in entire wheat. Every other dish must be governed accordingly. Wheat is the standard of grains and the bread from heaven for man."[80] And again: "Wheat is the staff of life, while fruit and vegetables are excellent eliminators, but not nourishment strictly speaking."[81]

Thus, we find with Ha'Nish, too, the now-familiar themes of dietary effects on body, mind, and spirit; the negative effects of meat; and the importance of foods like grains. The macrobiotic authors who follow also consider grains as the most important food. Yet unlike Ha'Nish and others, they sound the first notes of a different evaluation of animal foods that includes a positive effect.

MACROBIOTIC PHILOSOPHY

Macrobiotics is defined as "the way of health, longevity, and happiness in the large sense, through the view and application of the cosmological understanding of life."[82] It represents a modern movement that has spread from Japan throughout the world. The Japanese doctor Ishitsuka Sagen was responsible for reviving the traditional practices that led to macrobiotics. George Ohsawa, a student of Sagen, was the first to bring macrobiotics to the West and is considered the father of Western macrobiotics. Michio Kushi was one of Ohsawa's foremost students. Both Ohsawa and Kushi add valuable contributions to the understanding of diet's holistic effects.

The Writings of George Ohsawa

George Ohsawa was especially instrumental in defining the macrobiotic attitude toward diet, outlining three key ideas. The first is the order of the universe and the biological basis of religious teaching in the East. Philosophy in the East involves the art of teaching the order of the universe, and Eastern religions apply this understanding to human biology and physiology. Diet is important because it points the way to happiness, health, and freedom. The West, according to Ohsawa, has failed to understand this dimension of Eastern religion as well as its significance. The loss of Western religion's authority, he says, results from a lack of attention to this dimension, leading to the disappearance of "peace, freedom, health, and happiness."[83]

Ohsawa's second key idea is of grain as the principle food. He calls it strange that the West lacks such a basic concept that is of primary consequence in the East. Grain is so revered that the Upanishads considered it as a symbol of God. Cereals, he continues, are the true foundation of existence and one of the defining features of civilization (with fire and salt). They are the absolute key to well-being.[84]

His third key idea concerns knowledge about diet's effects, not just on the body but on human nature:

> Thousands of foods and the manner of their preparation . . . can change the individual human constitution, the intellectual tendency, the social behavior, the sexual inclination, and consequently the whole human destiny, as well as the nature of society.[85]

We heard something similar with the Pythagoreans. The issue with animal foods is a clear perception of the effect on the distinguishing characteristic between humans and animals—the human ability to think:

> Macrobiotics is not the kind of vegetarianism which is merely sentimental. If animal foods are to be avoided, it is for the purpose of preserving and improving man's ability to *think*. Animal glands produce hormones which are good for animals, unaccustomed to thinking. Their center of sensitivity, however, is not at all developed like ours.[86]

Finally, however, Ohsawa indicates that it is not necessary to avoid animal foods completely because the qualitative effect depends on quantity, and the philosophical principles of *yin* and *yang* can be used to achieve balance. Yin and yang describe the qualities relating to a dualistic conception of nature (in contrast to the Hindu threefold guna conception of sattva, rajas, and tamas discussed in chapter 1). Yin is expansive and cool and yang contractive and warm. As applied to foods, fruits and vegetables (except seaweed) are considered yin and most animal foods yang (milk, however, is also considered yin and, along with sweets, spices, and alcohol, more yin than other foods). Ohsawa writes:

> In the final analysis, however, there is no need to fear animal products. All depends on *quantity*, for quantity changes quality . . . you can Yinnize or neutralize food that is too Yang (animal products) and avoid the fatal domination of lower judgement (cruel, violent, slavish, delinquent) over higher thinking.[87]

Through Ohsawa and his delineation of macrobiotics, we hear a clear articulation of the effect of diet on the entire human nature, not just on the body. In addition, we hear a more precise explanation of why grains consistently appear on recommended food lists—they are the *principle* food, and at least in the East are considered divine-like in significance. We also hear the affirmation of the potentially detrimental effect of animal foods, but with the qualification that the effect can be controlled. These basic macrobiotic understandings lead to Michio Kushi's further elucidations.

The Writings of Michio Kushi

Along with his wife, Aveline, Michio Kushi cofounded the Kushi Institute, a macrobiotic educational center in Becket, Massachusetts. He was a leading figure in the US movement until his death in 2014. Following the essence of macrobiotic philosophy, Kushi asserted that diet is the origin of happiness or unhappiness at all levels—physical, mental, and spiritual—and that knowledge of this is the key to personal and collective destiny.[88]

One of Kushi's important contributions is a more scientific explanation of nutritional effects, beginning with the effect on the chakras and the blood. The chakras are traditionally understood as invisible energy centers in the body controlling physiological, mental, emotional, and spiritual activities. They are affected by the quality of the blood; and blood quality, in turn, is affected by food. Traditional dietary practices are rooted in this understanding. Foods create a particular blood quality that affects the chakras and the cells, organs, tissues, brain, and nervous system; and the cumulative effect influences behavior, consciousness, emotions, perceptions, thought, and worldview. Different human reactions to external stimuli relate in this way to diet.[89]

Another key concept for Kushi involves bodily systems and their functions. The digestive and respiratory systems consume "physical food"; the nervous and meridian systems (the invisible energy circuitry of the body) consume the "spiritual food" of radiations, vibrations, and waves that relate to the immediate environment and infinite time and space. Spiritual food is consumed continuously and limitlessly, but physical food at intervals and in limited quantities. Both kinds of food complement and oppose one another. Quantity is a determining variable. More consumption of material food means less consumption of spiritual food and vice versa.

Whether the food is animal or vegetal in origin is another important factor; animal food limits perception while vegetal food expands it:

> The consumption of animal food tends to limit our perception to the immediate environment, and to inhibit our awareness and receptivity to the unlimited scope of infinite time and space. . . . The consumption of vegetable-quality food tends to broaden our mental and spiritual view, and lessen our concern for small matters of the relative world.[90]

The reception of spiritual food further depends on regulating physical food variables such as combination, frequency of consumption, cooking method, quality, and variety (here we see the "artistic" practice of applying Oriental philosophy to diet). Differences among people result from differences in these variables.

The right combination of yin and yang foods, however, is especially important because too much of either causes imbalance. Too much yang animal food causes "egocentric and aggressive" attitudes toward the world; yet excess yin food (vegetables, fruit, hot spices, and alcohol) results in defensive withdrawal. Both extremes produce symptoms of "fear and exclusivity," yet in different ways; and both must be balanced to stabilize mental and spiritual functions:

> The more yang category of food produces a more aggressive and offensive attitude, while the more yin food produces a more defensive and self-excusing tendency. The former contributes more towards a materialistic view of life, the latter a more otherworldly view. Both these ways of thinking and acting are imbalanced, ultimately leading to sickness and unhappiness. By avoiding excess yang and yin qualities of food, our health and judgment remain strong and clear. By eating primarily whole grains and vegetables, with small supplemental amounts of other types of foods, and observing the seasonal order and other principles of environmental balance, we remain in the middle—centered and grounded. The macrobiotic dietary approach produces . . . physical strength and vitality as well as mental and spiritual balance.[91]

In this way, macrobiotics reveals a differentiated approach to the question of animal versus vegetal foods—too much of either causes imbalance. Understanding the interaction of yin and yang and other factors like preparation, quality, and quantity is the key to balancing between the extremes. Such an understanding seems to represent something new in our spiritual dietary explorations, yet perhaps it is implied in the Bhagavad Gita's concern for nourishing effects that are holistic.

Kushi continues that applying dietary knowledge is the key to solving all physical, mental, and spiritual disorders:

> Through proper eating, our blood and body will become sound and whole. Mental and spiritual well-being will naturally follow. Without any special preventive measures other than diet, we are able to maintain our physical health, suffering no

serious sickness or disability. Without any other special mental or psychological training, we are able to establish a sound mentality, experiencing no delusions or other mental disorders. . . . Without any special education, we are naturally able to develop a spirit of love for other people and of harmony with our environment.[92]

Macrobiotics is based on specific dietary principles, yet their application is meant to be not rigid or static, but flexible. Kushi outlines three different stages: 1) recovering from physical and mental sickness; 2) maintaining health; and 3) developing and realizing one's dream. The first stage requires strict adherence to recommendations until health and balance are restored. The second allows more flexibility according to individual need and adaptation to the environment. The third stage involves intuition in the pursuit of one's dream. In this stage, the "art" of applying knowledge about food effects is put toward the service of "freedom":

- "To be spiritual and intuitive, eat vegetable-quality food including whole cereal grains, beans, vegetables, and fruits with the minimum possible amount of animal food.

- "To be social and businesslike, eat mostly vegetable-quality foods including grains and beans, cooked in a standard way, in a wider variety of methods with the addition of a small volume of animal food.

- "To perform heavy physical labor, eat more volume of food, including whole cereal grains, beans, vegetables, and animal food, richly cooked, as well as a larger volume of liquid.

- "To be more intellectual, eat whole grains, beans, and vegetables with the occasional addition of a small volume of animal food and fruits.

- "To be more sensitive and aesthetic, eat mostly vegetable-quality food, including raw salad. Fruits may be added, as well as a little more liquid and a small volume of animal food if desired.

- "To be physically active and sportive, eat regularly. To be mentally active, eat less volume.

- "To be violent and warlike, eat more animal food and sugar, alcohol or drugs, with a variety of food prepared in a disorderly fashion."[93]

Kushi also links agricultural practice to holistic effects on the human being.[94] Natural organic agriculture produces stronger foods better able to create health and limitless spiritual development. Chemical agriculture, which is highly yin (expansive), increases crop size and volume, but with a corresponding decrease in strength, vitality, and taste (yang qualities) while also depleting soil. Consuming such food leads to degeneration and the yin qualities of tallness, weakness, shorter memory, and larger facial features such as noses and mouths. Natural organic agriculture reflects the consciousness of connectedness with the environment and not feeling called to subdue, improve, or redesign, as seen in the extreme with genetically modified crops. Natural agriculture restores domesticated crops to a freer and wilder original state through deliberate methods of weeding, tilling, fertilizing, spraying, and seeding. This kind of agriculture reverses biological degeneration and nourishes both physical and psychological health and limitless spiritual development, including capacities for "insight, foresight, imagination, telepathy, and other extrasensory perception."[95]

A final point to Kushi's work involves the food pyramids and pie charts he created for different geographical and climatic regions.[96] Pyramids show recommendations for monthly and weekly consumption and pie charts proportion recommendations by weight for daily consumption. Most of the pyramids recommend animal foods for monthly use optionally and fish and seafood for more frequent use. Exceptions are:

- Africa—game, insects, birds, and fish and seafood are recommended for weekly use.

MONTHLY, WEEKLY, and DAILY CONSUMPTION

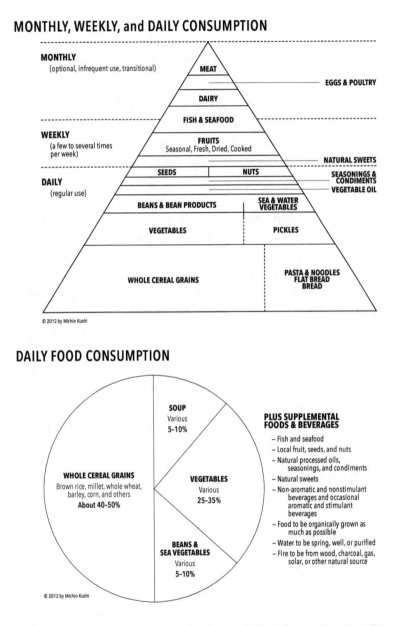

MONTHLY
(optional, infrequent use, transitional)

MEAT

EGGS & POULTRY

DAIRY

FISH & SEAFOOD

WEEKLY
(a few to several times per week)

FRUITS
Seasonal, Fresh, Dried, Cooked

NATURAL SWEETS

SEEDS | NUTS

DAILY
(regular use)

SEASONINGS & CONDIMENTS
VEGETABLE OIL

BEANS & BEAN PRODUCTS | SEA & WATER VEGETABLES

VEGETABLES | PICKLES

WHOLE CEREAL GRAINS | PASTA & NOODLES FLAT BREAD BREAD

© 2012 by Michio Kushi

DAILY FOOD CONSUMPTION

SOUP
Various
5–10%

WHOLE CEREAL GRAINS
Brown rice, millet, whole wheat, barley, corn, and others
About 40–50%

VEGETABLES
Various
25–35%

BEANS & SEA VEGETABLES
Various
5–10%

PLUS SUPPLEMENTAL FOODS & BEVERAGES

– Fish and seafood
– Local fruit, seeds, and nuts
– Natural processed oils, seasonings, and condiments
– Natural sweets
– Non-aromatic and nonstimulant beverages and occasional aromatic and stimulant beverages
– Food to be organically grown as much as possible
– Water to be spring, well, or purified
– Fire to be from wood, charcoal, gas, solar, or other natural source

© 2012 by Michio Kushi

FIGURE 2.1. Macrobiotic pyramid and pie chart for temperate regions including North America, Europe, Russia, China, and East Asia, and moderate regions in Southern Africa, South America, Australia, and New Zealand (in the pyramid fish and seafood can be chosen weekly or monthly, or for vegans, not at all; the pie chart shows recommended proportions by weight, with grains making up 1/4 to 1/3 of a plate and vegetables and beans the rest), *The Book of Macrobiotics*, Michio Kushi with Alex Jack, 296–97.

- Cool Climates (semi-polar regions including southern Cana-da, Iceland, Scotland, Scandinavia, Mongolia, and Siberia)—meat, poultry, eggs, and dairy are recommended for weekly use, optionally.

- Cold Climates (arctic region of Alaska, Northern Canada, Greenland, Northern Russia, Antarctica, and other polar cli-mates)—meat, dairy, wild birds, eggs, fish, and seafood are rec-ommended for regular daily use and make up about 60 percent by weight of the accompanying pie chart.

As these pyramid and pie chart guidelines suggest, flexibility is the key. Biological and spiritual evolution is the guiding dietary princi-ple, but other factors also come into play: "climate and environment, season and weather, social and cultural tradition and custom, ethical and environmental considerations, and finally . . . age, sex, gender, activity level, and personal condition and needs."[97]

In summary, we can say that Kushi's macrobiotic conception is both holistic and flexible. He considers a full range of dietary effects on the body, mind, and spirit; and although he cautions against ani-mal foods, qualifications such as quantity, activity, and climate make consumption acceptable or even necessary. He is the first of our au-thors to sound a warning about excess vegetal (yin) foods and to stress the ideal of "balancing in the middle." The teachings of Rudolf Steiner that follow elaborate on these themes and on the personal considerations that come into play.

ANTHROPOSOPHY AND DIET: RUDOLF STEINER

Rudolf Steiner (1861–1925) was a physicist with a PhD who also claimed the clairvoyant perception of spiritual realities. Turning his scientific training to these realities, he founded *Anthroposophy*, meaning the "science of the human" or "wisdom of the human be-ing," a movement dedicated to fostering the direct perception of the spiritual world through consciousness training and articulating the relationships between the human being, nature, the cosmos, and evolution. Steiner's numerous books (over fifty titles) and lectures (some six thousand) provide profound insights into diverse fields such as agriculture, art, economics, education, medicine, philosophy, religion, science, spirituality—and nutrition.

Although not the most modern of our authors, Steiner is treated last because of the depth of his insights and his ability to frame ideas scientifically. He corroborates much that has been discussed but details more fully the reasons for many spiritual dietary teachings while also revealing new perspectives.

As with many topics, Steiner's references to nutrition are scattered throughout his works. His lecture "Problems of Nutrition" is reviewed in detail because of the conceptual framework it offers for understanding dietary spiritual effects.

Steiner begins by critiquing a materialist understanding of nutrition that focuses on replenishing nutrients to the body. His intent, in contrast, is to clarify nutritional effects on spirituality, which requires reference to a fourfold paradigm of human nature:

1. a physical-mineral body (the kind of body possessed by everything in the mineral kingdom);

2. an etheric or life body (the kind of body possessed by the plant kingdom in addition to the physical body);

3. an astral body carrying sensations, feelings, and instincts (the kind of body possessed by the animal kingdom in addition to physical and etheric bodies); and

4. an ego or "I" unique to the human being, representing the spiritual nature and making self-awareness and freedom possible.[98]

According to Steiner, the ego's evolutionary task is gradually to take control of the various bodies and their functions. Its influence, however, depends on astral activity, and astral activity in turn is affected by food. The presence or lack of dietary fat illustrates how the relationships work.

When fat is lacking, the ego and the astral body work together to create it. When fat, however, is consumed, the inner ego and astral activity are restricted with resulting negative spiritual consequences:

> Inner activity signifies the unfolding of the actual inner life. When a man is forced to produce . . . fat on his own, then through . . . inner flexibility, the ego and the astral body become master of the physical and etheric bodies. . . . He is made free and thus becomes lord over his body. Otherwise, as a spiritual being he remains a mere spectator.[99]

In this way, creating fat signifies increased activity and gaining mastery over the etheric and physical bodies. A physiological corollary to the increased activity Steiner describes can be seen in the increased metabolic activity resulting from the conversion of carbohydrate to fat, which requires a lot of energy (see chapter 7 for discussion of thermic effect and basal metabolic rate).

Another dietary effect with spiritual consequences involves the astral influences that come with animal foods, a theme touched on by previous commentators. Steiner provides a different explanation of the potentially negative effect: humans have the capacity to express the characteristics and qualities found in the animal world by exerting their own astral bodies, yet when these characteristics and qualities come through food, astral activity remains constrained. A vegetarian diet, in contrast, stimulates astral activity:

> In the food we consume from the animal kingdom, we not only take into ourselves the physical meat and fat of the animal but also the product of its astral body. . . . When through a vegetarian diet, we enlist the virginal forces of our astral body, we call forth our whole inner activity. In a meat diet part of this inner activity is forestalled.[100]

Such comments suggest advocacy for a vegetarian diet. Yet the totality of Steiner's views about vegetal and animal foods is more complex. While it is important for humans to gain mastery over inner processes, they are also called to participate actively in the world, which requires qualities such as stamina, courage, and even aggressiveness, and meat is helpful to those who lack the inner strength:

> A man may not yet find himself strong enough to entrust everything to his astral body and may have to fall back upon the support of a meat diet. . . .

> That men are to become progressively freer while at the same time needing qualities that they can acquire with the help of impulses found spread out in the animal kingdom, has induced them to resort to nourishment in animal food.[101]

Meat in fact, Steiner asserts, correlates with aggressive and war-like behavior and a vegetarian diet with a peaceful nature, but there are good reasons for choosing a mixed diet, because vegetarianism works for some people but not others:

> Militant nations . . . generally . . . eat meat. Naturally, there are exceptions. [A] preference for an exclusively vegetarian diet will . . . prevail among people who have developed an introverted and contemplative existence. . . . Nevertheless, it is not without reason that a mixed diet has become acceptable to many people. To some extent it had to happen. We must admit, however, that even though a vegetarian diet might indeed be the correct one for some people purely for reasons of health, the health of others might be ruined by it.[102]

Steiner, like Michio Kushi, reinforces the potential need for meat by stressing balance between the inner and outer life. An extreme meat diet stifles inner activity, stimulating a worldly orientation and leading to narrow vistas; a vegetarian diet, on the other hand, stimulates inner activity and independence and leads to wider horizons. Yet people must be concerned with both the inner and outer and not become impractical.[103]

Elsewhere Steiner indicates that some, if not most, people lack the strength to create fat due to heredity, and so for them a vegetarian diet is inadequate.[104] Here he finds echo with others: Mary Enig, a nutritionist and biochemist, notes that some people need dietary cholesterol because the liver cannot synthesize enough (dietary cholesterol is considered a fat because it is fat soluble and carried in the body by fat; trace amounts exist in vegetable oils, yet the only abundant dietary source is animal tissue).[105] Sally Fallon Morell, president of the Weston A. Price Foundation, adds that "vegetarians and especially vegans risk deficiencies in complete protein, especially the sulphur-containing amino acids, long-chain fatty acids (AA, DHA, EPA), vitamins B_{12} and B_6, fat-soluble vitamins A, D and K_2, and the minerals iron, calcium, iodine, and zinc."[106]

Despite the caveats about meat's potential benefits, Steiner stresses the advantages of vegetal foods and the disadvantages of meat. Carried to an extreme, meat consumption leads to dogmatism and the inability to transcend the boundaries of one's environment. He predicts that, in the future, people will realize the value of vegetarianism for widening horizons, particularly in application to science.[107]

Yet Steiner also voices caution about vegetarian diets. Unless the forces they create are used wisely, harm can result:

> Certain forces will be changed from material ones into spiritual ones. If however they are not used, they will work in a detrimental way and can even impair the activity of the brain. If such a person works in a bank or is an ordinary intellectual he can do himself great harm unless he can take in spiritual ideas with the forces that have become available through his vegetarian mode of life. So the person who becomes a vegetarian must change to a more spiritual life, otherwise it were better he keep to meat. His memory could become impaired, certain parts of his brain could be impaired, etc.[108]

Steiner's qualification is to combine vegetarianism with spiritual life, and some of the teachings previously cited (such as the Lankavatara Sutra) do relate vegetarian recommendations to those on a spiritual path (we are left wondering if Adolph Hitler, an infamous vegetarian, went wrong because of the lack of a healthy spiritual life).

Considering the pros and cons that Steiner outlines of both vegetarian and meat diets, which is the proper course? He responds that an instinctive and gradual turning away from meat is preferable to following abstract principles. The knowledge spiritual science provides can lead to aversion: eventually, one begins to feel that meat becomes burdensome to the body.[109] In this vein, Steiner tells the story of a patient who asks his vegetarian doctor about giving up meat. The doctor asks the patient if he eats cats and dogs, to which the patient replies with disgust. The doctor then responds that when he feels the same disgust for meat, he should give it up.[110]

Steiner does not limit remarks about spiritual dietary effects to meat and vegetarianism. Other discussions involve alcohol, coffee, tea, milk, beans, and potatoes.

Alcohol usurps the ego by stimulating forces that otherwise depend on the ego's function and control. The effects of alcohol may seem desirable, but it creates subservience by substituting for ego activity.[111]

Coffee helps the nervous system function logically in a concentrated way, but at the expense of curtailing the exercise of inner strength. Yet Steiner asserts that the effect can be beneficial because doing everything on one's own is not always necessary.[112] He also expands on coffee's other advantages and disadvantages: it strengthens logical thinking, but in a compulsive, not an independent, way; those who want to think for themselves need to develop their own soul forces.[113] Yet coffee is recommended for the kind of logical thinking that is particularly relevant to anthroposophical training:

> For those who wish to ascend to the higher regions of spiritual life, it [coffee] is not amiss. . . . As citizens of the earth we sometimes need this drink according to individual circumstances and it must be emphasized that coffee, despite all its faults, can contribute to the increase of stability. Not that it should be recommended as a means of developing stability. . . . If, for example, someone undergoing anthroposophical development has the tendency of letting his thoughts stray in the wrong direction, we need not take it amiss if he stabilized himself with coffee.[114]

Tea works in an opposite way, "tear[ing] thoughts asunder," making them "scattered, light, witty, and brilliant." This is why diplomats prefer it.[115] But the effect is undesirable for cognitive training because the imagination is stimulated but not "adherence to the truth and solid facts."[116] And yet—Steiner notes that the tendency may not become manifest if the person possesses sufficient inner resistance.[117] Here we hear an echo (see chapter 1) of the notion that guna qualities represent tendencies, but not necessarily specific effects. Multiple variables can come into play, including inner strength, and we can assume that such qualifications apply to other purported food effects.

Milk, Steiner writes, is only partially an animal food and does not fully express animal qualities. For this reason it is valuable to those who want to give up meat but are insufficiently strong to rely on their own astral bodies. Everyone can benefit from milk, Steiner asserts. Not only does it stimulate regular forces, but living on it exclusively for a period of time results in extra strength and healing forces.[118]

As for beans, we have already heard (in the section on Pythagoras) that they are predominately composed of protein and that protein digestion relates to mental image creation. Steiner recommends eating neither too much nor too little protein. Too much can lead to an overabundance of mental images and becoming overwhelmed by them. As already noted, Steiner relates such an effect to the Pythagorean saying about refraining from beans.[119]

We previously heard from Otoman Ha'Nish that foods like potatoes that ripen underground have a negative effect on consciousness and intelligence. Steiner supports this view. Potatoes, he says, are an inferior food. They require a lot of digestive effort, but digestion continues beyond the digestive tract, resulting in a general weakening. Potatoes nourish the lower part of the head and stimulate thinking, but the kind of thinking that is materialistic and quick, not deep or long lasting. They fail to nourish the head's middle part, which is the true seat of intellectuality and spirituality. Overconsumption as a result leads to soul and spiritual impoverishment. Potatoes are, Steiner emphasizes, the true source of the materialism of the times.[120]

In the conclusion to the lecture "Problems of Nutrition," Steiner reiterates the goals of promoting human freedom, independence, and potential through diet. Yet he also reiterates the caveat that applies to vegetarianism in particular: some people are capable of it, but others not. This is why diet is always an individual question.[121]

Thus concludes the presentation of Steiner's thoughts on nutrition, although he has much more to say. He echoes the virtues of vegetarianism and the vices of meat eating, as have others, but ultimately he emphasizes the need for balance and the dangers of each, in a way similar to Michio Kushi. Steiner's insights into pros and cons are particularly revealing. Vegetarianism stimulates inner activity and thereby promotes spiritual development. Yet the ability for this activity varies, and the forces that are mobilized must be channeled correctly or harm results. Steiner's comments about the benefits of meat are the first to suggest that the appeal has as much to do with need as with desire. Such a notion is undoubtedly controversial and important to highlight. The distinction between desire and need is a topic to which we will return. Steiner's remarks about alcohol, coffee, and tea provide insight into their appearance on prohibition lists, although he finds value at least with coffee. The remarks about milk also support its high status as a sattvic food supreme.

Lastly, I want to reemphasize the importance Steiner gives to individual considerations. Chapter 1 discussed qualifications about meat relating to social role or activity as well as to climate. Macrobiotic teaching similarly raised the issue of climate and other individual matters. Steiner stresses individual considerations by revealing in more detail the benefits of meat as well as the danger of a vegetarianism divorced from spiritual practice. We will return to the importance of individual considerations and the difference between desire and need in chapter 5, which explores more deeply religious attitudes toward vegetarianism.

NOURISHING THE SPIRIT AND THE SATTVIC DIET

Chapter 1 ended with the question of the sattvic diet, the kind of diet chosen by a person of sattvic temperament that nourishes the mental, vital, and physical forces together. In the present chapter, we have heard the voices of diverse traditions with dietary teachings whose particular focus is spiritual effects. What do those voices say about diet and nourishing the spirit?

The first point to emphasize is the general consensus that diet does have effects beyond the body upon the mind and spirit. Such assertions may seem surprising, but they are a perennial theme across all cultures. Explanations may be difficult to articulate, understand, or accept, but the theme is nevertheless universal and represents spirituality's unique contribution to nutrition.

As for assertions about dietary effects and the consequences for the sattvic diet, there is a similarity and even consensus among these teachings, but to a point. All agree that a vegetarian diet can be helpful to spiritual development and a meat diet harmful, but then other complicating considerations come into play. There are a host of individual factors to consider, such as age, gender, social role, bodily ability, ego strength, spiritual practice (or the lack thereof), climate, and other factors as well, such as food quality, quantity, preparation, and agricultural practices. Also important is the notion of balancing the inner and outer life, as articulated by macrobiotic authors and by Rudolf Steiner as well. Steiner's teaching also hints at the notion of evolutionary development.

A poignant, paradoxical, and even perplexing example of the role played by individual considerations and the clash between the ideal and the real is the case of the present Dalai Lama, Tenzin Gyatso. The Dalai Lama is an acknowledged spiritual master and a public advocate for vegetarianism, yet he has been known to eat meat occasionally on the advice of his doctor. As a result, both he and the doctor have been criticized and even maligned.[122] Is this the case of a Tibetan lama eating meat for warmth, or of a constitutional bodily weakness despite the best intentions, or even, perhaps, of divine irony?

Chapter 1 raised the question of whether meat can be part of the sattvic diet. The sum of considerations in the present chapter suggests that meat can have a beneficial health role, even from a spiritual point of view. Chapter 5 will take up this topic in more detail.

As for other foods, stimulants like alcohol, coffee, tea, and spices consistently appear in a negative light (although some positivity about coffee is expressed), and potatoes and beans are highlighted more than once for potentially negative effects. With all such indications, variables such as quantity and frequency of consumption are important to bear in mind in addition to individual considerations. Alcohol will be the special focus of appendix B. Foods like grains, fruits, vegetables, and dairy are consistently mentioned in a positive light, but again, even the recommendation for a vegetarian diet comes with cautions.

The present chapter does not represent all that there is to say about vegetarianism, in general or from a spiritual point of view. Its particular emphasis has been on grounding the notion of spiritual effects as represented by particular teachings. We will hear more about vegetarianism in the chapters ahead.

Our point of view about the sattvic diet, however, is holistic, and in addition to concerns about spiritual effects, we are concerned with effects on the mind and body as well. The following chapter turns our attention to some views about effects on the mind, specifically.

3
NOURISHING THE MIND: ORTHOMOLECULAR MEDICINE AND WESTON PRICE

The holistic perspective of the teachings in chapter 2 do include the dimension of the mind. They speak about nutritional effects on attitude, disposition, intellectual power, philosophical view, reasoning, social consciousness, and spiritual horizon. Mostly these effects are related to animal or vegetal foods as food categories, but some individual foods are highlighted (for example, onions, garlic, and potatoes); and the issue of quality also comes up in distinguishing between fresh and nonfresh meat and the general effects of different agricultural practices.

The teachings in the present chapter focus on mental effects related to quality in a more specific sense by highlighting the effects of toxins, devitalized foods, parental nutrition, and nutrient-depleted soils. These teachings are holistic, too, in the sense that physical health effects are also acknowledged. But our special interest here is the contribution they make to a deeper understanding of the effect between food quality and the dimension of the mind.

ORTHOMOLECULAR MEDICINE: B VITAMINS AND WHOLE FOODS

The word *orthomolecular* signifies "correct molecules" (Gk., *ortho*, "correct"). Linus Pauling, one of the pioneers of orthomolecular medicine, defines orthomolecular psychiatric therapy as "the treatment of mental disease by the provision of the optimal molecular environment for the mind, especially the optimum concentrations of substances normally present in the human body."[1]

Orthomolecular medicine traces its origins to the use of nicotinic acid (niacin, or vitamin B₃) to treat pellagra, a vitamin deficiency disease that causes physical illness as well as psychosis. Nicotinic acid has cured hundreds of thousands of pellagra patients not just of physical symptoms but of psychoses as well.[2] Tracing the development of niacin's use, Pauling writes, "The discovery in 1937 that niacin is the pellagra-preventing vitamin soon led to its trial in controlling mental disease in patients *not* suffering from pellagra."[3] He continues that researchers reported success using doses of 300–1500 milligrams per day compared with pellagra-related use of 13 milligrams per day.

Megavitamin therapy (i.e., larger than normal doses) is the corollary of orthomolecular theory and resulted from continuing studies with niacin. One researcher studying the use of niacin to treat patients with mental and physical deterioration described "striking improvement in mental health as well as physical health" on doses of 1 to 5 daily grams of niacinamide (an alternate form of niacin). Megavitamin therapy then began to be used to treat schizophrenia with success,[4] and since such pioneering work with niacin, other vitamins, minerals, and nutritional substances have been studied and found effective for correcting psychological problems.[5]

Dr. Abram Hoffer, the "father of orthomolecular psychiatry," describes orthomolecular medicine as representing a paradigm shift and a radically different perspective constituting the "third wave" of nutritional medicine.[6]

In the first wave, which lasted thousands of years, people learned through experience which foods and plants caused sickness and which led to health and healing. The second wave began in the nineteenth century, when foodstuffs were broken down into constituent macro- and micronutrients, resulting in the insight that vitamins prevented disease. This insight, however, was resisted because of the then-prevalent idea that bacteria caused disease. The isolation of vitamins along with their synthesis and proven safety did allow them to be used in small amounts in order to prevent deficiency diseases. Beyond that, however, they were considered worthless. According to Dr. Hoffer, this remains the prevalent view, despite the accumulation of a rich body of literature since the 1930s attesting to the success of megavitamin doses to treat disease beyond deficiency issues.

The use of megavitamin doses represents the third wave of nutritional medicine and is based on the following principles:

- The best diet is inadequate for many, especially in the face of stress.

- Optimum amounts of vitamin supplements are necessary depending on the degree of stress.

- Many nondeficiency diseases respond well to optimum doses.

- "Best practice" in medicine includes the proper use of vitamin supplements along with the best diet.

Orthomolecular proponents also focus on diet. Foods adulterated with toxic chemicals, processed and refined foods lacking nutrients, and foods causing allergic reactions all have adverse effects on mental functioning through the medium of brain biochemistry.[7] Hence, along with megavitamin therapy, a careful monitoring of diet has become a standard part of orthomolecular practice.

With a stress on diet and megavitamin treatment (and the use of conventional drugs, depending on circumstances), the orthomolecular approach has become an established part of psychiatric practice.[8] The International Schizophrenia Foundation explores the treatment and prevention of mental illnesses using orthomolecular medicine.[9] The orthomolecular movement includes a journal (published for over forty years) and an annual international conference.[10]

Yet orthomolecular theory and practice have not been unanimously accepted. An American Psychiatric Association Task Force Report in 1973 criticized orthomolecular research and claims.[11] Although it was rebutted at the time,[12] little has changed. Current critics include the American Psychiatric Association and the National Institute of Mental Health. A *Wikipedia* entry reads that "there is no evidence that orthomolecular medicine is effective."[13]

Proponents, in turn, claim "educational bias and effective censorship": medical textbooks exclude pioneering orthomolecular work from the 1930s through the 1950s; and the National Library of Medicine, the largest medical library in the world, excludes the *Journal of Orthomolecular Medicine* from its electronic database.[14] One orthomolecular proponent adds that medical research disfavors low-tech approaches like the orthomolecular treatment for alcoholism, and pharmaceutical companies lack the motivation to investigate addiction treatments that cannot be patented.[15]

This continuing controversy, however, is no reason not to take orthomolecular medicine seriously, for it claims to know what nourishes the mind and brain. In addition, we seek the synthesis and the harmony among different points of view. Whether orthomolecular views accord with others will soon enough become apparent.

Three important concepts have resulted from the orthomolecular understanding of the effects of nutrition on the mind:

1. The body and mind are a two-way, interacting continuum.

2. Vitamin and mineral nutrients are the "right" molecules for proper brain functioning.

3. Whole foods are also important.

The Body-Mind Continuum

Orthomolecular medicine focuses on physical correlates to mental processes that work through the biochemical environment of the brain.[16] In doing so, it understands the word *psychosomatic* dynamically, not in a one-sided way.

Although the theory of psychosomatic interaction became a standard part of psychotherapy in the twentieth century, stress was placed on the mind's influence on the body despite the concept referring to a two-way process.[17] Much of the resistance to orthomolecular medicine from psychology and psychiatry is attributed to a

different understanding of the word *psychosomatic*.[18] The orthomolecular emphasis on two-way interactions and the biochemical aspect
of mental activity attempts to reintroduce balance. Critics, however,
have criticized orthomolecular proponents for overly stressing the
biological side.[19]

Vitamin and Mineral Nutrients as the "Right" Molecules

The "right" molecules of orthomolecular practice contrast with
"wrong" molecules that impair functioning. Adulterated, refined,
and processed foods provide "wrong" molecules because they are
missing important nutrients and have harmful added chemicals.[20]
Conventional drug therapy follows a similar approach to orthomolecular medicine by changing the brain's chemical environment, yet
it provides "wrong" molecules that have harmful side effects:

> Professionals who close their minds to the Orthomolecular
> concept are actually using it when they prescribe tranquilizers,
> psychoenergizers, and antidepressants. They, too, are prodding
> enzyme production; they, too, are in pursuit of the right mole-
> cules, for which they are using the wrong molecules, as demon-
> strated by the appalling list of side reactions to the potent drugs
> they employ.[21]

Vitamin and mineral supplements, in contrast, are safe and provide
the "right" molecules for proper functioning.[22] Conventional drugs
and "non-intact," processed foods provide "wrong" molecules and
result in impaired functioning.

The Importance of "Whole" Foods

Orthomolecular treatment focuses on the use of megavitamins along
with dietary control, yet proponents have increasingly emphasized
"whole" foods as the most important source of "right" molecules. The

histories of using vitamins therapeutically and treating hypoglyce-mia (low blood sugar) illustrate the thinking behind the emphasis on whole foods.

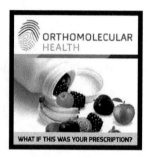

FIGURE 3.1. Orthomolecular medicine's prescription: vitamins.

Beriberi, a nervous disorder relating to B_1 deficiency, had been linked by researchers over time to faulty nutrition. Refined carbohy-drates like white rice, whose outer hull with essential nutrients had been removed, seemed to be the cause. The nutrients in the hulls were isolated, duplicated, and then marketed as a cure for beriberi in the form of a synthetic vitamin pill. Yet the vitamin itself was neces-sary only because essential nutrients had been refined from the hulls in the first place![23]

Hypoglycemia, or low blood sugar, affects the brain's chemical balance and leads to mental dysfunction. Refined carbohydrates once again, like flour, rice, and sugar, are widely recognized as the cause. In the past, treatment focused on eliminating refined foods and eating a low-carbohydrate diet to stabilize blood sugar and brain functioning.[24] Orthomolecular proponents Hoffer and Walker came to recognize, however, the importance of whole and unprocessed foods themselves instead of a special diet because intact carbohy-drates (whole-grain bread and brown rice) did not cause problems.[25]

Practitioners have emphasized food quality to varying degrees, and yet the trend toward whole foods has become evident. In dis-cussing the therapeutic use of vitamins, Carlton Fredericks writes:

> Some Orthomolecular psychiatrists . . . have been achieving
> excellent responses to very low doses of vitamins and miner-

als when given in the form of concentrates from natural [food] sources. Such concentrates offer these nutrients in the company of other [trace] substances normally accompanying them in foods. It is scientifically possible that Nature knows—and we do not yet know—how to create "fellow travelers" which vastly increase the effectiveness of essential nutrients. That is why vitamin supplements are never used as a license for poor dietary habits; they are supplements, not substitutes.[26]

Hoffer and Walker emphasize again and again the importance of food quality:

The real villains [of ill-health and degenerative disease symptoms both physical and psychological], the catastrophic deterioration in the quality of our food, is ignored. As long as food processing continues to strip out essential nutrients, there will be no letup in the creation of chronic ill-health.[27]

They even state in all capital letters, "USE WHOLE FOODS WHENEVER POSSIBLE."[28] Such foods are superior because knowledge about vitamin and mineral requirements is incomplete. Foods in the natural state contain all the essential nutrients and in the right amounts:

Natural foods in our optimum diet have incorporated elements from their surroundings during the period of growth and development. It is quite presumptuous of Man to think that he can tamper with nature, given our present state of nutritional information. Only our unprocessed foods offer the proper quantities of mineral nutrients.[29]

Are whole foods, then, the ultimate treatment for mental dysfunction? Hoffer and Walker respond that the prevalence of "junk" diets and the delay in applying vitamin therapy have resulted in an increased vitamin need (i.e., the use of megadoses) to treat conditions not clearly related to deficiency, such as psychoses and schizophrenia. They state emphatically, however, that people should turn to megavitamin doses only after good nutrition has proved ineffective.[30]

In summary, orthomolecular medicine has contributed three important concepts to understanding the relationship between diet and the mind:

1. the two-way interaction of psychosomatic processes spotlighting nutrition's importance for the mind;

2. the effect of "right" and "wrong" molecules on brain functioning; and

3. intact "whole" foods as the best source for "right" molecules.

Whole foods themselves, orthomolecular medicine teaches, have the capacity to correct imbalance and promote proper mental functioning, and for this reason they are to be preferred.

The stress of orthomolecular medicine on whole foods and the negative effects of refined grains are of special interest to us because spiritual teachings cite grains as a principle food and sattvic food supreme. As such, these teachings consider grains the basis of health, not to mention the basis of a vegetarian diet. Thus it is important that the effect be healthy, not harmful, and that the reputation of grains remains intact, not maligned. The focus on whole foods is based on research and makes intuitive sense. Yet we shall see that there are criticisms against whole grains, too, and so it will be necessary to return to these themes and to reconsider them in more detail later.

WESTON PRICE: INTERCEPTED HEREDITY AND SOIL QUALITY

Weston A. Price (1870–1948) breaks new ground in the understanding of the relationship between diet and mind by raising issues about parental diet and soil quality. As does orthomolecular medicine, Price warns about refined foods, but in the context of psychological effects on the next generation. Nutrient-depleted soils become an issue because even intact foods themselves, if they are nutritionally inferior, can cause impaired functioning.

Price was a respected dentist and researcher and author of the influential book, *Nutrition and Physical Degeneration*.[31] Through his

60

practice, Price became convinced that the cause of dental caries is less important than what prevents it. Suspecting nutrition's role, he sought out healthy groups with sound teeth to study their dietary habits, traveling to different parts of the world over a period of years. Invariably, he found that traditional foods promoted vigorous health and minimal tooth decay. If, however, modern refined foods were adopted, both general health and dental health declined.

Among the people Price studied, diet affected not only health and the incidence of caries but tooth spacing, the shape of the mouth arch, and facial proportions as well. The traditional diets of local foods eaten for generations created well-formed teeth, broad and symmetrical arches, and well-proportioned faces; modern diets created crooked teeth, narrow arches and nose passages, and elongated and distorted faces.

Price observed structural differences between parents and children, but also between older and younger siblings in the same family. Older children might have shown no degenerative effects, but younger children born after a familial shift to modern foods showed disturbances. If parents reverted to a traditional diet, however, subsequent children showed no malformations. The numerous photographs in Price's book dramatically depict such contrasts and changes.

Price concluded that facial and dental structures relate to effects on the human embryo resulting from parental diets. A traditional diet affects embryos in a positive way, producing sound structures, but modern diets in a negative way, leading to malformed structures. Price noted the awareness in some cultures of the importance of parental nutrition and the prescription of special foods for prospective parents, such as animal organ meat, fish and fish oil, fish eggs and sperm, high-quality dairy products from cows fed on fresh young grass, and green vegetables.[32]

The relationships Price observed between diet and facial and dental effects led him to link these effects to mental health and functioning. Research by others had shown that dental-arch malformations were much higher among delinquents, criminals, the mentally disabled, epileptics, and the insane than among the general population.[33] Price hypothesized that the faulty nutrition causing dental and facial malformations was also causing brain and personality disorders.[34] He argued that not only faces and mouth arches, but also the behaviors of many inmates in state penitentiaries, showed evidence of such injuries.[35]

The correlations led him to propose a new factor influencing behavior and individuality besides the environment and normal heredity—namely, *intercepted heredity,* or adverse fetal effects resulting from parental nutrition. Consequently, he questioned whether delinquents and criminals should bear full responsibility for their actions. In addition, he asserted that a better social environment would not compensate for germ plasma defects that resulted from prenatal nutrition.[36]

Down syndrome demonstrates the relationships Price postulated between diet and mental functioning. Unusual facial features and impaired mental functioning are part of the syndrome, which is associated with deficient pituitary gland activity. The pituitary, which is found at the base of the brain, is related to facial and dental-arch shape, and adverse pituitary effects were part of the developmental disabilities that research had linked to vitamin E deficiency. Noting that modern, refined flour had largely lost its vitamin E through removal of the germ, Price hypothesized that a maternal lack of vitamin E could result in Down syndrome in fetuses.[37]

Price's work with a sixteen-year-old Down syndrome patient suggested support for his hypothesis. When the mouth arch was widened with a dental appliance, dramatic results ensued. Within four months, the boy had grown three inches and a moustache had begun to show; the genitals developed, along with a sense of modesty; and intellectual capacity, independence, and displays of affection improved. When the appliance became dislodged, a relapse occurred, but once it was restored, the boy's condition improved again.[38] The appliance apparently was stimulating the pituitary gland, whose functioning had been impaired, according to Price's hypothesis, through embryo effects related to parental diet.

Such experiences led Price to assert that thinking is as biological as digestion, and brain embryonic effects as biological as club feet.[39] He concluded that, from conception, the protoplasmic germ of the mentally and morally impaired is abnormally organized.[40] The cause is not defective genes or environmental influences, but intercepted heredity—impaired fetal germ plasma caused by deficient parental nutrition.

Price added, however, that deficient nutrition was not necessarily the result of poor food choices among the people he had studied, as for example in eating processed foods. He pointed to a deeper cause in the relationship between nutrition and soil quality. His discussions about forebrain development demonstrate this additional dimension.[41]

The forebrain, and especially the human forebrain, signifies a higher evolutionary development compared with many lower animals. Lower animals are ruled by automatic instinctual responses and are virtually unable to learn. Forebrain development, however, allows learning and the operation of intelligence, such as controlling the sex instinct and appetite through reason and mental inhibitions.[42] Such capabilities, however, depend on sound forebrain structure, and Price asserted that its development depends on healthy embryonic development and in turn on parental nutrition. Forebrain injury leads to a decreased ability to express inhibitions as well as to character disturbances, delinquency, and even mental retardation.

Yet the influence of parental diet on forebrain functioning and the embryo also relates to the soil from which food comes. Price pointed to statistics indicating that a large percentage of prominent American scientists had come from the Midwest, which is known for rich soil quality, and that school children in the Texas Panhandle, also known for rich soil, showed superior intelligence. He noted, moreover, that the area around Hereford in the Panhandle was known for a low incidence of dental caries, and his own data demonstrated that cows fed on Panhandle-area pastures produced high-quality milk and cream.[43] He also pointed to the fact that, in the 1930s and 1940s, farms were being abandoned because of the inability to maintain cattle herds on farmland soils.[44] He predicted that the decrease in food quality resulting from impoverished soil would become the most serious problem of the future and result in a host of health-related effects.[45] (In addition to the soil depletion pointed to by Price in his own time, a macrobiotic review of government statistics between 1975 and 1997 indicates an average 25–50 percent decline in vitamin and mineral contents among many fruits and vegetables.)[46]

Critics may well object that the evidence for Price's assertions is pretty thin: correlations between facial features and mouth arch shape, hypothetical embryo and forebrain disturbances related to an assumed vitamin deficiency, and correlations between soil quality, prominent scientists, and children's intelligence. In fairness to Price, I should say that I have summarized his findings from various chapters of his book, which documents in much more detail, including photographs, the fullness of his work on diet and health. My next chapter elaborates on this work. In any case, the cumulative evidence Price presents is logically consistent, arguably commonsensical, and certainly worthy of serious consideration.

In his concluding chapter, Price eloquently sums up all he has learned about the relationships between diet and health, hoping to point to solutions for problems like delinquency and mental retardation:

- Native and modern peoples share similarities: some are physically and mentally healthy, and others are physically and mentally disturbed.

- The most important variable among natives is contact with a modern demineralized and devitalized diet.

- The cause of physical malformation and mental disturbance is intercepted heredity due to faulty nutrition, a cause that can be prevented.

- The force in plant and animal protoplasm passed on by diet to human protoplasm is a small but powerful force, similar to or perhaps identical with atomic energy.

- Native cultures show intelligence, purpose, and the wisdom-filled intention of living in harmony with this force and with nature: "LIFE IN ALL ITS FULLNESS IS THIS MOTHER NATURE OBEYED."[47]

For Price, obedience to Mother Nature meant heeding the laws of nutrition as they relate to health and mental health and living in harmony with them. This meant then and means now avoiding refined, processed, and minerally depleted foods that lead to adverse physical and psychological effects.

Nourishing the Mind and the Sattvic Diet

We have heard both orthomolecular medicine and Weston Price link mental disturbance with refined foods and refined grains in particular. The negative effect of refined grains is a cause for concern, and we will meet it again in the following chapter. Yet I want to reiterate that even whole grains have a problematic dimension. They will be treated at more length in chapters 6 and 8.

I also want to note again that Weston Price takes the issues of diet, health, and mental health deeper in two senses. First, beyond individual diet, he focuses on the importance of parental diet for the sound inheritance that is necessary for health (a dimension to which Rudolf Steiner alludes in mentioning inherited constitutional weaknesses). Second, beyond the adverse effects of refined foods, Price points to the importance of the soil for making even whole foods fully nourishing (a dimension Michio Kushi touches on in differentiating agricultural practices). These deeper levels of consideration are beyond individual control and add more complexity to the understanding of diet, health, and the sattvic diet.

At this point, we can say that wholeness for foods like grains appears to be an important criterion for a diet to be considered sattvic, as is soil quality, and that the sattvic diet is not only an individual but also a social concern. All such points come up again in the chapters ahead. The following chapter, however, shifts to the specific question of nourishing the body.

4

NOURISHING THE BODY: ANCIENT AND MODERN PARADIGMS

Diet's effect on the body and physical health seems common-sensical compared with its effects on the mind or spirit. Our holistic spiritual paradigms in chapter 2 speak about bodily effects, yet details are sparse and mainly concern effects on the blood and nervous system and, through them, ultimately on the realm of spirit. In the present chapter, we hear primarily the voices of modern paradigms about diet and physical health. Interestingly, the different evaluations of vegetal and animal foods presented in chapter 2 regarding spiritual effects are repeated here with regard to the body. Many modern paradigms trend away from animal foods and toward vegetal ones on the basis of alleged health effects, yet a strong countermovement challenges their point of view. In the quest for understanding the sattvic diet, now in relation to bodily health, this debate is important to pursue. We begin with a brief look at two ancient teachings.

ANCIENT TEACHINGS OF THE FAR AND NEAR EAST

A commentary in the famous *Yellow Emperor's Classic of Medicine* reads: "The five grains are used to nourish, the five fruits to assist, the five animals to fortify, the five vegetables to fulfill."[1] This succinct teaching ascribes special roles to the different types of food, and yet all are understood to work together. Of special interest is the nourishing role assigned to grains, which are mentioned first. Perhaps their nourishing function and primary position reflect the notion of principle food that we heard in chapter 2. The five grains, however, are also interpreted to include beans, so perhaps a more accurate statement would read, "The five grains and beans are used to nourish . . ." Of special interest also is the fortifying role given to animal foods, which are clearly seen as a source of strength. Perhaps this role is considered secondary in importance to grains. Yet the teaching is holistic with respect to the different groups of foods, and the four it mentions—grains/beans, fruits, animal foods, and vegetables—remain the focus of nutritional attention today.

A significantly different ancient teaching is found in the first chapter of the biblical book of Genesis:

> See, I have given you every plant yielding seed that is upon the face of all the earth, and every tree with seed in its fruit; you shall have them for food.
>
> (Gen. 1:29)

This verse includes only vegetal foods. Animal foods are missing. Yet the ninth chapter of Genesis subsequently includes them:

> Every moving thing that lives shall be food for you; and just as I gave you the green plants, I give you everything.
>
> (Gen. 9:3)

This biblical dietary teaching, and the important change that takes place between the first and ninth chapters of Genesis, will be taken up in more detail in chapter 5. The point now is that both ancient teachings—the *Yellow Emperor's Classic of Medicine* and the Bible— accord with one another. Both serve as past examples in different cultural contexts about the food that nourishes; and in each, both animal and vegetal foods are included.

MODERN PARADIGMS AND THE TREND TOWARD VEGETAL FOODS

For most of human history, diet has been considered part of the cultural legacy passed on from generation to generation.[2] It is even asserted that, in the past, nutrition was chosen on the basis of a reliable "instinctual feeling"[3] (echoing Sri Aurobindo's remark, quoted in chapter 2, about the vital normally being the safest guide to health). Yet it is also claimed that today science, the government, and special interests have replaced these influences, resulting in disorientation, a focus on nutrients and the latest research, and a diversity of views. We will certainly see such claims reflected in the dueling guidelines, plates, and pyramids that follow. Yet the glimmer of orientation that can be discerned despite conflicting claims is the common trend toward vegetal foods among institutional paradigms. We begin with the United States Department of Agriculture (USDA).

USDA: From Five Food Groups to *MyPlate*

Critics claim that the USDA pays more heed to food producers and the animal-foods lobby than to public health and scientific research. Yet policy changes over time show a clear trend away from animal foods toward vegetal foods.

In the first half of the twentieth century, USDA educational efforts focused on nutritional deficiencies.[4] From 1916 to 1942, various food guides appeared with different numbers of food groups—five in 1916, twelve in 1933, and seven in 1942.[5] In 1956, the "basic four" appeared:

1. dairy

2. animal foods, legumes, and nuts

3. vegetables and fruits

4. grains

Guidelines recommended a 2-to-1 ratio of plant to animal foods.

In later years, attention shifted away from nutrient deficiency to dietary overabundance due to the rise in chronic diseases linked to an overconsumption of fats, cholesterol, refined carbohydrates, and sodium.[6] The US Senate's McGovern Committee Report of

1977 recommended less meat, eggs, and dairy and more complex carbohydrates (fruits, vegetables, and whole grains), influencing subsequent policy.[7] In 1992 the first *Food Guide Pyramid* was released.

The 1992 pyramid changed the number of food groups from four to six—dairy became a separate group, and the group for fats, oils, and sweets was added. Daily recommendations also changed. The plant-to-animal foods ratio became 3 to 1 or 4 to 1, depending on minimum or maximum servings. The accompanying food guide, however, stressed that the food groups comprised a whole: each provided different necessary nutrients, and good health required foods from all of them.[8]

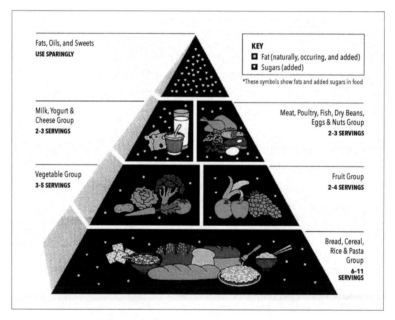

FIGURE 4.1. The first *Food Guide Pyramid*, United States Department of Agriculture, 1992.

Meat was not necessarily recommended daily, as the protein group also included beans, seeds, and nuts. The guide also spotlighted health concerns related to animal foods and mentioned that "some" grains should be whole. In short, the 1992 paradigm showed an increased stress on plant foods compared with the previous "basic four."

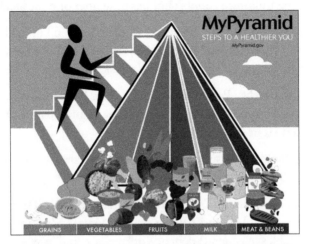

FIGURE 4.2. The *MyPyramid* food guide, United States Department of Agriculture, 2005.

In 2005, the USDA updated and reissued the food pyramid as *MyPyramid*. Although it was visually different from the 1992 pyramid, the food groups were much the same. The 2005 food guide, however, showed significant changes. The whole-grains recommendation increased to "one-half" of the total consumed, and calcium sources other than dairy also appeared.

The *2010 Dietary Guidelines for Americans*, released in January 2011, emphasized healthier food choices, which meant

- more nutrient-dense foods such as vegetables, fruits, and whole grains; fat-free and low-fat dairy; seafood, lean meats, and eggs; beans, peas, nuts, and seeds; and

- less sodium, saturated and trans fats, added sugars, and refined grains.

The *2010 Guidelines* also announced the imminent arrival of a "next generation" pyramid, which turned out to be a plate.[9]

Released in June of 2011, *MyPlate* emphasized the goals of the *2010 Guidelines* by depicting fruits and vegetables as one-half of the plate, protein as less than the other half, and dairy as an off-plate complement. Some details about the different groups and headings follow:

71

- **Fruits**: fruit juice counts (but has little fiber or none at all).

Important Messages: "Focus on whole fruits"; fill up half of the plate with fruits (and vegetables); daily recommended amount depends on age, sex, and level of physical activity.

Health Benefits: Potential reduced risk for bone loss, some types of cancer, type 2 diabetes, heart disease, high blood pressure, kidney stones, and obesity.

- **Vegetables**: five subgroups—dark green, starchy, red and orange, beans and peas, and others.

Important Messages: "Vary your veggies"; fill up half of the plate with vegetables (and fruits); daily recommended amount (of vegetables in general) depends on age, sex, and level of physical activity; see weekly recommended amounts for each subgroup; beans and peas have excellent amounts of protein and also count as part of the protein foods group.

Health Benefits: Potential reduced risk for bone loss, some types of cancer, type 2 diabetes, heart disease, high blood pressure, kidney stones, and obesity.

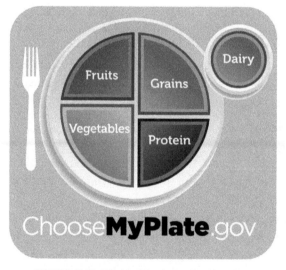

FIGURE 4.3. *MyPlate*, United States Department of Agriculture, 2011.

- **Grains**: divided into whole and refined; look for the "enriched" label with refined grains (but they still lack fiber).

  Important Message: "At least half of all grains eaten should be whole grains."

  Health Benefits: Whole grains may help with weight management and reducing the risk for constipation and heart disease; grain vitamins and minerals also have other important health functions.

- **Protein foods**: include beans, eggs, meat, nuts, peas, poultry, seafood, and seeds; a protein variety benefits health and nutrient intake; choose lean and low-fat meat and poultry because of potential health risks associated with saturated fat and cholesterol.

  Important Messages: "Vary your protein routine"; daily recommended amount depends on age, sex, and level of physical activity.

  Health Benefits: Protein helps to build blood, bones, cartilage, enzymes, hormones, muscles, skin, and vitamins.

- **Dairy**: choose fat-free or low-fat; excluded are products with little to no calcium such as cream cheese, cream, and butter; included are calcium alternatives such as greens, fish, and soy as well as calcium-fortified breads, cereals, juices, nondairy milks, and soymilk.

  Important Messages: "Move to low-fat and fat-free dairy"; daily recommended amount depends on age.

  Health Benefits: Dairy is a primary source of calcium, potassium, and vitamin D; calcium builds bones and teeth and maintains bone mass; potassium can benefit healthy blood pressure; vitamin D helps to maintain calcium and potassium levels; dairy can also help to lower blood pressure and to reduce heart disease and type 2 diabetes risk. (The caveats are that saturated fat and cholesterol levels in whole-milk dairy can have adverse health implications; a high fat content increases calories.)

- **Oils** (fats that are liquid at room temperature): contain essential nutrients but are not a food group. Sources: plants and fish; most are high in monounsaturated and polyunsaturated fats and low in saturated fats; hydrogenation turns vegetable oils into solids at room temperature.

  Important Messages: Daily allowance depends on age, sex, and level of physical activity; daily foods may provide enough (cooking oil, fish, nuts, and salad dressings); solid vegetable fats (trans fats) increase risk of heart disease; limit oil intake to balance calorie intake.

  Health Benefits: Polyunsaturated oils are the source of the "essential fatty acids" necessary for health; oils are also a major source of vitamin E.[10]

Reviewers praised the *2010 Guidelines* and *MyPlate* for improvements, but they also voiced criticisms. The more severe questioned the continuing prominence of animal foods despite the health risks, the continuing influence of meat and dairy lobbies, and the discrepancy between the alleged emphasis on plant-based foods and food subsidies favoring animal-food production.[11]

The USDA released its newest guidelines—the *2015-2020 Dietary Guidelines for Americans*—in January of 2016. Noteworthy is the emphasis on healthy eating patterns "across the lifespan" in contrast to the previous focus, by the USDA's own admission, on food groups and nutrients. Key recommendations for a healthy eating pattern repeat the advice for each food group cited above as well as limiting saturated fats and trans fats (less than 10 percent of daily calories for saturated fat), added sugars (less than 10 percent of daily calories), and sodium (less than 2,300 milligrams daily). Recommendations also emphasize that young and old alike meet the *Physical Activity Guidelines for Americans* released by the US Department of Health and Human Services. One critique of the 2015–20 guidelines states that they ignore the advisory committee's recommendations (submitted in February of 2015) for emphasizing food sustainability in the interest of planetary health and reducing the consumption of red meat and sugary drinks for human health.

The sustainability issue involves the lower environmental impact of producing plant-based foods versus animal foods in terms of energy costs, greenhouse gas emissions, and land and water use. The purported explanation for excluding these focuses is the influence of the meat and soda lobbies.[12]

Despite any and all critiques, the trend of the USDA toward emphasizing plant over animal foods is evident. The various institutional paradigms that follow lack the history to show similar changes, but they nonetheless demonstrate the same emphasis on plant versus animal foods.

Oldways's Traditional Diet Pyramids

Oldways is an organization dedicated to the health benefits of traditional diets. Together with the Harvard School of Public Health and the European Office of the World Health Organization, Oldways introduced a *Mediterranean Diet Pyramid* in 1993 in response to the USDA's 1992 pyramid.

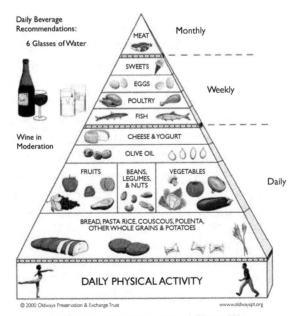

FIGURE 4.4. The *Mediterranean Diet Pyramid*, Oldways, 1993.

75

The concept for the *Mediterranean Diet Pyramid* emerged from the famous Seven Countries Study conducted by Ancel Keys in the late 1950s and the 1960s.[13] The study found that people eating traditional diets, particularly in the southern Mediterranean area, had significantly lower rates of mortality and chronic disease.

The Oldways paradigm criticized USDA guidelines for four reasons:

1. equating all fats and recommending minimum consumption;

2. equating all carbohydrates and recommending maximum consumption;

3. failing to differentiate among protein sources; and

4. failing to provide guidance about alcohol and exercise (subsequent *MyPyramid* and *MyPlate* paradigms did include exercise guidelines).[14]

In contrast, the *Mediterranean Diet Pyramid* made the following changes:

- It distinguished healthy "unsaturated" fats (from fish, nuts, seeds, avocados, olive oil, and other plants) from animal saturated fats. It did so by separating beans, legumes, and nuts into one group occupying a large "daily" foods tier, together with vegetables and fruits. Olive oil (mostly monounsaturated) was given its own "daily" tier lower and wider than the animal-foods groups. The fish tier was lower and wider than poultry, eggs, and meat tiers. The pyramid deemphasized fish, poultry, and eggs by relegating them to the pyramid's "weekly" portion section (placements show fish preferred to poultry and poultry preferred to eggs). The pyramid also relegated red meat, the most problematic of the saturated fats, to the topmost "monthly" tier.

- It differentiated plant proteins from animal proteins, which it deemphasized. Beans, legumes, and nuts were given their own tier.

The pyramid placed animal foods higher, onto smaller tiers.

- It visually provided guidelines for alcohol consumption (moderate), water intake (6 glasses daily), and physical exercise (daily).

- Lastly, the *Mediterranean Diet Pyramid* also placed grains onto the bottommost tier, like the 1992 USDA pyramid, but in contrast emphasized "whole" grains.

Among animal foods, dairy was the only one recommended daily (in low to moderate amounts) in the form of cheese or yogurt (i.e., cultured products considered more beneficial and more easily assimilated).

Oldways also released other pyramids: an *Asian Pyramid* in 1995, a *Latin Pyramid* in 1996, a *Vegetarian Pyramid* in 1997 (updated to include vegan guidelines in 2013), and an *African Heritage Pyramid* in 2011. The details of each differ, but the basic principles are the same: whole grains, vegetables, and fruits as daily fare, and other foods less frequently and in lesser amounts.

In 2008, Oldways updated the *Mediterranean Diet Pyramid* (other pyramids have been or will be updated). The new pyramid combines all plant foods onto the bottommost tier along with olive oil, herbs, and spices (for health and taste). Plant foods have been put into one group visually "to emphasize their health benefits."[15] The fish tier (now including shellfish) is lower, recognizing the benefits of regular consumption; cheese and yogurt are combined into one group with eggs and poultry; and meats and sweets are also combined. Although the previous pyramid recommended "whole grains," the new pyramid recommends "mostly whole." Consumption frequencies have also slightly changed. Plant foods are now an "every meal" recommendation (previously, they were a daily recommendation); fish "often, at least two days or weekly" (previously, weekly); cheese and yogurt "moderate portions, daily to weekly" (previously, daily); poultry and eggs "moderate portions, every two days or weekly" (previously, weekly); and meats and sweets "less often" (previously, sweets weekly and meats monthly).

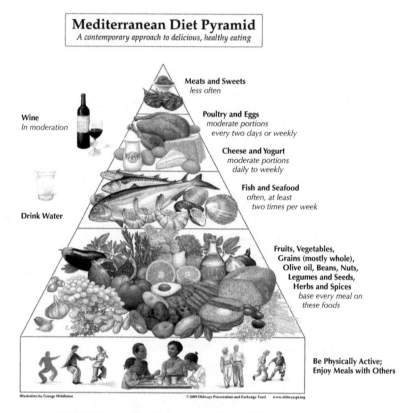

Mediterranean Diet Pyramid
A contemporary approach to delicious, healthy eating

Meats and Sweets
less often

Wine
In moderation

Poultry and Eggs
*moderate portions
every two days or weekly*

Cheese and Yogurt
*moderate portions
daily to weekly*

Fish and Seafood
*often, at least
two times per week*

Drink Water

Fruits, Vegetables,
Grains (mostly whole),
Olive oil, Beans, Nuts,
Legumes and Seeds,
Herbs and Spices
*base every meal on
these foods*

Be Physically Active;
Enjoy Meals with Others

FIGURE 4.5. The updated *Mediterranean Pyramid*, Oldways, 2008.

Oldways summarizes the Mediterranean eating pattern in the following way:

- Abundant plant foods, minimally processed, seasonably fresh, and locally grown

- Olive oil as the primary fat

- Total fat between 25–35 percent of daily calories; saturated fat 7–8 percent

- Daily small amounts of cheese and dairy (low and nonfat may be preferred)

- Twice weekly fish and poultry (low to moderate amounts; research suggests that fish may be somewhat preferred) and up to seven eggs weekly (including as a part of recipes)

- Fresh fruit as regular dessert; other sweets no more than a few times weekly

- Red meat a few times a month (leaner may be preferable)

- Regular physical exercise

- Optional moderate wine consumption with meals (1–2 glasses for men; 1 for women)[16]

Oldways adds that the healthfulness of this kind of diet has been corroborated by years of research.

In summary, we can say that Oldways, like the USDA, emphasizes plant over animal foods and especially deemphasizes high- and saturated-fat animal foods. The updated combination of all plant foods onto one tier, however, deemphasizes the previous importance given to grains as the only occupant of the bottommost food tier. *MyPlate* evidenced a similar change by equating grain and vegetable portions. We shall see that this same pattern of diminishing the status of grains holds with other paradigms as well.

Harvard's Healthy Eating Plate and Pyramid

The Harvard School of Public Health (HSPH) has also released pyramids and a plate. Previously it had collaborated with Oldways in releasing the first *Mediterranean Diet Pyramid* in 1993. After the USDA's *MyPyramid* appeared in 2005, HSPH released its own *Healthy Foods Pyramid* and subsequently updated it in 2008. HSPH released its own *Healthy Eating Plate* in 2011, a few months after the USDA's *MyPlate* appeared.[17]

(Due to the required fee, HSPH's *Healthy Eating Plate* and *Healthy Eating Pyramid* have not been reproduced. To view the images, see HSPH's website. The *Healthy Eating Plate* is divided into four quadrants. The quadrants on the left half are labeled "Vegetables" on top and "Fruits" on the bottom, in proportions of approximately two-thirds to one-third, respectively. Each has accompanying text. The quadrants on the right half are labeled "Whole Grains" on top and "Healthy Protein" on the bottom, both in equal proportions and each with accompanying text. At the top left corner of the plate is a cruet labeled "Healthy Oils," with text about oils, and at the top right is a glass labeled "Water," with text about drinks. At the bottom left corner of the entire image is an icon of a person in motion labeled "Stay Active!")

HSPH has been a long-time critic of the USDA. It claims that the USDA's policies neglect the latest scientific evidence, are beholden to powerful interest groups, and, most importantly, neglect the healthiest food choices. HSPH's critique of *MyPlate*, for instance, cites the USDA's failure to distinguish between healthier grain and protein choices and its promotion of dairy consumption at every meal despite the health risks. Further, *MyPlate* recommends whole grains only 50 percent of the time; other recommendations fail to distinguish, for example, easily digested potatoes (that spike blood sugar) from other, healthier vegetables, and no distinction is made between healthy and unhealthy fats.

Harvard's *Healthy Eating Plate*, in contrast, addresses all the above issues. The guidelines to the plate assert that, despite widespread dietary confusion, sound advice can be succinctly stated:

> We recommend eating mostly vegetables, fruit, and whole grains, healthy fats, and healthy proteins. We suggest drinking water instead of sugary beverages.... It's also important to stay active and maintain a healthy weight.[18]

A ten-point list provides more detailed recommendations:[19]

1. "Choose good carbs, not no carbs. Whole grains are your best bet." Carbohydrates are important energy sources for bodily functioning and physical activity; the type is more important than the amount. Healthiest sources: whole grains, beans, fruits,

and vegetables minimally processed that provide vitamins, minerals, fiber, and important phytonutrients. Whole-grain bran and fiber slow digestion and help to regulate blood sugar; fiber also helps to lower cholesterol and eliminate wastes and may help to prevent blood clots; whole-grain phytoestrogens and essential minerals may help to prevent some cancers. Unhealthier carbohydrate sources: highly processed and refined foods (white bread, pastries, and sodas, which digest easily, interfere with weight control, and contribute to disease).[20]

2. "Pay attention to the protein package. Fish, poultry, nuts, and beans are the best choices." The accompanying elements in animal and plant proteins make the difference: healthy or harmful fats; fiber or hidden salt. Steak has lots of saturated fat; ham has less but lots of sodium. Wild salmon is low in saturated fat and sodium, but rich in healthy omega-3 fats; poultry, beans, and nuts are also better choices. Eggs have nutrient benefits despite the cholesterol; moderate consumption (up to one daily) is recommended, but diabetes and heart-disease sufferers should limit yolks to three per week.[21]

3. "Choose healthy fat, limit foods high in saturated fats, and avoid foods with trans fat. Plant oils, nuts, and fish are the healthiest sources." Fats are important to health, but type matters; "good" unsaturated fats (mono- and polyunsaturated fats) are found in vegetable oils, nuts, seeds, avocados, and fish (especially oily fish such as salmon and canned tuna); "bad" trans fats made from partially hydrogenated oil are found in processed foods, baked goods, deep-fried foods, margarines, and snack foods. (Many products have now eliminated them; ask in restaurants. With packaged foods, check nutrition-facts labels for trans fats and check the ingredients for partially hydrogenated oil.) Limit high-saturated-fat foods like red meat, butter, and cheese.[22]

4. "Choose a fiber-filled diet rich in whole grains, vegetables, and fruits." Fiber (indigestible carbohydrate) helps to regulate blood

sugar and check hunger. Soluble fiber (dissolvable in water) lowers cholesterol; insoluble fiber prevents constipation. Fiber also helps to prevent heart disease, type 2 diabetes, diverticular disease, and breast cancer. Best sources: whole fruits, whole vegetables, whole-grain products, beans, and nuts.[23]

5. "Eat more vegetables and fruits. Go for color and variety—dark green, yellow, orange, and red." Variety and quantity are both important. Fruits and vegetables positively affect blood pressure, blood sugar levels, digestion, the eyes, and the risk of heart disease and some types of cancer; beneficial effects increase with increased consumption. Potatoes digest quickly; limit consumption.[24]

6. "Calcium is important. But milk isn't the only or even best source." Healthy bones need calcium. Dairy can prevent osteoporosis and colon cancer, but increase the risk for prostate and possibly ovarian cancer; dairy is also high in saturated fat, and the high vitamin A content can actually weaken bones; limit dairy and choose no-fat and low-fat products. Good alternative calcium choices: leafy green vegetables, baked beans, fortified soy milk, and supplements with both calcium and vitamin D.[25]

7. "Water is best to quench your thirst. Skip the sugary drinks and go easy on the milk and juice." Best choice: calorie- and sugar-free water; general guide for water consumption: 15 cups for men, 11 for women; coffee and tea (without sweeteners) are healthy too. Limit diet drinks, fruit juice, and milk. Moderate alcohol consumption is healthy for some, not all. Avoid sugary drinks, sports drinks, and energy drinks.[26]

8. "Eating less salt is good for everyone's health. Choose more fresh foods and fewer processed foods." Salt is a mixture of sodium and chloride; the body needs a small amount of sodium for essential functions, but too much leads to high blood pressure, heart disease, and stroke. Almost 70 percent of Americans risk developing salt-related health problems; fifteen hundred milligrams daily is the recommended goal for everyone. Tips for reducing consumption: eat fewer processed and prepared foods

and more fruits and vegetables; use salt substitutes and healthy fats and oils; prepare meals yourself; use cooking methods like searing, sautéing, and roasting.[27]

9. "Moderate drinking can be healthy—but not for everyone. You must weigh the benefits and risks." The dose determines whether alcohol is a tonic or poison. Moderate drinking may increase colon and breast cancer risks but also benefits cardiovascular health, which is important in middle age, and it lowers diabetes risk. Latest US consensus on moderate drinking: two drinks daily for men and one for women (one drink: 12 oz. beer, 5 oz. wine, or 1½ oz. hard liquor). Drinking to improve health is unjustified—exercise and healthier eating are better choices.[28]

10. "A daily multivitamin is a great nutrition insurance policy. Some extra vitamin D may add an extra health boost." A healthy diet is more important than vitamins, yet multivitamins can fill in deficiencies. Benefits outweigh the claims for risks; stick to recommended doses. People in latitudes north of San Francisco (37° 47'), or not getting fifteen minutes of sunshine daily, are more likely to be deficient in vitamin D. A moderate dose is safer than a high dose.[29]

HSPH's *Healthy Eating Pyramid* preceded the *Healthy Eating Plate*, and HSPH asserts that the pyramid won't go away, as the two are complementary—the pyramid is the shopping list for the plate's healthy meal prescription. Neither specifies daily servings or portion sizes, but foods lower down on the pyramid are emphasized in approximate proportions to plate sections.[30]

(The *Healthy Eating Pyramid* has five tiers. The bottom-most tier is labeled "Daily Exercise and Weight Control" and has images of sports equipment on the left, feet on a scale in the middle, and a plate on the right. The next higher tier has three sections: "Vegetables & Fruits" on the left, "Healthy Fats/Oils" in the middle, and "Whole Grains" on the left; accompanying text to the right details healthy oils and whole grains. The next tier is equally divided between "Nuts, Seeds, Beans & Tofu" on the left and "Fish, Poultry & Eggs" on the right. The next higher tier has images of cheese, a "low fat" milk carton, and a cup of—presumably—yogurt with a spoon and the label "Dairy (1–2 servings a day) or Vitamin D/Calcium Supplements." The tier at the tip of the pyramid is slightly detached from the underlying tiers and contains various images; accompanying text to the right speaks of using meat, butter, refined grains, potatoes, sugary drinks, sweets, and salt sparingly. To the left of the pyramid are icons of a wine bottle and glass recommending moderate use and a vitamin container with the recommendation for a daily multivitamin and extra D for most people.)

Lastly to note is the claim that the data of long-term health studies involving the eating habits of nurses and male health professionals show a better outcome for those in line with HSPH's guidelines than for those in line with USDA guidelines.[31]

In sum, HSPH follows the pattern previously seen of emphasizing vegetal foods and deemphasizing animal ones, especially animal fats. Yet its deemphasis on grains goes further by increasing vegetables to a larger portion of the plate paradigm. The paradigm that follows justifies the challenge to grains' preeminent status.

PCRM's Power Plate

Power Plate is a paradigm introduced by the Physicians Committee for Responsible Medicine (PCRM). Although strikingly similar to the USDA's *MyPlate* and HSPH's *Healthy Eating Plate*, *Power Plate* preceded both by over a year (PCRM, in fact, lobbied the USDA to replace *MyPyramid* with a plate paradigm).[32] The concept for *Power Plate*'s four food groups goes back to PCRM's "New Four Food Groups," proposed back in 1991 as an alternative to the USDA's "Basic Four."

PCRM is another long-time critic of the USDA, claiming that it neglects research showing that vegetarians are healthier than animal-foods consumers, and vegans (eating no animal-food products) even more so.[33] The claim is made that PCRM's plant-based diet is adequate not only for sustaining good health but for reversing as well chronic diseases like type 2 diabetes, cardiovascular disease, and some types of cancer, potential benefits acknowledged by the American Dietetic Association and the Academy for Nutrition and Dietetics.[34] For these reasons, PCRM asserts that vegetarian, plant-based foods should be the focus of the daily diet, with animal foods optional at best, and then only in small amounts.

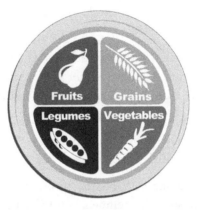

FIGURE 4.6. The *Power Plate*, Physicians Committee for Responsible Medicine, 2010.

The following message accompanies the *Power Plate* graphic:

> The plant kingdom provides excellent sources of the nutrients once only associated with meat and dairy products—namely, protein and calcium.
>
> The Power Plate is a no-cholesterol, low-fat plan that supplies all of an average adult's daily nutritional requirements, including substantial amounts of fiber. In 2011, the USDA revised its recommendations with MyPlate, a plan that reduces the prominence of animal products and vegetable fats. But because regular consumption of such foods—even in lower quantities—poses serious health risks, PCRM recommends instead the Power Plate, based on the New Four Food Groups.[35]

Like other recent paradigms, *Power Plate* also provides no recommended servings or portion sizes. Similar to the trend among other paradigms to readjust plant food proportions, and like the latest *Mediterranean Diet Pyramid*, PCRM equalizes them all, claiming that no evidence exists to support any preference (e.g., for grains).[36] Dietary advice simply focuses attention on the four food groups, emphasizes variety, and provides maximum flexibility for individual choice. Below are some accompanying guidelines:

- Grains: rich in B vitamins, fiber and other complex carbohydrates, protein, and zinc. "Build each of your meals around a hearty grain dish." [37]

- Vegetables: rich in nutrients such as beta-carotene, calcium, fiber, iron, riboflavin, and vitamin C. Choose a variety. Dark green ones are especially good nutrient sources.[38]

- Fruit: rich in beta-carotene, fiber, and vitamin C. Citrus, melons, and strawberries are high in vitamin C. Choose whole fruit over fruit juice with less fiber.[39]

- Legumes, including peas, beans, lentils, chickpeas, baked and refried beans, soy milk, tempeh, and tofu: a good source of B vitamins, calcium, fiber, iron, protein, and zinc.[40]

- Carbohydrates: provide energy, especially for the brain ("the only carbohydrate-dependent organ"). A high, unrefined, complex-carbohydrate diet (whole grains, beans, vegetables, and fruits) has no adverse health effects.[41]

- Protein: required for building, maintaining, and forming body tissues. Nine protein amino acids (the essential amino acids) must be obtained from the diet. Protein deficiency is rarely seen; the healthiest diets are moderate in it. A variety of plant foods, in quantities sufficient to maintain weight, provides sufficient protein.[42]

- Fatty Acids: omega-3 and omega-6 fatty acids are important for all tissue functioning and to prevent liver and kidney disorders, reduced growth, skin dryness, decreased immunity, atherosclerosis, heart disease, stroke, other disease conditions, and even depression. The body can synthesize most needed fats from the diet except the essential linolenic and linoleic fatty acids used to create omega-3s and omega-6s, which must be consumed; the proper ratio of omega-6 to omega-3 fatty acids in the body (between 1:1 and 4:1) is also important, but the consumption of processed foods and oils results in an imbalance in favor of omega-6s. Most diets have adequate omega-6s, but all people need a rich daily source of omega-3s (especially flaxseeds and walnuts, but also beans, fruit, nuts, seeds, vegetables, and whole grains).[43]

- Fiber: soluble fiber helps to control blood sugar and reduce cholesterol; insoluble fiber helps to eliminate bodily wastes and is related to cancer prevention. A varied plant diet provides both kinds. Fiber is found only in plant foods.[44]

- Calcium: protects the bones. But retaining calcium in the body is an important issue. To do so, exercise regularly, consume adequate vitamin D (which controls calcium use), avoid excess salt (which increases calcium loss), get protein from plant sources (because animal sources leach calcium), and don't smoke. The most healthful calcium sources are greens (except for spinach, which allows less absorption) and beans; other good sources are calcium-fortified juices such as orange and apple.[45]

- Iron: important in small amounts for healthy blood cells. Abundant in plant foods such as beans, dark green vegetables, dried fruits, blackstrap molasses, nuts and seeds, whole grains, and enriched breads and cereals.[46]

- Vitamin D: essential for developing healthy bones. Sunlight is the natural source; fortified grains, orange juice, soy and rice milks, and a multivitamin all provide it.[47]

- B_{12}: deficiency can lead to fatigue, weakness, digestive disturbances, anemia, and other blood and nervous system disorders. B_{12} is found mainly in animal foods, but a multivitamin and variety of vegan foods can provide it, including fortified cereals, soy milk, meat analogues, and nutritional yeast.[48] (Michio Kushi expands this list to include fermented foods like miso, shoyu, tempeh, natto, and some sea vegetables; he also notes that eaters of a predominately plant-based diet can produce B_{12} in the intestines.)[49]

In sum, PCRM's indications, like those of previous paradigms, emphasize plant foods, but they go further by questioning the value of animal food and endorsing veganism. In addition, PCRM affirms a lack of evidence to justify preferring one type of plant food over another (such as grains, our so-called "principle" food).

Summary: The Trend toward Vegetal Foods

The paradigms and discussions above show evidence of the issues mentioned at the outset as problems of the day regarding diet—accusations of special-interest influence, a focus on research and nutrients, and divergent views. Despite differences, the underlying motive of all paradigms is to promote health. Animal foods, fat, and grains are particular issues of concern. Nutrient research, in fact, has helped with understanding the benefits and the adverse effects of particular foods; and nutrient knowledge, indeed, is of special concern for vegetarians and vegans in order to find alternative sources for nutrients such as vitamin B_{12} that are otherwise available only from animal foods. Recommendations for vitamin supplements reflect the view that today's foods are insufficient to cover nutritional needs due to food quality (we hear the echo of previous authors) or even stress.

Another paradigm, the *Healing Foods Pyramid*, created by the Department of Integrative Medicine at the University of Michigan, focuses on food as a source of "healing and nurturing" rather than of energy.[50] Unique features include water as the foundation tier, chocolate as part of an "accompaniments" tier toward the top, an empty "personal space" at the very top for individual choice (and occasional indulgence), and a consistent recommendation for organic products. Also noteworthy are tips for decreasing intestinal gas from legumes (more on this issue later) and a recommendation for whole soy products because of health problems associated with processed soy (soy protein isolate, soy protein concentrate, hydrolyzed soy protein, and texturized soy protein).

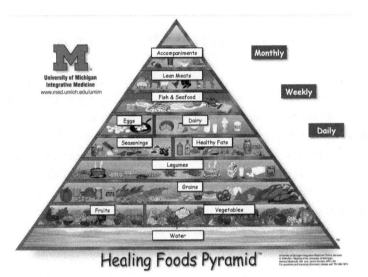

FIGURE 4.7. The *Healing Foods Pyramid*, Department of Integrative Medicine, University of Michigan, 2010.

Despite the differences among them, though, all the above paradigms have the following features in common:

- An emphasis on plant carbohydrate foods

- An emphasis on whole, minimally processed foods (in the cases of grains and soy products)

- A deemphasis on animal foods

- A special deemphasis on fat, and especially saturated animal fat

As for deemphasizing fat, PCRM asserts that the body can synthesize most needed fatty acids. Readers will recall from chapter 2, though, that when Rudolf Steiner speaks about the self-synthesis of fat and the spiritual benefits thereby, he also speaks of the inability of some, if not most, people to achieve this synthesis in sufficient amounts.

The discrepancy between a hypothetical and an actual ability is an important one to keep in mind as we turn to opposing views about the value of animal and plant foods for nourishing the body.

The Case for Fat and Meat Nutrition

As mentioned, this chapter reengages the debate in chapter 2 about animal and vegetal foods concerning spiritual effects, but now with a special focus on the body and bodily health. A few spiritual teachings cited in chapter 2 supported the nourishing quality of animal foods, including meat, based on beneficial spiritual and psychological effects; the witnesses that follow in the present section similarly argue that such foods are healthy for the body. Indeed, one witness raises the question of whether the diet can be fully nourishing without them. Reflecting on these views is essential for gaining a comprehensive perspective.

Vilhjalmur Stefansson: Fat and Meat as Superior Foods

Vilhjalmur Stefansson (1879–1962) was an explorer and ethnologist who lived among the Eskimos for over a decade at the beginning of the twentieth century.[51] His book *Not by Bread Alone* documents his experiences with eating the traditional, predominately flesh-based diet (meat and fish) of the Far North. Stefansson recounts that upon arriving, his attitude epitomized the typical prejudice of the times about needing a diverse diet of plant and animal foods for good health (and the less meat, the better).[52] Gradually, however, his beliefs and tastes changed. He began not only to accept but to value the standard diet of boiled and even decayed fish (which he compared to fermented cheese), realizing that such a diet was not only healthy but never boring. He concluded that, except for the short time needed to adapt to digesting unfamiliar food, disavowing such a diet or finding it distasteful was largely a matter of psychological or sociological conditioning.

After his time in the field, Stefansson documented his experiences in journal articles and books that generated both interest and skepticism, leading to a year-long study beginning in 1928 at New York's Bellevue Hospital. Both Stefansson and another explorer lived on a diet consisting solely of fat and meat in proportions determined by individual taste.[53]

Despite predictions of disaster and the inability to maintain such a diet for a long time, Stefansson and his fellow explorer concluded the experiment in good health and spirits. The presiding physician, Dr. Eugene Du Bois, wrote:

> The evidence is ample and incontrovertible. . . . The textbooks on nutrition are still narrow in their viewpoints. They do not seem to realize the great adaptability of the human organism and the wide extremes of diet that are compatible with health.[54]

The prejudices of modern dietetics are one of Stefansson's central themes. He encountered these prejudices in himself, then in his fellow explorers, and finally in a medical establishment that remained resistant to contrary evidence.

In documenting his experiences with meat, he cites the example of pemmican, a food originating with the Plains Native Americans made of finely shredded meat covered with fat. Stored and carried in skins, pemmican was especially useful for long trips because it combined maximum energy with minimum bulk and weight and provided sufficient protein for optimal health. Fur traders and explorers regarded it highly, including the artic explorer Admiral Robert Peary, who considered it an essential (a *sine qua non*) for polar expeditions.[55]

One of pemmican's reputed virtues was protection against scurvy, a vitamin C–deficiency disease. Such an idea was considered controversial at the time because nutritional theories focused on the protective qualities of vegetables and fruits.[56] Yet despite the apparent contradiction, examples abounded of Native American travelers, fur traders, and explorers living healthily and scurvy free on pemmican for long periods of time.

In *Not by Bread Alone*, Stefansson reflects on the evolutionary transition from animal foods to a diet combining both animal and vegetal foods, whereby carbohydrates become increasingly valued and fat devalued. Long ago, some tropical human ancestors gathered vegetal matter, including fruits and nuts, for food and also nourished themselves on small creatures. Outside the tropics, humans were primarily hunters and, secondarily, gatherers of insects, worms, shellfish, dead fish, and animals. This general animal-foods dependence lasted from one to several million years. The agricultural age that followed has lasted approximately five to ten thousand years, but Stefansson argues that we are still adapting to this relatively new diet. The incentive, however, is clear: more people can live from the food fed to animals than from the animals themselves.[57]

Yet despite this continuing transition to a mixed diet, Stefansson asserts that meat and especially fat have always been considered superior foods. He claims to have experienced this among the natives of the Far North, and he notes the biblical passages praising fat, such as the feast God makes available of "rich [i.e., fatty] food filled with marrow" (Isaiah 25:6). Fat, says Stefansson, was considered the "best, among men and gods, in most religions and in all countries." Among the Hebrews, suet, or the pure fat of animal sacrifices, was considered the richest part and reserved for God (Leviticus 3:3, 9, 17; 7:3, 23); and Stefansson points out that God shows preference for meat and fat by accepting Abel's but not Cain's offering.[58] As we hear in Genesis,

> In the course of time Cain brought to the LORD an offering of the fruit of the ground, and Abel for his part brought of the firstlings of his flock, their fat portions. And the LORD had regard for Abel and his offering, but for Cain and his offering he had no regard.
>
> (Gen. 4:2–5)

In this historical and cultural context stretching back millions of years, Stefansson says, people prized meat and fat because those foods were considered highly nourishing. He continues that, since the agricultural revolution, attitudes and foods themselves have changed. In Western European history and literature, fat's former status as a luxury and delicacy has declined in proportion to sugar's increased availability and evaluation. The word *greasy* may have negative connotations today, but in Shakespeare's time the connotation was positive. Similarly, fat-describing words such as *blubber* have taken on a negative connotation; but the word *rich*, which previously referred only to fat, now includes the quality of sweetness. Statistics from 1791 to 1940 (Stefansson's book was published in 1946) show the dramatic rise in sugar consumption, which parallels fat's decreasing valuation.[59]

Stefansson speculates that although people have been trimming fat from meat, the taste for fat has not decreased. Contemporary statistics of the time showed fat consumption to have been increasing since 1912, especially in the form of hidden fats in various animal and vegetable foods.[60]

Stefansson continues that the plentiful availability and cheapness of starches and sugar has affected the negative valuation of fat. In his view, protein is what is essential to the diet, and fat and carbohydrate are interchangeable supplements. As inexpensive carbohydrates have been replacing previously abundant fats, attitudes toward fat have been changing as well.

This cultural history is the backdrop, Stefansson feels, to the skepticism he had encountered about the healthiness of meat and fat despite anthropological and scientific evidence to the contrary. This skepticism was partly due to historical and cultural amnesia about humans having existed for millions of years on animal meat and fat. Yet it was also reinforced by the evolution toward accepting and valuing inexpensive carbohydrate foods made readily available through the agricultural revolution.

Another crucial influence on changing attitudes Stefansson highlights is the effect of mixing carbohydrates and fats. He asserts that while a diet of proteins and fats remains healthy, the inclusion of carbohydrates causes problems. He speculates that carbohydrates interfere with fat metabolism and reports receiving corroboration from a Harvard professor, who indicated that protein accelerates fat metabolism and thereby precludes difficulty.[61] Stefansson's speculation, in fact, is supported by current knowledge of the body's metabolic preferences—carbohydrates and proteins are metabolized first, before fats. As a result, diets that mix carbohydrates and fats easily lead to storing the fat, resulting in weight gain and other more serious problems.[62] The effect of mixing carbohydrates and fats will be discussed in more detail later in the chapter.

In brief, Stefansson is the first of the authors in this chapter vigorously to contest the health effect of meat and fat, albeit in the qualified sense of total dietary makeup, and he is not alone.

Weston Price and Animal-Fat Activators

We revisit Weston Price and his research into traditional diets, this time with a focus on physical health. Price, too, contests negative claims about animal foods and fat, having found not only that animal-based diets are healthy, but that animal-fat "activators" are essential for nutrient absorption. His work also challenges the trend toward vegetal foods and especially vegan diets, for Price found in addition that plant-based diets with few, if any, animal products lead to nutritional deficiencies and fail to promote health in the way that diets containing animal foods do.

Price's views, as the last chapter indicated, grew from his experiences as a dentist and researcher. He had decided that the cause of dental caries—whether a lactobacillus or an acid-producing strep—was less important than the "something missing" that prevented caries in healthy people.[63] As a result, he voyaged around the world, searching out healthy populations without disease. He found them among "primitive" populations, which did not mean that they were "uncivilized," for he also found them among isolated mountain and village dwellers in Switzerland and the Outer Hebrides islanders. What it did mean, however, was that they subsisted primarily on traditional foods.

These isolated groups possessed several common features: a very low incidence of caries, well-formed dental arches, broadly proportioned faces—and vigorous health. Yet caries, deformed arches and facial features, and impaired "physical, mental, and moral health" soon followed if the groups adopted Western refined and processed foods. Price also found, however, that symptoms of disturbance could be reversed by readopting traditional diets. When parents of children with disturbances did so, subsequent offspring became symptom free.

No single diet, however, was the "key" to robust health. The diets of healthy groups varied greatly. Some were high in protein and fat and based almost entirely on animal foods or fish; others contained various mixtures of plant and animal foods. But all these diets produced healthy teeth, broad dental arches, well-proportioned faces, and excellent health.

Price concluded that fat-soluble animal "activators" were essential to healthy diets, hypothesizing that they facilitated nutrient absorption. Yet the activators themselves were not the entire story. His analyses found that native foods were extremely high in vitamins and minerals—much higher than typical modern recommendations. Thus he cited food and soil quality as important issues. A discussion of Price's primary points follows:

Caries is a disease of modern civilization and a symptom of an underlying nutritional deficiency. The incidence of caries has risen dramatically in modern times, but was virtually unknown in the past. Among those on traditional diets, incidence was very low to nonexistent, yet it dramatically increased after exposure to modern, refined, and processed foods. See table 1 on page 96 for percentage summaries for caries based on the number of teeth examined.

As the primary variable for Price's studies was the type of diet, he concluded that food quality was either causing or preventing decay. He also found that changing to a healthy diet could reverse the symptoms of caries without treatment: decay stopped, and a veneer filled over the cavity, making the tooth whole again. For this to happen, he hypothesized that the quality of the saliva bathing the cavity must improve, and that animal-fat substances were primarily responsible for effecting this change.[64]

Diet affects individual health, as the presence of caries demonstrates. Yet through reproduction, parental diet affects the germ embryo, fetal structures, and subsequent health, including mental health. Caries are the most dramatic and immediate manifestation of improper nutrition. Equally dramatic, however, if not more significant, is the appearance of well- or malformed dental arches and faces, which points to hereditary effects prior to birth. On a traditional-foods diet, parents give birth to children with well-formed arches and broad faces. On a diet of modern refined foods, children's arches become narrower, the teeth crowded and crooked, and faces underdeveloped in significant ways (pinched nostrils, for example, making nose breathing difficult and shifting breathing emphasis to the mouth). These manifestations result not from genetic traits passed on from parents to children but from a parental diet that either nourishes healthy embryo formation or not. Embryo effects also manifest in stature, the shape of the hips (affecting reproductive ability), and the form of the brain (affecting intelligence, personality, and morality, as discussed in chapter 3). Different children of the same parents show different effects depending on parental prenatal diet. Price also noted that the folk wisdom of many na-

TABLE 1. WESTON PRICE'S PERCENTAGE SUMMARIES FOR CARIES		
	TRADITIONAL DIET PERCENTAGE	MODERN DIET PERCENTAGE
Swiss villagers	4.6	29.8
Gaelic islanders	1.2	30.0
Far North Indians	0.16	21.5
Seminole Indians	4.0	40.0
Melanesian islanders	0.38	29.0
Polynesian islanders	0.32	29.0
African tribes	0.20	6.8
Australian Aborigines	0.00	70.9
New Zealand Maori	0.01	55.3
Malays	0.09	20.6
Coastal Peruvian Indians	0.04	40.0+
High Andes Indians	0.00	40.0+
Amazon Jungle Indians	0.00	40.0+

tive cultures dictated special foods prior to marriage, and before and after conception, to stimulate healthy embryo development (high-quality dairy and green vegetables; animal organ meats; fish and fish oil; and fish eggs for women and fish sperm for men).[65] The photographs reproduced in his book of the facial structures of different people are one support for his claims; he also pointed to rising social rates of disease, juvenile delinquency, criminality, and impaired mental functioning as well.

A variety of diets, including primarily animal-based diets, provide sound health. The variety of diets that Price found healthy is surprising—from an almost exclusive use of animal foods to a mix of animal and plant foods:

- Swiss villagers: high-vitamin dairy products, whole rye bread, meat approximately once a week, and vegetables in season

- Outer Hebrides islanders: sea foods, oat cakes and porridge, marine plants, and limited seasonal vegetables

- Eskimos and Indians of the Far North: sea and land animal tissues (especially animal organs), limited vegetables, and limited seeds

- South Sea islanders: sea animals, marine and land plants, limited seeds, and lily roots or taro

- African natives: cattle tribes—primarily milk, blood, and meat supplemented by plants; agricultural tribes—domestic animals (organs), freshwater foods, insects, and plants

- Australian Aborigines: large and small wild animals, wild plants, and fresh-water marine life when available

- New Zealand Maori: marine animals, birds and plants, marine bird eggs, land birds, tree and plant seeds, and vegetables (especially fern root)

- Plains natives of North and South America: organs and tissues of wild animals, various plant foods, and fresh- and saltwater life when available

97

- Coastal natives of the Americas: sea and plant life

- Amazon Jungle natives: freshwater life, small animals and birds, and wild plants and seeds

Particularly striking is the positive health effects of almost exclusively animal-food diets, as with Eskimos and Indians in the Far North and African cattle tribes. Price noted that African Nilotic cattle tribes had superb physiques, were extremely brave and mentally astute, and consistently dominated other tribes.[66]

The essential dynamism in all healthy diets is the liberal presence of good-quality, fat-soluble animal foods. Price called these fat-soluble foods "activators," meaning that they catalyze the absorption and use of nutrients. He divided activator foods into four groups: 1) dairy products from cows, camels, sheep, oxen, and yaks; 2) animal organs and eggs from animals and birds, both wild and domesticated; 3) sea animal life; and 4) small animals and insects. Price noted that some peoples used activators from more than one group and that the source was irrelevant as long as the supply was adequate and the quality good.[67]

The importance of animal organs is particularly interesting. Price recounted the story of lions unable to breed in captivity until a specialist observed a wild lion eating organs after a kill and then abandoning the carcass. When organ meat was subsequently introduced to captive lions, the breeding problem was solved. Another story involved a prospector of the Far North suffering from sudden blindness. He encountered an old Indian who diagnosed the problem. The Indian then caught a fish from a nearby stream and instructed the prospector to eat the eyes and tissues around the eyes. Within a few hours, the prospector's vision had begun to improve.[68]

Price added that, for modern life, seafood and dairy might be the most convenient and useful sources of animal-fat activators, and milk the best source of all because minerals in milk are quickly absorbed. He also outlined a method for concentrating butter activators through melting, allowing crystallization, and finally separating the potentized oil with a centrifuge. Price asserted, however, that the inclusion of dietary activators was no health guarantee, noting that despite drinking whole milk, one might develop tooth decay if the vitamin content was insufficient. His numerous food analyses indicated that vitamin content varied considerably depending on season and, perhaps most importantly, soil quality. The quality of animal feed and the soil ultimately determined the effectiveness of activators.[69]

A plant-based diet without animal-fat activators fails to promote effective health. Price noted that he had not found a single group of primitives with excellent health who lived just on vegetal foods. As for those who abstain from animal foods for ethical reasons, he wrote:

> I have found in many parts of the world most devout represen-
> tatives of modern ethical systems advocating the restriction of
> foods to the vegetable products. In every instance where the
> groups involved had been long under this teaching, I found
> evidence of degeneration in the form of dental caries, and in
> the new generation in the form of abnormal dental arches to an
> extent very much higher than in the primitive groups who were
> not under this influence.[70]

These are sobering comments, especially with respect to vegan diets excluding animal foods. At stake is the health not just of individuals but of offspring as well. The statistics that Price cites for agriculturalist African tribes do suggest a higher incidence of caries compared with those who include animal foods.[71] He wrote that one such agriculturist tribe was not as well built, lacked courage and resourcefulness, and was dominated by others.

Sally Fallon Morell, president of the Weston A. Price Foundation, notes of Price's work:

> His main discovery was very high levels of [fat-soluble] vita-
> mins A, D and K_2 in traditional diets—something impossible
> to achieve on a vegetarian diet. These vitamins come from
> nutrient-dense animal products like organ meats, butter, egg
> yolks, fish eggs, fish liver oils, and animal fats. These were the
> sacred foods, considered essential for having healthy chil-
> dren.[72]

We should, however, acknowledge Price's critics, who argue that his research lacked the detail that would allow for more rigorous analysis and that he had preconceived notions about "healthy savages" that distorted his views. The criticism about lack of detail is valid; we do not know, for example, the composition of the vegetarian diets Price deemed unhealthy. Yet the accusation of prejudice is difficult to reconcile with his reputation as a scientist.[73]

Food quality depends on vitamin and mineral content, but ultimately on soil quality. Price emphasized again and again that the problem with modern foods is the removal of important vitamins and minerals. Much of the vitamin E in wheat is lost by removing the germ through milling. Yet even much of the nutritive value of whole grain flour could be lost through oxidation. Price recounted the story of his encounter with an old Indian grinding corn. When Price suggested using larger wheels to increase efficiency, the Indian shook his head in negation. When Price asked about keeping the ground flour for three days, the Indian shook his head again. When Price asked why, the Indian replied "Something lost." Price's own recommendation was to grind flour fresh and use it as soon as possible. As for milk, he wrote: "Unless hay is carefully dried so as to retain its chlorophyll, which is a precursor of vitamin A, the cow [feeding upon it] cannot synthesize the fat-soluble vitamins."[74]

In addition to these problems with nutritive content is the additional problem of soil quality. As the previous chapter notes, Price related the high incidence of Midwest scientists and the high academic performance of Texas Panhandle children to rich soil. His analyses of different foods showed vastly different nutrient levels attributable to soil quality. For this reason, he recommended nutrient consumption in vastly greater amounts than normally recommended because the quality of foods was unreliable. In the 1930s and 1940s, he warned about the increasingly visible effects of soil depletion and its relationship to healthy foods, and he predicted that, in the future, reduced food quality due to depleted minerals in the soil would become an almost insurmountable problem.[75]

One final item of note regards the dietary guidelines of the Weston A. Price Foundation. Among the emphases are whole, unprocessed foods; animal foods, including organ meats from pasture-fed animals; wild fish, fish eggs, and shellfish; full-fat milk products, preferably raw or fermented (see chapter 8); the liberal use of animal fats such as butter; a cod-liver oil supplement for the fat-soluble vitamins A and D; fresh fruits and vegetables, preferably organic; carefully prepared whole grains, legumes, and nuts (see chapter 8); lacto-fermented vegetables, fruits, beverages, and condiments; and homemade soup stocks from animal and fish bones. See the foundation's website for more detail.[76]

In summary, Price reaffirms the importance of unrefined foods and emphasizes soil quality, too, but he also refocuses attention on the relative merits of animal and vegetal foods. Not only were animal foods sufficient for promoting health among some primitives, but diets devoid of them led to impaired health. These claims may seem paradoxical in light of the trend of modern paradigms and even many of the spiritual teachings cited in chapter 2. Yet they echo the teachings of others, including the Bible and the *Yellow Emperor's Classic of Medicine* as cited at the beginning of the chapter. There will be more to say about this debate later.

The Low-Carbohydrate Movement and Pyramid

The witness of Vilhjalmur Stefansson and Weston Price prepares the way for considering the low-carbohydrate movement and its focus on animal foods as an alternative prescription for health. Besides Stefansson and Price, much scientific evidence supports the low-carbohydrate view.

The roots of the movement go back to the end of the eighteenth century, when a low-carbohydrate diet was prescribed for diabetes and subsequently became the standard treatment in the 1800s.[77] As early as 1825, a low-carbohydrate diet was associated with weight loss,[78] and the link was further strengthened through the influence of William Banting's "Letter on Corpulence Addressed to the Public" published in 1863. In fact, until the 1950s, many prominent hospitals and institutions used low-carbohydrate diets as the standard treatment for weight loss.[79]

Here we must reflect that low-carbohydrate diets had been the standard treatment for diabetes during the nineteenth century and the standard treatment for obesity until the 1950s. Obesity and diabetes are closely related diseases. Obesity can lead to diabetes and to other chronic diseases as well, including heart disease. Obesity is the first symptom of a metabolic disorder in a similar way to dental caries (perhaps obesity is the second symptom after caries). That low-carbohydrate diets—diets with a high meat and fat content—were used to treat obesity and the related more severe condition of diabetes as well is a counterintuitive fact for a modern perspective on diet and disease to ponder carefully.

In the late twentieth century, low-carbohydrate diets like the Atkins Diet were maligned as fad diets and even considered dangerous. This attitude must have been due, at least partly, to a sudden onrush of cultural amnesia, for as we have seen, low-carbohydrate diets were standard disease treatments until the 1950s.

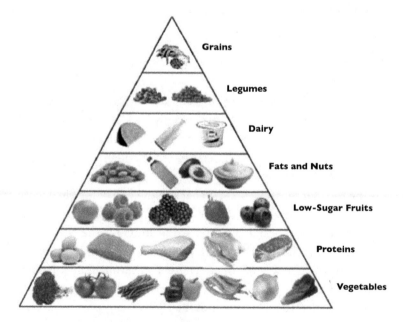

Figure 4.8. An example of a low-carbohydrate pyramid, Steve Aycock, 2012.

The prestige of low-carbohydrate diets had begun to change after the 1950s through the influence of the fat hypothesis of disease,[80] stimulated by Ancel Keys's famous Seven Countries Study (previously mentioned in the discussion of the USDA paradigms).

Here we must again pause and consider the irony that the previous *cure* for disease (meat and fat diets) had suddenly become a potential *cause*, and the previous cause (carbohydrates) had suddenly become the cure. How could this be? The greater irony is that there is truth to both perspectives: carbohydrates can cause but also cure, and the same is true of fats. Again, how could this be? We will soon return to these issues.

The influence of the fat hypothesis of disease also accounts to some extent for the trend away from animal foods that we have observed in modern paradigms. Yet despite this change, the low-carbohydrate movement remains a vital nutritional and social force. At the peak of its popularity in the early 2000s, approximately 18 percent of US Americans were using a low-carbohydrate diet[81] (and this means that 20 percent or less of the caloric intake comes from carbohydrate foods).[82] Yet low-carbohydrate diets vary. Two influential such diets—the Atkins and the Paleo-style[83]—are widely divergent. Atkins focuses on weight loss. Initially, it restricts carbohydrates in order to stimulate the use of dietary fat for bodily fuel. Later stages can include more carbohydrates to the extent that fats are reduced (chapter 7 reviews the Atkins Diet at greater length). Paleo-style diets are lifestyle diets that focus on lean meat protein (reviewed at greater length in chapters 6 and 7). Both diets, however, agree that animal foods are fundamentally healthy. Scientific evidence concurs with them (and with Vilhjalmur Stefansson and Weston Price as well): besides being effective for weight loss, low-carbohydrate diets reduce the symptoms of other disease conditions such as diabetes and heart disease.[84]

We have almost arrived at the point of resolving the paradox of carbohydrates and fats as both the cause and cure of disease, but first it is important to review the Blood-Type Diet, which offers some significant perspectives.

THE BLOOD-TYPE DIET

The Blood-Type Diet, developed by naturopath Dr. Peter D'Adamo, offers a unique view on conflicting claims about the value of animal and vegetal foods (fats and carbohydrates) by claiming that suitability depends on blood type,[85] the kind of individual consideration we heard so much about in chapters 1 and 2.

The Blood-Type Diet's philosophy is based on the timing of each type's evolutionary appearance and correlations to shifting dietary trends. Type O, posited by Dr. D'Adamo as the first type to appear, was dominant during the hunter-gatherer phase of human history when animals were the primary food. Type O's abundant stomach acid digests animal protein well. Type A became more prevalent during the transition to the agricultural revolution. Type A secretes less stomach acid, and so vegetal foods suit it best. Type B developed later, along with animal domestication. "B" is said to stand for the balance between types O and A. Type B thrives on a combination of animal and vegetal foods, including dairy. Type AB was the last to appear, about a thousand years ago. As the blend between types A and B, type AB shows characteristics of both, yet has its own unique identity and dietary needs.

Food recommendations are also based on other factors such as lectin reactivity, the body's response to lectin proteins in foods that find their way into the blood. Different types react to various lectins differently, so the foods suitable for one type are not necessarily suitable for others. Other digestive peculiarities also come into play. In general, a high-protein meat diet suits blood-type O the best (type O is present in about 45 percent of the US population) and a vegetarian diet type A (present in about 40 percent of the US population).[86] Types B and AB combine both diets to varying degrees but also show individual preferences. Recommendations comprise sixteen food groups (meat and poultry, seafood, dairy and eggs, etc.) broken down into "highly beneficial," "neutral," or "avoid" recommendations for each blood type. "Highly beneficial" foods are considered to act medicinally, "neutral" ones merely in a nourishing way, and "avoid" foods poisonously. The summary below for meat/poultry and cereal foods show similarities among the types, but mostly differences:

TABLE 2. D'ADAMO'S RECOMMENDATIONS FOR MEAT, POULTRY & CEREALS BASED ON BLOOD TYPE				
MEAT & POULTRY	TYPE O	TYPE A	TYPE B	TYPE AB
Highly Beneficial	Beef, lamb, mutton, veal, venison	None	Goat, lamb, mutton, venison	None
Neutral	Chicken, goat, turkey	Chicken, goat, turkey	Beef, turkey, veal	Goat, lamb, mutton
Avoid	Pork	Pork, beef, lamb, mutton, veal, venison	Pork, chicken	Pork, beef, chicken, veal, venison
CEREALS	TYPE O	TYPE A	TYPE B	TYPE AB
Highly Beneficial	None	Amaranth, buckwheat, oats	Millet, oats, rice, spelt	Amaranth, millet, oats, rice, rye, spelt
Neutral	Amaranth, buckwheat, kamut, millet, oats, rice, spelt, teff	Barley, corn, kamut, millet, quinoa, rice, sorghum, spelt	Barley, quinoa	Barley, quinoa
Avoid	Barley, corn	Teff	Amaranth, buckwheat, corn, kamut, rye, teff	Buckwheat, corn, kamut, teff

It is worth noting that despite a general caution across all types against wheat products, sprouted Essene Bread (also called Manna Bread) rates as highly beneficial for all, and Ezekiel Bread as highly beneficial for types B and AB and neutral for types A and O. This is due to sprouting, which destroys lectins, and to other beneficial live enzymes in the breads. (Sprouting and other methods for dealing with problematic lectins will be a topic in chapter 8.)

Another noteworthy feature of the Blood-Type Diet is the associations made between type and personality: type O is considered as more aggressive and individualistic; type A as more quiet, sociable, and cerebral; type B as more energetic than A, but less conformist and also less confrontational or purposeful than O; and type AB as somewhat enigmatic and even "flakey." The traits are thought to reside in each type as a kind of genetic coding, and recommended diets are meant to support the basic underlying personality. Thus, animal foods support type O's aggressive personality, and vegetarian foods type A's more docile nature.

In these brief descriptions of the Blood-Type Diet, there is much to highlight. Foremost is its ability to bridge the carbohydrate–fat debate by affirming both sides to some extent, but relative to different types: animal foods, or a low-carbohydrate diet, works best for some; and vegetal foods, or a low-fat diet, for others. Such distinctions apparently work—Dr. D'Adamo reports an 85 percent satisfaction rate among all types with thousands of patients. One critic attributes such success to the placebo effect; Dr. D'Adamo counters that all of the diets are healthy by any measure.[87]

Thus, the Blood-Type Diet supports both sides of the carbohydrate–fat debate, and additionally it brings to the fore individual considerations. Readers will recall that such considerations came up in chapters 1 and 2, ultimately determining the possibility of considering meat as part of the sattvic diet. For both reasons, we can affirm the Blood-Type Diet, and also for the associations it makes between diet and personality—meat associated with an aggressive nature and vegetal foods with a more docile one. Such associations we have heard earlier from spiritual teachings and from Weston Price, too.

Where a spiritual perspective differs, however, is regarding the intention of reinforcing personality through diet—for example, type O's aggressive nature with meat. Within a spiritual perspective, human freedom, personality malleability, the possibility of biological adaptation (see chapter 8), and spiritual evolution are important concerns. Rudolf Steiner speaks of the unsocial character of special diets and appetites and indicates that developing a tolerance for disagreeable foods strengthens the human organization.[88] Perhaps Michio Kushi expresses these concerns most succinctly by outlining various diets for eating "according to one's dream" (chapter 2).

The Blood-Type Diet's value may lie in the distinction that can be made between curative and lifestyle diets. If the purpose is to alleviate disease or imbalance, then "resetting the metabolic clock" by aligning each blood type with a genetically inclined diet may well be appropriate and beneficial (which is the reported effect). Once well-being has been restored, however, the effects of different diets in the interest of spiritual evolution are important factors to keep in mind. There will be more to say about these matters in the chapters ahead.

THE CAUSE OF DISEASE: CARBOHYDRATES, FATS, OR EXCESS CALORIES?

During the second half of the twentieth century, the cause of increasingly prevalent chronic diseases such as obesity, diabetes, and heart disease became a major concern. We have heard of the therapeutic use of low-carbohydrate diets until the mid-1950s. After that time, the fat hypothesis began to eclipse the carbohydrate hypothesis in importance. One factor was the well-known diabetologist Elliott Joslin's dismissal of the carbohydrate hypothesis in the early part of the twentieth century. His reason was the low incidence of diabetes in Japan despite a diet high in carbohydrates. Another factor was the influence of Ancel Keys's Seven Countries Study beginning in the late 1950s that correlated heart attack and stroke risk with blood cholesterol levels.[89] Readers will recall that the Oldways paradigms such as the *Mediterranean Diet Pyramid* discussed earlier in the chapter took their impetus from Keys's study. For its part, the American Heart Association (AHA) first opposed the fat hypothesis but by 1960 had changed its position. The AHA began to endorse a low-fat diet not only for heart disease but for weight control as well.[90] This signified linking fat with the fundamental cause of chronic disease, since obesity was considered the beginning of many disease conditions. When the US government's McGovern Committee Report of 1977 officially endorsed low-fat diets, they became a standard part of official recommendations, food pyramids, and dietary guidelines. The hearings themselves had represented a kind of war between low-carbohydrate and low-fat proponents.

Dr. Atkins testified in favor of the fundamental healthiness of fat and in favor of low-carbohydrate diets. In addition, Campbell and Cleave's work documenting the link between Western chronic diseases and refined carbohydrates (asserted also by Weston Price) supported the low-carbohydrate view.[91] Yet despite conflicting evidence, it was the fat hypothesis and the importance of low-fat diets that became emphasized.

The carbohydrate hypothesis, however, did not disappear completely. Paradigms and recommendations had begun to emphasize whole grains and the harmful effects of refined sugar. The USDA's continuing promotion of animal products among its recommendations (to the displeasure of many) also can be understood as resistance to the fat hypothesis. Yet public sentiment for low-fat diets became dominant, and the reputation of low-carbohydrate advocates like Dr. Atkins suffered until studies emerged vindicating animal foods and low-carbohydrate diets (scientific evidence mattered, not the previous tradition of using low-carbohydrate diets therapeutically!).

How can the emphasis on low-fat diets be understood, considering that evidence existed to support both the low-fat and the low-carbohydrate sides? What comes to mind is the de facto acceptance of carbohydrates as the most important source of food calories since the agricultural revolution, as pointed out by Vilhjalmur Stefansson, prejudicing the debate in favor of carbohydrates and against fats. As for resolving the debate more fairly, what also comes to mind is Stefansson's assertion that the true cause of trouble is mixing carbohydrates and fats.

In trying to convince the medical establishment of the fundamental healthiness of meat and fat, Stefansson hypothesized that carbohydrates interfere with fat digestion, a hypothesis supported by his Harvard doctor friend. Present-day research into food metabolism also bears him out. The body prefers to digest and utilize carbohydrates (and proteins) first before fats. Fat are used only if the total number of calories consumed is insufficient to meet immediate energy needs. Otherwise, fats are stored, and storing fat turns into a caloric nightmare: gram for gram, fats have about twice as many calories as carbohydrates and proteins, and storing them costs less energy, which means that a little goes a long way toward gaining weight.[92]

Complicating the matter is the less filling effect of refined carbo-hydrates. They "trick" the body into consuming more, and if fats are part of the mix—which is usually the case—then fats are more likely to get stored.[93]

A further complication involves the metabolism of refined car-bohydrates, as described by *metabolic syndrome*, the name given to a host of symptoms underlying many disease conditions. Refined carbohydrates digest quickly and turn into glucose or blood sugar. The body responds by secreting insulin, which stimulates cells to take up and use the glucose for fuel—glucose being the body's pre-ferred fuel—and to store fat. When glucose, however, chronically floods the blood, the system begins to break down. Cells become resistant to insulin and fail to utilize glucose or to store fat effi-ciently. Chronic hunger results because glucose is being poorly uti-lized. Consequently, more food is ingested, glucose continues to flood the system, insulin continues to be secreted, fats accumulate, weight gain ensues, and eventually glucose is eliminated through the urine, a symptom of the next and more serious phase of distur-bance, namely diabetes.[94]

So, which is to blame in such a scenario, carbohydrates or fats? If either is absent, the problem is largely resolved, which is why low-carbohydrate diets limiting carbohydrate intake, and low-fat di-ets limiting fats, both work (see chapter 7 for more detail). And that is why some refuse to take sides in the debate and focus instead on "excess calories" as the causal factor.

The excess-calories view is the logical extension of Vilhjalmur Stefansson's hypothesis, not to mention the fairer assessment of the reality. Various government agencies and the American Dietetic As-sociation represent this view.[95] Its basic position is that it is impos-sible to determine which factor is the primary cause of conditions like metabolic syndrome.[96] Both factors (and possibly others) work together, resulting in the view that the best approach to chronic dis-ease is not eliminating carbohydrates or fats, but controlling calo-ries. If calories remain within the limit of immediate bodily needs, everything will be metabolized safely.

To be fair, the institutional paradigms previously reviewed have the "low-calories" approach at heart in that fats are not demonized completely. But recommendations do emphasize limiting them (lean meat and low- or no-fat dairy recommendations), which is understandable because carbohydrate diets are the cultural norm and also because fats have caloric disadvantages. Yet from the perspective of low-carbohydrate proponents and fat-lovers, the attitude of institutional paradigms toward fat amounts to food discrimination.

Unhealthy fats, however, have also contributed in a justifiable way to the ascendency of the low-fat emphasis. Scientific research (not such a bad thing, after all) has uncovered that polyunsaturated fats and the omega-6 fatty acids found in vegetable oils, oxidized cholesterol and fats, partially hydrogenated oil, and damaged fats such as trans fat have been linked to heart disease and associated plaques and inflammation.[97] Trans fats also lead to insulin-binding in the blood and to high blood glucose levels and weight gain.[98] All the above fats do have harmful effects and are an important part of the disease-causing picture. Yet animal fats and saturated fat have been expressly vindicated.[99] This should come as no surprise in light of the history of the therapeutic use of low-carbohydrate diets, the low-carbohydrate movement itself, and the work of Weston Price and Vilhjalmur Stefansson. Research also shows that grain-fed animals have an unhealthier omega-3 to omega-6 fatty-acid ratio compared with animals fed on grass.[100] (Here the important factor is not fat or meat but feed.)

So, what does this all mean for the carbohydrate–fat debate? Excess calories are the fairest view to take about the cause of disease, not carbohydrates or fats. Healthy and unhealthy carbohydrates and fats, however, do need to be distinguished from one another.

NOURISHING THE BODY AND THE SATTVIC DIET

As I mentioned in the book's introduction, learning that meat and fat are fundamentally healthy foods came as a surprise to me. There are, of course, a host of issues to consider, such as the carbohydrate–fat mix, unhealthy fats, and even the quality of meat as it depends on animal feed. Yet all in all, it seems clear that meat and fat are healthy bodily foods.

This conclusion joins with similar ones in the two previous chapters. Other factors do come into play, such as quantity, as emphasized by macrobiotic authors. All in all, from a holistic point of view, a mixed diet with some animal food seems preferable to a low-carbohydrate diet with excessive amounts, or to a low-fat diet with minimal amounts. These, however, are ultimately personal questions requiring individual determinations. (Chapter 7 takes up the pros and cons of low-carbohydrate, low-fat, and low-calorie diets in more detail from a spiritual point of view.)

As for vegetal foods, refined carbohydrates are revealed as unhealthy for the body, just as chapter 3 revealed them to be unhealthy for the mind. Whole carbohydrates are potentially healthier—we will hear of their critique in chapter 6 and the possible resolution of the critique in chapter 8. Even in healthy forms, however, carbohydrates have the potential to cause trouble in diets mixed with fats. This is always something to keep in mind regarding mixed diets.

The importance of grains in the whole form, however, begs the question of why wholeness is also not an important criterion for dairy. The general concern, of course, is total calories, especially in mixed diets, and limiting fat instead of carbohydrate seems expedient. Yet reducing the fat quantity should work just as well. The *Mediterranean Diet* paradigm and the Seven Countries Study point to the traditional practice of including small quantities of animal foods with meals. Claude Aubert does so as well, and he further indicates that as little as 2 percent boosts vegetable protein assimilation synergistically.[101] The satiating effect of whole, full-fat dairy in limited amounts and whole-grain products with their bulk argues against excessive calorie accumulation. An overall healthier effect from the use of dairy in the whole form seems intuitive. In fact, recent research (that magic word) indicates that low-fat dairy is not healthier than full-fat dairy, and full-fat may even be healthier![102] Part of the reason given is the satiating effect of full-fat dairy suggested above, which may help to control weight gain. There will be more to say about traditional practices and dairy in chapter 8.

A significant and even surprising indication at the moment, however, is Weston Price's suggestion that animal food in some form is *necessary* for physical health. This is in harmony with the similar suggestions of some teachings regarding spiritual health, yet certainly at odds with the vegan *Power Plate* paradigm of the Physicians Committee for Responsible Medicine (PCRM) in particular, which is the logical outcome of the modern vegetal foods trend. In response to such a suggestion, PCRM and vegans might well point to the vibrant health they enjoy. Price, however, would ask about the health and physiological structures of offspring, measures that offer an objective way to assess the validity of the claims he makes.

Price's suggestion about the importance of animal foods is at odds not only with *Power Plate* but with the biblical diet cited in the first chapter of Genesis before it introduces meat in its ninth. Hence it is important to turn to religious traditions once again in order to assess in greater depth their attitude toward vegetarianism. We will see that this investigation leads deeper into the topic of diet and spirituality and into the mysteries of human and world evolution as well.

5

VEGETARIANISM RECONSIDERED

Weston Price's suggestion that animal food is not only conducive but necessary to physical health leads us to consider more deeply the question of vegetarianism from a religious and spiritual point of view. Chapter 2 explored this topic, but its primary focus was the spiritual effects of diet, which necessarily brought up the issue of meat. The teachings it cited from a variety of traditions are unanimous in asserting that diet does have spiritual effects, but views on vegetarianism are less than unanimous. Most support it, but the Mosaic dietary laws allow some forms of meat, and only the macrobiotic tradition and Rudolf Steiner support vegetarianism with caution while supporting animal foods as well to some extent. The present chapter reviews the attitudes of religious traditions as a whole on vegetarianism.

A survey of the major traditions reveals a remarkably mixed picture. In the Far East, Hinduism supports vegetarianism, yet with qualifications; Buddhism's two major traditions—the Hinayana and Mahayana—are largely at odds, one opposing and the other supporting vegetarianism; Jainism requires vegetarianism; Sikhism rejects it. Among the Abrahamic traditions of the Near East (Judaism, Christianity, and Islam), vegetarianism plays no outwardly significant role, yet an undercurrent of varying degrees of strength underlies the entire tradition.

In short, we see an overall ambivalence, undoubtedly due to the host of individual considerations raised in chapters 1 and 2. Foremost among them is the question of whether meat represents a desire or a need. At the root of this question is the notion that human development requires animal food, at least initially. We have heard this notion from Rudolf Steiner and, more indirectly, from macrobiotic authors; Weston Price hints of it as well. The present chapter addresses this same theme, beginning with the Hindu tradition.

HINDUISM

The Laws of Manu are cited as India's earliest writings advocating vegetarianism while condemning "the entire social and economic structure of meat eating . . . as spiritually impure."[1] Yet a closer look reveals a more complex picture: the laws not only distinguish between sanctioned and unsanctioned meat eating, but they also reveal the cultural importance of ritual sacrifice. To fully understand texts like the Laws of Manu and other religious teachings involving sacrifice, it is first necessary to understand the significance of sacrifice in ancient cultures. Important themes that emerge are memorializing a deity whose death is responsible for world creation and sustaining the world order that has come into existence.

Animal Sacrifice

Ritual blood sacrifice has played an integral role throughout human history and is linked to cultivator or agricultural cultures. Its meaning is twofold: to memorialize a sacrificed deity from whose body all life arises, and then to renew divine energy by returning blood—the source and symbol of life—back to the divine world.

Myths abound about deities slain by other deities or who sacrifice themselves for the sake of earthly and universal life. Examples are the Aztec deity Nanahuatzin, who sacrifices itself for the sake of universal life, and the Indonesian deity Samyam Sri, who is killed by gods and from whose body rice and grasses grow for human nourishment (see appendix A). In effect, "life proceeds from death," and this principle is fundamental for understanding ritual sacrifice. In the myths, food crops spring from the body of the slain deity, and sacrifice renews the memory and power of the myth and demonstrates human dependence on the deity's sacrifice as well as appreciation for it. Consuming the sacrifice also signifies communion with the deity and the assimilation of divine attributes, including the power to survive death, just as the slain deity is understood to survive and live in another existence.

The accompanying notion of renewing divine energy through the sacrifice signifies mutual dependence between gods and human beings. Just as the deity shed blood for the sake of life, so too do humans shed blood to revitalize the gods and keep universal energy in circulation. In the Durga festival of the Indian goddess Kali, animals are sacrificed and their blood buried to renew nature's strength and fertility; similarly, the Aztec Snake Woman yields nature's fertility only through blood sacrifice (appendix A). In this way, the gods are able to sustain earthly and universal life. In addition, ritual sacrifice was thought to sustain deceased ancestors, and adverse effects were considered to result from failing to perform such rituals.[2]

Humans, animals, and grain effigies were sacrificed. Over time, emphasis appears to have shifted from humans to animals and then to vegetal effigies that used the fruits of the field (we heard that Pythagoras himself eschewed blood sacrifices).[3] Sacrificing humans seems abhorrent to today's sensibilities, but human sacrifice appears to have been a universal practice rooted in the understanding of a sacrificed deity. Yet it is important to note that the ancient Avestan people believed that Angra Mainyu, the evil spirit, was responsible for sacrificial killing, whose domain in the beginning was solely the province of the gods.[4] We will return to this point later.

The picture that emerges is that offering and consuming sacrifices were integral parts of cultural understanding and identity. Ritualization within a religious context allowed hallowing both the sacrificial act and the accompanying consumption of flesh. Consumption outside of this context was considered sinful:

> The good who eat . . . the sacrifice, are released from sin; but evil are they and enjoy sin who cook (the food) for their own sake.

> From food creatures come into being, from rain is the birth, from sacrifice comes into being the rain, sacrifice is born of work; work know to be born of Brahman, Brahman is born of

the Immutable; therefore is the all-pervading Brahman established in the sacrifice.

(Bhagavad Gita, 3:13–15)[5]

In this Bhagavad Gita selection, we see the understanding of sacrifice as sustaining the universal creator Brahman and the order of the universe; eating flesh is allowable only in this sacred context.

The ideas above relate to ritual sacrifice in all cultures: it memorialized and recreated a sacred event, and it also allowed meat consumption, which was otherwise sinful.

Here we can raise the question of whether such a mythological complex was of human or divine origin, which is to say, does it represent a projection of the human mind to justify the desire—or base craving—for meat, or does it represent instead a divine injunction within strict guidelines to control a human desire shading into need? We can also ask if humans would conclude on their own that eating meat outside of a hallowed context is sinful. Much depends on the answers to such questions.

The notion of the sinfulness of eating meat at all is arguably the first hint of the vegetarianism impulse in Eastern traditions. Ambivalence toward blood sacrifice, and even rejecting both it and the consumption of meat, were later developments. To understand the genesis of these developments, it is necessary to outline the evolution in Indian culture from Vedic to subsequent times.

From Vedism, to Brahmanism, to Hinduism

Animal sacrifice was a central part of the Vedic culture developing in India after the incursion of peoples from present-day Iran around 1500 BCE.[6] Sacrifice was seen as necessary for maintaining harmonious relations between the gods and society.

Over time, the Vedic focus on sacrifice and ritual as outlined in the Vedas evolved into Brahmanism. Brahmanism divided society into four classes: *Brahmans* were the priests and teachers; *Kshatriyas* the warriors, nobles, and administrators; *Vaishyas* the merchants, farmers, artisans, and commoners; and *Sudras* the servants. At first, movement from class to class was upwardly mobile, with priesthood open to everyone. Yet as the rituals increased and became more complex, the Brahmans became a specialist and hereditary class,[7] a development, however, that created social tension.

Concurrently, religious thought was becoming more philosophical as reflected in the Upanishad texts. Ideas emerged like that of the *atman* (the universal self and unchanging core of the human being), the atman's merging into *Brahman* (the supreme deity), and the identity between the atman and Brahman. Personal experience of that identity was said to end reincarnation, or the cycle of rebirth.[8]

Other developing ideas related to *karma* (destiny or fate) and the determination of karma. It began to be seen as having less to do with preforming rituals and more to do with individual behavior.[9] Other important developing ideas were *ahimsa* (nonviolence); the links between karma, violence, and reincarnation and between nonviolence and a meatless diet; *moksha*, or liberation from the cycle of death and rebirth; and meditation instead of sacrifice as the means for liberation.[10] All these ideas contributed to increasing interest in asceticism, to the development of Buddhism and Jainism as alternative philosophies and lifestyles, to the rejection of ritualism and Brahmanism, and to a focus on achieving release from *samsara*, the cycle of death and rebirth.[11]

Brahmanism in response developed the doctrine of the *ashramas*, or four successive life stages, each with its own function and goals:[12]

- The student (*bramacharya*), whose goal was righteousness (*dharma*)

- The married householder (*grihastha*), whose goals were righteousness, wealth (*artha*), and pleasure (*kama*)

- The hermit or forest dweller (*vanaprastha*), whose goals were righteousness and preparing for liberation (*moksha*)

- The wandering ascetic (*sannyasa*), whose goals were righteousness and achieving liberation[13]

The last two stages were not required but chosen,[14] and they were typically understood as the time for seeking liberation and practicing yoga, meditation, and asceticism (which also implied strict vegetarianism).[15] Moving immediately from the student to the wandering stage was possible, but it depended on the cumulative effect of past lives.[16] Practically speaking, few chose to withdraw immediately from the world,[17] as withdrawal was frowned upon because fulfilling one's obligations to the gods and ancestors through sacrifices and begetting sons was important.[18]

During this time of ideological change (500–0 BCE) Hinduism took shape, having inherited the legacy of the Vedas and Brahmanism as well as interest in personal karma and liberation. All such diverse and contradictory impulses were responsible for creating conflict.[19] It is within this cultural context that teachings such as the Laws of Manu appeared and need to be understood, particularly in regard to eating meat and vegetarianism.

The Laws of Manu

Chapter 2 in this book related that the Mosaic dietary code specifies the creatures that are allowable and forbidden for consumption. So, too, do the Laws of Manu. Its own list, however, is more extensive (see the Laws, chapter 5, verses 5–25). Following the list are rules for eating and avoiding meat (verses 26–56). Significantly, all these indications apply to "twice-born men"—those who belong to the upper three classes in Hindu society.

The rules can be roughly divided into two parts. The first part (verses 26–42) focuses on lawful contexts for eating meat. Such consumption is allowed when prayers are recited and when performing a religious rite or when one's life is in danger. The verses state that the gods will that life be sustained through eating creatures, and there is no sin in doing so in compliance with the law. In fact, when people partake in rituals involving sacrifice, *not to consume meat is sinful*. Slaughtering for the sake of sacrifice is not really considered slaughter in a negative sense, because sacrificed creatures will be reborn to a higher existence.

Meat consumption outside of such religious contexts, however, is considered sinful. When faced with the desire, one should make and consume butter or flour effigies instead. Illustrative verses from the Laws of Manu follow:

27. One may eat meat when it has been sprinkled with water, while Mantras [are] recited, when Brahmanas desire (one's doing it), when one is engaged (in the performance of a rite) according to the law, and when one's life is in danger.

28. The Lord of creatures (Pragapati) created this whole (world to be) the sustenance of the vital spirit; both the immovable and the movable (creation is) the food of the vital spirit.

30. The eater who daily even devours those destined to be his food, commits no sin; for the creator himself created both the eaters and those who are to be eaten (for those special purposes).

33. A twice-born man who knows the law must not eat meat except in conformity with the law; for if he has eaten it unlawfully, he will, unable to save himself, be eaten after death by his (victims).

35. But a man who, being duly engaged (to officiate or to dine at a sacred rite), refuses to eat meat, becomes after death an animal during twenty-one existences.

37. If he has a strong desire (for meat) he may make an animal of clarified butter or one of flour, (and eat that); but let him never seek to destroy an animal without a (lawful) reason.

39. The slaughtering (of beasts) for sacrifices is not slaughtering (in the ordinary sense of the word).

40. Herbs, trees, cattle, birds, and (other) animals that have been destroyed for sacrifices, receive (being reborn) higher existences.

The second part of relevant verses (43–56) focus on the importance of *ahimsa*, or nonviolence or injury. One should not injure or harm animals in any way. Injury in the context of the law (i.e. religious rites), however, is not considered injury at all. Harming animals outside the law, especially to seek the "increase of one's own flesh" by eating them, is a grave sin and results in bad karma. Eating meat itself is not sinful, yet still it is best avoided:

43. A twice-born man of virtuous disposition, whether he dwells in (his own) house, with a teacher, or in the forest, must never, even in times of distress, cause an injury (to any creature) which is not sanctioned by the Veda.

44. Know that the injury to moving creatures and to those destitute of motion, which the Veda has prescribed for certain occasions, is no injury at all; for the sacred law shone forth from the Veda.

45. He who injures innoxious beings from a wish to (give) himself pleasure, never finds happiness, neither living nor dead.

48. Meat can never be obtained without injury to living creatures, and injury to sentient beings is detrimental to (the attainment of) heavenly bliss; let him therefore shun (the use of) meat.

52. There is no greater sinner than that (man) who, though not worshipping the gods or the manes [spirits of the dead], seeks to increase (the bulk of) his own flesh by the flesh of other (beings).

56. There is no sin in eating meat, in (drinking) spirituous liquor, and in carnal intercourse, for that is the natural way of created beings, but abstention brings great rewards.

In sum, the Laws of Manu condemn meat consumption only outside of religious contexts. Written at the time when cultic life was being challenged in favor of individual salvation and ahimsa, they walk a fine line between affirming meat consumption within a limited sacrificial context on the one hand, and affirming ahimsa, or nonviolence, on the other. They reflect the understanding that sacrifice sustains the world, which includes the sustenance of human beings through eating meat, but also the understanding that this practice is not the ideal. The attitudes of the times are shifting, yet meat consumption is still allowable and beneficial as long as it remains within a sacred context.

The Anusasana Parva

We see many of the above themes in the next Hindu text, the *Anusasana Parva*, or "Book of Instruction." The Anusasana Parva is part of the Mahabharata, like the Bhagavad Gita, and it also appeared, like the Laws of Manu, at a time when Hinduism was evolving to a complex reality that challenged traditional Vedic morality and ideas.[20]

The sections below from the Anusasana Parva invoke the name of Manu once (in section 115), suggesting a familiarity with Manu's laws and harmony with their principles. Some themes echo the Laws of Manu, but differently. Below is a summary of relevant points from sections CXIII–CXVI (113–116):[21]

- Compassion is the highest good and highest form of religion, higher than observing rituals (and higher than meditating, subjugating the senses, doing penance, and obeying authorities) (section 113).

- Abstaining from eating meat is the highest form of compassion (114).

- The taste of meat is addictive, and giving it up to observe the high vow of abstinence is difficult (115).

- The benefits of abstinence include health, longevity, the friendship of all creatures, the favor of the gods, and freedom from karmic consequences (115).

- Religious practice for householders (focusing on performing acts and rituals) is different from practice for those who seek emancipation (115).

- Meat hallowed with mantras and properly sanctified is pure (115).

- In the past, those seeking karmic benefit after death performed sacrifices with seeds (instead of meat) (115).

- Abstaining from meat for even a short time has meritorious effects (115).

- Eating meat benefits the exhausted, the sick, the thin, and the weak, and those addicted to sex (!). It promotes development and strength and is superior to all other foods (116).

- Eating meat also has numerous disadvantages (killing animals to eat them provokes their fear and animosity and may lead to being killed by them; it also has negative consequences for human rebirth); abstention from cruelty and showing compassion to all living creatures is the highest form of religion (116).

The above summary, however, fails to convey the emphasis throughout the entire text on compassion and abstention from cruelty and eating meat.

These verses from the Anusasana Parva do, though, clarify several things about meat consumption in Hindu society: First, they show the distinction made between householders (in the second stage of life), for whom meat eating represented a norm because of its benefits, and hermits and ascetics (in stages three and four), for whom abstention represented the highest form of practicing compassion. The verses also suggest the distinction between Brahmans, for whom meat eating was not generally allowed, and the three other classes of Hindu society (the *Kshatriyas, Vaishyas,* and *Sudras*—or again, briefly, the warriors, merchants, and servants), from whom the rigors of the Brahman diet would not be expected. In addition, we hear of the possible use of effigies (seeds) instead of animals (reminding us again of Pythagoras), suggesting that it was sacrifice itself—but not necessarily animal sacrifice—that was important for universal and social cohesion. Lastly, we see an arguable distinction being made between the desire and the need for meat. Its taste can become addictive and make abstinence difficult, yet it promotes development and strength. Chapter 2 noted a similar tension between desire and need in the teachings it cited, and we will continue to see that such a distinction provokes controversy. Both sides of the dichotomy are important for understanding diverse attitudes toward eating meat among religious and spiritual teachings as a whole.

In sum, we can say that excerpts from the Laws of Manu and the Anusasana Parva show qualified support for vegetarianism in the Hindu tradition. Abstention from meat represents the highest form of compassion, but consumption is allowed in religious contexts. Current statistics in India show this same qualified support: The number of lacto-vegetarians (those who consume dairy) and ovo-lacto-vegetarians (eggs and dairy) together is approximately 30–40 percent of the total Hindu population.[22] Vegetarianism is more common among Hindu Brahmans (about 55 percent) than among other social groups.

BUDDHISM

Philosophical speculation in the Upanishads began to loosen the hold of ritual on religious practice and stimulated yearning for union with Brahman and release from *samsara*, the cycle of death and re-birth. Such developments led directly to Buddhism.

Arising about 500 BCE, Buddhism rejected sacrifice completely and made *ahimsa*, or the practice of nonviolence, a cornerstone of its ethical teaching.[23] From the beginning, vegetarianism was an important part of ahimsa practice and discipline. Yet adherents of the different Buddhist sects dispute the strictness of applying ahimsa to eating meat.

The original Theravada tradition claims that Buddha himself ate meat when received as alms and also allowed monks and nuns to do so, and he specifically refused to prohibit meat and fish consumption when the monk Devadatta proposed it.[24] Theravadans point to various texts (cited below) to support this point of view.

Proponents of the later-appearing Mahayana tradition challenge such claims, pointing to sutras such as the Lankavatara Sutra (reviewed in chapter 2) that reflect a prohibition on meat, in line with the fundamental doctrine of ahimsa.

This debate among Buddhists appears to be irreconcilable. Today about half of all Buddhists worldwide are vegetarians, and the other half are meat eaters.[25] Habits depend on geographical location and tradition. Yet even within traditions, different practices and points of view exist.[26]

Daisetz Suzuki, the translator of the Mahayanan Lankavatara Sutra, notes the likelihood of early Buddhists' eating meat and says that advocacy for vegetarianism was a later response to criticism (the chapter on diet and meat eating in the Lankavatara Sutra was a later addition).[27] Followers of Jainism, in particular, criticized Buddhists for the seemingly inconsistent way of applying ahimsa.[28]

Followers of the Theravadan Buddhist tradition justify a less rigid stance on the basis of scriptures such as the Jivaka and Amaghanda Sutras. In the Jivaka Sutra, a disciple goes to the Buddha, saying he has heard that animals are being slaughtered for the Buddha's sake and asking him to respond. The Buddha replies:

> Jivaka, those who speak thus, do not truthfully speak about what has been said or done by me, but misrepresent me with what is untrue and quite contrary to the actual facts. . . .
>
> Jivaka, I say there are three occasions in which meat should not be eaten; when it is seen, heard or suspected that the living being has been killed for sake of a bhikkhu [an ordained male disciple]. I say: Meat should not be eaten on these three occasions.
>
> I say that there are three occasions in which meat may be eaten: when it is not seen, not heard, and not suspected, that the living being has been killed for sake of the bhikkhu, I say: Meat may be eaten on these three occasions.[29]

In the context of this passage, wandering monks may accept the offering of meat alms as long as slaughter does take place on their behalf. According to John Kahila, this exemplifies the Buddhist "Middle Path" (between the extremes of strict asceticism and sensory gratification).[30]

In the Amaghanda Sutra, the question of defilement (*amaghanda*) is taken up. In a series of seven verses, the Buddha enumerates what defiles and contrasts such things with the final words of each verse "but not the eating of flesh":

- Destroying living beings, killing, cutting, binding, stealing, lying, fraud and deceit, worthless reading, and adultery

- Unrestrained sensual enjoyment, greediness for sweets, impurity, skepticism, injustice, and obscurity

- Roughness, harshness, backbiting, treachery, unmercifulness, arrogance, and stinginess

- Anger, intoxication, obstinacy, bigotry, deceit, envy, grandiloquence, pride and conceit, intimacy with the unjust

- Defaulting on debts, wickedness, slander, deceit, and counterfeiting

- Unrestrained behavior toward living creatures, intending to injure them after taking what belongs to them (presumably their lives), wickedness, cruelty, harshness, and disrespect

- Greediness toward living creatures, hostility, offensiveness, and evilness[31]

All these things defile—"but not the eating of flesh." We are reminded of the Gospel passage in which Jesus emphasizes the defiling effect of evils exiting the heart but not that which enters the mouth (Mark 7:14–15; a passage that we shall revisit later).

The Mahayana tradition, in turn, points to discourses like the Mahaparinirvana Sutra (purportedly Buddha's last) that foretell of rationalizations like those of the Jivaka Sutra, stressing once again that eating meat is incompatible with Buddhist doctrine. A summary of relevant points from the Mahaparinirvana Sutra follows:[32]

- Those close to the Buddha do not eat meat, even if given as alms.

- Eating meat destroys "the attitude of great compassion."

- Buddha allowed meat after a threefold examination (cited in the Jivaka Sutra) to help striving ones overcome the habit, yet he intended the habit to be broken.

- Rules of discipline were established with particular individuals in mind; those closest to the Buddha, however, should abstain from meat.

- Meat eaters are a source of terror to animals.

Returning to the Theravadan view, Venerable S. Dhammika reports that the Buddha prescribed meat broth to cure certain illnesses.[33] Bhikku Ariyesako, the compiler of the Vinaya Sutra, a Theravadan text also disputed (as is the Jivaka Sutra) by Mahayanans, asserts that the sutra refers to meat eating approximately twenty-six times, sometimes casually, thereby suggesting the credibility of the verses. One reference says that the Buddha refused to accept Devadatta's aforementioned proposal to prohibit flesh on the grounds that food is pure unless specifically killed for the monks' benefit. Ariyesako affirms the likelihood that eating meat was common during Buddha's time and became prohibited only later through Mahayanan teaching. He speculates that the Mahayanan Tathagatagarbha doctrine (about all sentient beings having the power to become a Buddha) was responsible, as well as the influence of Chinese Taoism.[34] John Kahila suggests that the Mahayanan attitude stems from the development of monastic life, which primarily affected the Mahayanan tradition. Monks in monasteries were no longer dependent on alms and were able to prepare their own special food.[35] Samanera Kumara Liew notes that the entire Tipitaka (the Theravadan Buddhist canon written in Pali) shows no evidence of the Buddha's advocating vegetarianism. Also, Liew questions the assumption that meatless diets are more spiritually wholesome, considering that farming, industry, and modern life in general all cause the destruction of life. He suggests that moderate and mindful eating, which the Buddha did recommend, are more important considerations.[36]

The final word goes to Philip Kapleau, a Mahayanan representative doubting the veracity of the Theravadan Vinaya Sutra.[37] After citing the arguments against the Theravadan position and in favor of the Mahayanan view, he concludes that sutra authority alone cannot be decisive. In keeping with the Buddha's teaching, truth must be grasped directly and rest on an innate sense of moral goodness and compassion.[38]

Kapleau's last points are noteworthy for our own inquiry. We want to consider first all points of view before trying to grasp the inner truth about spirituality, diet, and the controversial topic of vegetarianism.

JAINISM

Of India's major religious traditions, Jainism is the most extreme with regard to dietary attitude. Mahavira (599–527 BCE) was the person responsible for revitalizing the ancient Jain religion. Like Buddha, Mahavira was among the "reformers" of the middle part of the first millennium BCE who were strongly opposed to animal sacrifice. He made *ahimsa*, or nonviolence, the foremost of five ethical vows for Jainist monks and the first of ethical rules for the laity.[39]

As the foremost of Jainist ethical rules and vows, ahimsa applies equally to animals and humans. Meat is forbidden and a vegetarian diet (i.e., lacto-vegetarian) is mandatory. Honey is also forbidden because harvesting honey is considered a form of violence, and fermented foods are forbidden, too, in order to avoid harming microorganisms. Moreover, Jains do not eat root vegetables, tubers, onions, or garlic, because uprooting plants may cause injury and small bulbs are understood as living beings with the power to sprout. Some Jains are vegans and avoid dairy because milk production can also be considered a form of violence. Jains criticize both Hindus and Buddhists for laxness in applying ahimsa.[40]

The Jainist attitude toward diet is reflected in the Akaranga Sutra. One part enumerates seven categories of living beings according to their creation and senses, adding that all experience pain or pleasure. Then the reasons for killing animals are enumerated, including for sacrificial purposes, along with the assertion that those injuring them do not comprehend or renounce their sinful acts. "Reward-knowing sage[s]," however, do comprehend and renounce, and they should not act sinfully toward animals nor cause or allow others to do so.[41] Another part of the sutra sums up succinctly the Jainist attitude:

> The first great vow, Sir, runs thus:
>
> I renounce all killing of living beings, whether subtile [sic] or gross, whether movable or immovable. Nor shall I myself kill living beings (nor cause others to do it, nor consent to it). As long as I live, I confess and blame, repent and exempt myself of these sins, in the thrice threefold way, in mind, speech, and body.[42]

The strictness of the Jainist attitude is reflected by the fact that, among major religious traditions, Jainism is one of the smallest. The latest survey estimates that there are about 5.2 million Jains in India and approximately another two hundred thousand in the rest of the world.[43]

SIKHISM

Established in the fifteenth century CE, Sikhism is the most recently appearing Indian religion under consideration. Sikhs understand their religion as a "progressive religion well ahead of its time," rejecting "blind rituals" such as the fasting, vegetarianism, and yoga associated with celibacy and renunciation. Instead, normal family life is emphasized.[44]

Sikhs acknowledge the similarities and differences between Sikhism and other major religions, but they reject Jainism completely because of its asceticism, extreme practice of ahimsa, and unhygienic life style.[45] Jainism puts animals and humans on the same level and applies ahimsa equally to both; Sikhism, on the other hand, puts animals, plants, and minerals on one level, separating humans from all three. Thus Sikhs are neutral toward the question of eating meat, even though some sects oppose it. The ten historical Sikh Gurus (the only recognized authorities besides Sikh scripture) advocated a simple diet, neither excluding nor including meat.

According to the Guru Granth Sahib scripture, arguing about diet while ignoring meditation and spiritual wisdom is foolishness (recall the contrast between this assertion and the Hindu Anusasana Parva, which values compassion toward animals over meditation). Arguments against animal foods are also hypocritical because plants, too, can suffer. The Guru Granth Sahib cites the custom of the gods to sacrifice the rhinoceros and feast on it. Those who avoid meat are not only hypocrites, but also blind:

> Those who renounce meat, and hold their noses when sitting near it, devour men at night. They practice hypocrisy, and make a show before other people, but they do not understand anything about meditation or spiritual wisdom.
>
> O Nanak, what can be said to the blind people? They cannot answer, or even understand what is said.
>
> They alone are blind, who act blindly. They have no eyes in their hearts.[46]

The reference to "Nanak" is to Nanak Dev, the founder of Sikhism and the first of the ten Sikh Gurus. This passage stresses diet's relative unimportance compared with virtues like compassion toward humans, honesty, hard work, humility, and attention to God. Sikh temples do serve vegetarian food, but only in order to accommodate non-Sikhs.

Another distinguishing feature in Sikhism about diet is the practice of *jhakta* slaughter in contrast with the *kutha* practice of Muslims and Jews. Sikhs consider *jhakta* slaughter, which decapitates the head with one blow, to be the quickest and least painful way to administer death. *Kutha* slaughter, in contrast, slits the throat amidst prayers and is considered a slower form of death, representing the "blind ritual" avoided by Sikhism. Eating kutha meat is a sin for baptized Sikhs. (As we will hear more about later, Jews and Muslims would contest Sikh assertions, considering kutha slaughter to be most humane and painless if done properly.) Presently, and in the past, Hindus who eat meat eat jhakta-slaughtered meat.[47]

Today in India there are about 21.3 million Sikhs, representing about 1.9 percent of the total population.[48]

IN SUM, THE BALANCE of opinion in the East tilts toward favoring vegetarianism. Sikhism's opposition and Jainism's support offset one another, Buddhism is split, and Hinduism's qualified support tips the scale, however slightly. This picture accords with a general public impression linking Eastern traditions with the practice of vegetarianism. It contrasts sharply with that among the dominant religions of the West, who do not support vegetarianism, or even discuss it, in the same way. Nevertheless, in Western traditions an underlying vegetarian ideal continues to live as an undercurrent, albeit in varying degrees of vitality and force.

THE ABRAHAMIC TRADITIONS:
JUDAISM, CHRISTIANITY, AND ISLAM

The three Abrahamic religions of the Near East show some similarities and contrasts with Far Eastern traditions regarding all that has been discussed so far, yet they also complement the Eastern traditions in important ways.

As in Hinduism, we know in Judaism of an ancient form of ritual animal sacrifice, and like the Buddha and Mahavira, Jewish "renouncer prophets" arose to criticize temple sacrifice, although from a different perspective. As with later-appearing Buddhist and Jainist traditions, religious animal sacrifice abruptly ended with Christianity. And Islam, similar to Sikhism, appeared later and renewed ritual slaughter.

Yet the major difference between Far and Near Eastern traditions is the lack of a visibly abiding vegetarian tradition in the Abrahamic tradition. Although the first chapter of the Jewish Torah and the Christian Bible clearly articulates a vegan-vegetarian vision (Gen. 1:29), a meat-eating sanction soon replaces it (Gen. 9:3). Meat consumption then continues unabated throughout the histories of Judaism, Christianity, and Islam into modern times, albeit with individuals and groups who recall the vegetarian ideal and also with what can be identified as a vegetarian undercurrent—conditions surrounding meat consumption similar to the Laws of Manu, the observance of which was meant to guide and even limit consumption. Examining the context and the rationale for this undercurrent is important because of its significance to the vegetarian impulse.

Both Far and Near Eastern traditions, however, also complement one another in remarkable ways. The vegetarian focus in the Far East is consistently lacto-vegetarian, while the initial dietary command in the Book of Genesis (1:29) is vegan. In addition, Judaism interprets the subsequent meat-eating sanction that appears in Genesis 9:3 in a progressive evolutionary way not seen in the East. Another complementary aspect involves the mythology surrounding sacrifice and the progression from human to animal to plant sacrifices discussed at the chapter's beginning. Both the Laws of Manu (verse 37) and the Anusasana Parva (verse 115) refer to the sacrificial substitution of vegetal effigies for animals (seen also with Pythagoras). The traditions surrounding Jewish animal sacrifice, however, reflect the substitution of animals for humans. The context for this change is arresting the increasing degeneration resulting from the mythological Fall.

Judaism: The Fall and Establishing the Vegetarian Undercurrent

The history of the vegetarian impulse in the Abrahamic tradition begins with the Genesis vegan command, but the impulse becomes diverted all the way to cannibalism by the degeneration resulting from the Fall. Degeneration is checked by the meat-eating sanction of Genesis 9, along with a restrictive framework put into place for eating meat. Initially there are few restrictions, but they become many with the founding of the Jewish people, who have a special call to holiness through the Mosaic dietary laws.

Interpretations of these laws outline a vision of evolutionary development within which meat plays a necessary but transitional role. Consumption is not the ideal, and the dietary laws are meant to foster that awareness and energize a vegetarian undercurrent leading into the future. Judaism bears the brunt of the undercurrent's strictures, which are destined to continue throughout the Abrahamic tradition, but in milder forms. We begin at the beginning.

The Paradisal Vegan Command and Aftermath

The original human diet in the Abrahamic tradition is the vegan-vegetarian diet that is given in the Garden of Eden:

> See, I have given you every plant yielding seed that is upon the face of all the earth, and every tree with seed in its fruit; you shall have them for food.
>
> (Gen. 1:29)

Although at first glance this diet seems to include all plant foods, some suggest that the diet is actually "fruitarian," composed of grains, seeds, legumes, nuts, and fruit, whose consumption would preclude the destruction of life (a value similar to ahimsa in the Far East).[49]

An additional but enigmatic aspect to this vegetarian prescription, however, is that it also applies to animals:

> And to every beast of the earth, and to every bird of the air, and to everything that creeps on the earth, everything that has the breath of life, I have given every green plant for food.
>
> (Gen. 1:30)

Thus in Paradise, humans are meant to be fruitarian and animals herbivorous. Preying on other creatures or killing in any form does not exist. The dominion given to humans over other creatures (Gen. 1:28) occurs in the context of peaceful and harmonious relations among them. Abuse in any form does not exist.

The Fall and Expulsion from Eden occur in chapter 3 of Genesis. Adam and Eve are expelled for eating the forbidden fruit from the Tree of the Knowledge of Good and Evil. This act, or eating forbidden food, sets the Fall in motion. The first result is a change in consciousness, reflected by Adam and Eve becoming aware of their nakedness. Before turning them out, God tells Adam:

> Cursed is the ground because of you; in toil you shall eat of it all the days of your life; thorns and thistles it shall bring forth for you; and you shall eat the plants of the field.
>
> (Gen. 2:17–18)

This passage has been interpreted to mean that, after the sin of eating the forbidden fruit, plants also become part of the human diet, putting humans on a level comparable with animals (Gen. 1:30).[50] Before expulsion, however, another noteworthy event takes place: God makes garments of skin to cover Adam and Eve (Gen. 3:21), suggesting the first instance of animal sacrifice in order to clothe them.

The next development in the saga of the Fall comes with the story of Cain and Abel in chapter 4 of Genesis. Abel is a keeper of sheep and Cain a tiller of the earth. They both bring offerings to God, Abel of his sheep and Cain of the fruits of the earth—the first instance of sacrificial offering to the Divine. God accepts Abel's offering but not Cain's, and, as a result, Cain kills Abel—the first instance of human murder.

In chapter 6 of Genesis, we subsequently hear that "the earth was corrupt in God's sight and filled with violence" (Gen. 6:11). Richard Alan Young has described this violence as

> unrestrained and ruthless slaughtering of animals (and perhaps humans) and gorging on their flesh. A Jewish writing dating to the second century B.C. reads, "They all corrupted their way and their ordinances, and they began to eat one another" (Jubilees 5.2). The Genesis text implies that the guilt and destructive violence had spread to animals as well. The expression "all flesh" in the phrase "all flesh had corrupted its ways" (Gen. 6:12) refers to all that has breath (Gen. 6:17).[51]

The result of this violence and gorging is God's decision to destroy life through a flood, which comes in Genesis, chapter 7. Noah, his family, and the animals brought into the ark built at God's command are the only living creatures chosen to survive. The Flood marks the end of a long process of degeneration that culminated in cannibalism (about which we will hear more).

The Meat-Eating Sanction and Kashrut as the Middle Way

Only after disembarking from the ark after the Flood does Noah receive permission from God to eat creatures, which are now to live in fear of humans (in contrast to the harmonious relations existing in Paradise amid vegetarian diets):

> The fear and dread of you shall rest on every animal of the earth, and on every bird of the air, on everything that creeps on the ground, and on all the fish of the sea; into your hand they are delivered. Every moving thing that lives shall be food for you; and just as I gave you the green plants, I give you everything.
>
> (Gen. 9:1-3)

The permission to eat meat, however, is accompanied by a condition: "Only, you shall not eat flesh with its life, that is, its blood" (Gen. 9:4), which is to say that blood consumption is not allowed. The verse has been interpreted to mean that eating any part of the animal while it is still alive—something that was apparently practiced in antiquity—is not allowed, yet it is generally interpreted to signify a prohibition against the consumption of blood.[52] Verses 5 and 6 that follow make clear that shedding *human* blood is not allowed. Thus, the killing and consumption of animals is juxtaposed with the killing of humans, which is expressly prohibited.

A final note about the blood prohibition is that it is given to Noah, the new father of the human race after the Flood. The prohibition is one of the laws given to him and his sons that are considered binding for all of humanity. The more restrictive Mosaic laws that apply to the Jewish people come later, after the nation's founding.

But to return to the meat-eating sanction itself—why does God suddenly condone killing animals and eating their flesh, contradicting the Genesis 1 command and the seeming motive for sending the Flood as well? Various rabbis view the sanction as an intermediate stage accompanied by strict conditions until human moral growth has matured and the dawn of a brighter age.

The strict conditions referred to include the blood prohibition given to Noah, but especially the much stricter Mosaic dietary laws in Leviticus (11:1–47) and Deuteronomy (14:3–20) as well as the slaughtering laws of the oral tradition.[53] These restrictions apply to the Jewish people, specifically. The most relevant are the kashrut laws distinguishing allowable and forbidden creatures (see chapter 2) and prohibitions against consuming blood and fat.

The renowned first Chief Rabbi of pre-State Israel, Abraham Isaac Kook (1865–1935), provides the most comprehensive interpretation of the significance of the sanction and rules in a tract entitled, "A Vision of Vegetarianism and Peace."[54] Kook was motivated to address them because of the interest among Jews of the time in vegetarianism as a sign of the coming Messianic Age.[55] Below is a summary of Kook's most important points along with some comments:

1. *When the sanction was enacted, the lust for flesh was so overpowering that the eating of animals was permitted in order to prevent cannibalism.*[56] As controversial as this assertion may sound, we noted above the Jubilees 5:2 passage referring to the pre-Flood period that is interpreted to suggest cannibalism ("They all corrupted their way and their ordinances, and they began to eat one another"). Anthropological evidence advances the same conclusion of cannibalism as a prevalent part of the pre-Flood world.[57] Moreover, at this chapter's beginning, we noted the link between creation mythology and human sacrifice, which is acknowledged to have been widespread in ancient times and was typically replaced by effigies and by sacrificing animals instead.[58] In fact, the Bible also speaks of child sacrifice in Canaan

after the Hebrews settle there (Lev. 20:2; Deut. 12:31) and of the Israelites engaging in child sacrifice through the influence of their neighbors (Ps. 106:34–39).

2. *Our fallen state has led to the moral shortcoming of taking animal life. Human development requires physical exertion and at times a meat diet. A general prohibition on animal flesh would mean reverting to cannibalism when the craving became overpowering. Animals must pay the price, but not for all time.*[59] The notion of falling from grace into sinful corruption goes hand in hand with the dietary change from vegetarianism to eating meat. Asserting that meat represents a need beyond desire (or pleasure) may seem controversial, but it is nonetheless implicit in the sanction given to allow it. Rabbi Kook portrays meat as an overpowering craving, need, or requirement multiple times.[60] The distinction between desire and need is essential to understanding the question of vegetarianism from a spiritual perspective. We have touched on this issue before and will return to it. Kook's suggestion that prohibiting flesh would result in reverting to cannibalism has been challenged on the basis of studies of vegetarian societies and communities that show no such proclivity.[61] Yet there is a difference between vegetarian societies deliberately eschewing meat and general populations. Individual variables always apply, and Kook appears to have intuited that a general prohibition would lead to difficulty at least for some—see the next point.

3. *Justice toward animals is hidden "in the deeper layers of the Torah," as Kook puts it. To affirm the rights of animals presently is beyond the capacity of human moral development "except insofar as it doesn't overtax ... the force of human morality, in its weakened state, to sustain." Moral struggle overcomes the inclination for meat, but the time of conquest has not yet arrived. What is called for presently is moral activity focusing on human relationships.*[62] Rabbi Kook considered vegetarianism a high spiritual ideal but "beyond the grasp of most" at present. He was concerned that championing such an idealistic cause would involve deluding oneself about personal character defects, and taking on such austerities prematurely

could cause character defects to manifest in other ways.[63] Kook supported vegetarianism, but in a differentiated way: he reportedly ate meat himself only on the Sabbath and at religious festivals,[64] yet he disapproved of vegetarianism for his son[65] while supporting vegetarianism for his disciple Rabbi David Cohen.[66] Such differentiations allow for the need for meat, as does the meat-eating sanction. The prohibition against killing humans (Gen. 9:5–6) immediately following the meat-eating sanction (Gen. 9:4) underscores the priority given to human relationships. Kook emphasizes that righteousness toward animals must depend on having ordered human relationships first. The underlying logic is that such a struggle provides the necessary strength to overcome the lust for flesh, so as to be in a position to live in harmony with animals as well.

4. *The consumption only of animals close to human beings in nature is allowed to prevent a corrupting effect on human character. Their closeness to us evokes pity and compassion, but this is a weak expression of morality, not the perfected sense of justice that will be revealed in time:*

> [The] echo released by the moral voice shall not be the voice of weaklings, of ascetics and timid spirits, but the firm and joyous voice of life.[67]

Chapter 2 of this book addressed the subtle spiritual effects attributed to eating creatures prohibited by the Mosaic code. The distinction between a weak sense of compassion and a full sense of justice reflects Kook's evolutionary understanding of human strength as developing over time by first ordering human relationships.

5. *The blood and fat prohibitions remove the worst element of gluttony and sensual gratification from meat consumption. The fat prohibition also stimulates the strengthening of one's powers and emphasizes that meat consumption may be necessary but is still problematic.[68]* The sanction expressly prohibits blood out of reverence for life (Gen. 9:2). Yet the blood prohibition also

relates to sensual gratification, as does the fat prohibition. Kook's intended meaning about becoming stronger through the fat prohibition is unclear. Perhaps he means the strength that comes from suppressing the desire for fat, yet in his comments we also hear an echo of Rudolf Steiner's teaching (see chapter 2) of the inner strengthening that comes from creating one's own fat. The fat and blood prohibitions suppress sensual desire while allowing for meat's need. Both Kook and the meat-eating sanction and laws distinguish between suppressing desire and allowing for need.

6. *Through repeated practice over generations, Kook says that "the light that is hidden within these prohibitions and laws" will lead to perfection, and then humanity will turn to animals and realize harmonious life together with them. Awakened human sensibilities will even extend to the feed that is provided to animals, "expressing a permanent sense of compassion and justice" (Kook quotes Isaiah 30:24 about flavoring fodder with spices and removing the chaff).*[69] A moral force is set in motion through the practice of the kashrut laws that leads to perfected compassion and justice. This is the genius of the dietary code, which Kook affirms.

7. *This understanding comes from a moral sense linked to the divine source. Impatient morality detached from the source cannot tolerate it.*[70] Kook voices this thought in the context of transitioning to a higher state that first necessitates eating meat and even just wars. It serves as a fitting summary to all of Kook's thought—about the sanction, relationships with animals, relationships among human beings, and spiritual evolution.

Some final details about Judaism's meat-eating sanction involve the *shechita* slaughtering laws that are intended to minimize animal pain:

> Shechita is the most humane method of slaughter known to man. The procedure involves a traverse cut in the throat of the animal with an extremely sharp and smooth knife. Due to the sharpness of the knife and the paucity of sensory cutaneous

nerve endings in the skin covering the throat, the incision itself causes no pain. . . . The resultant massive loss of blood causes the animal to become unconscious in a matter of seconds.[71]

Rabbi David Sears adds that this assertion is borne out by scientific evidence and that the well-known animal scientist Temple Grandin suggests that reported variations may be due to experience and skill. Humane treatment prior to slaughter is also required.[72] Rabbi Samuel H. Dresner adds that the stringent requirements to be a *shochet*, or slaughterer, include piety, a thorough knowledge of slaughtering law, and an appreciation of the entire process that involves a "divine concession." These requirements protect against brutalization[73] (a concern raised by Annie Besant; see chapter 2).

To sum up, the Genesis meat-eating sanction and the related accompanying rules were meant to

- check human moral degeneration;
- satisfy the need for meat while curbing desire;
- limit harmful animal effects (from prohibited animals);
- hallow the act of eating and stimulate reverence for life; and
- pave the way for the return to a vegetarian future.

In Kook's view, the sanction and rules represent "the 'next best' alternative to vegetarianism."[74] Rabbi Dresner adds that, while others engage in diets for the sake of the body, "we have created a diet for the soul."[75] He further characterizes kashrut as the "third way" between the extremes of unbridled enjoyment and asceticism.[76] In fact, a facile distinction between vegetarians on the one hand and nonvegetarians on the other fails to capture kashrut's spirit—here, too, practitioners represent a third, middle way.

It is estimated that approximately one-sixth of American Jews practice kashrut.[77] Considering its purpose as a moral force meant to prepare the way for a vegetarian future, kashrut deserves wider attention from all meat eaters, Jews and non-Jews alike.

Challenging the Meat-Eating Sanction

Despite Judaism's sanction that allows meat, some commentators point to passages that seem to put consumption in a negative light (Num. 11:34 and Deut. 12:20–21), in effect questioning the righteousness of eating meat.[78]

Numbers 11, which takes place during the exodus from Egypt, recounts the dissatisfaction of the Hebrews with the manna provided by God for food and their desire for meat. In anger, God sends quail and also a plague, which kills those "who had the craving" (Num. 11:34).[79] Deuteronomy 12 describes the partial lifting of the restriction against making sacrifices outside the Temple in order to accommodate dispersion into the Promised Land. God gives the Israelites permission to eat meat "whenever you have the desire" (Deut. 12:20–21). The Jewish Encyclopedia refers to this as meat of "desire or luxury, not necessity." It continues that Deuteronomy 14:26 also deals with the desire of spending money on "oxen, sheep, wine, strong drink, or whatever you desire." The Encyclopedia then adds:

> The Rabbis, referring to Deut. 14:26, said: "The Torah teaches a lesson in moral conduct, that man shall not eat meat unless he has a special craving for it, and shall eat it only occasionally and sparingly."[80]

This important comment affirms the sanction to eat meat, yet it emphasizes the restraint on consumption as well. As we have seen, this is the intent of the entire kashrut system—to allow for need, but to curb desire. What pro-vegetarian commentators will dispute is the existence of a *need* for meat; they argue that it is only a matter of desire. As we have tried to demonstrate, no less an authority than Rabbi Kook affirms both. Likewise, this study asserts the reality of both the desire and the need for meat, two very different issues and another topic to which we will return.

Isaiah and the "Peaceable Kingdom"

Isaiah's visions of the "Peaceable Kingdom" are the next vegetarian-related milestone in the Jewish tradition. The first vision depicts humans and animals living together in peace and even lions eating straw:

> The wolf shall live with the lamb,
> the wolf shall lie down with the kid,
> the calf and the lion and the fatling together,
> and a little child shall lead them.
> The cow and the bears shall graze,
> their young shall lie down together;
> and the lion shall eat straw like the ox.
> The nursing child shall play over the hole
> of the asp,
> and the weaned child shall put
> its hand on the adder's den.
> They will not hurt or destroy
> on all my holy mountain;
> for the earth will be full of the
> knowledge of the LORD
> as the waters cover the sea.
>
> (Is. 11: 6–9)

Chapter 65 of Isaiah sounds similar themes, adding the important detail that fulfillment takes place at a time when the heavens and earth are renewed:

> For I am about to create new heavens and a new earth . . . the wolf and the lamb shall feed together, the lion shall eat straw like the ox. . . . They shall not hurt or destroy on all my holy mountain, says the LORD.
>
> (Is. 65:17, 25)

This notion of humans and animals living together harmoniously recalls the Genesis command of vegetarian diets not just for humans, but for animals, too:

141

> And to every beast of the earth, and to every bird of the air, and to everything that creeps on the earth, everything that has the breath of life, I have given every green plant for food.
>
> (Gen. 1:30)

Jews and Christians alike justifiably seize upon these visions as portraits of the "Messianic Age," or in the case of Isaiah 11:6–9, of "paradise regained"—a time when harmony is restored to disordered nature.[81]

The mystery of fulfilling the Messianic Age is deep enough for human beings, who at that time according to Rabbi Kook will have overcome both the desire and need for flesh. Yet in a sense the mystery is deeper still for "obligate carnivores" such as lions that lack the physiological capacity to digest vegetation.[82] Because human beings are able to digest and live from vegetal matter, the human need for meat may seem debatable. This need is not debatable, however, in the case of obligate carnivores.

The Jewish tradition speaks of animals not harming one another in the future because of an enlightenment and a sharing in human intellect and wisdom, as part of the spiritual elevation and perfection attained by all levels of creation. But the tradition also speaks of souls and animals falling into "forces of unholiness" as the result of the Fall, which will be rectified, and which involves a "new, exalted form."[83] Certainly such a form seems necessary for animals in order for them to become herbivores. The question remains as to what it means for human beings in order for them to overcome the need, overpowering craving, or desire for meat. This is a question about how to understand the effects of the Fall. Does it signify merely the disobedience of the will, which is the traditional understanding, or something deeper? We will return to this question, too.

Subsequent Jewish Vegetarian Threads to Modern Times

Animal sacrifice and slaughter initially took place only in the Temple and were administered by priests. These stipulations ensured a sense of thanksgiving to God for the gift of life and that all relevant rules were followed.[84] Yet some commentators (vegetarian apologists once again) point to utterances in the Psalms and among the prophets that seemingly repudiate temple sacrifice, implying the illegitimacy of everything surrounding meat consumption.[85] On the other hand, Richard Alan Young, himself a vegetarian supporter, argues that these criticisms are repudiating hypocrisy, not sacrifice—namely, the hypocrisy of performing prescribed rituals without a truly worshipful heart.[86]

Temple sacrifice continued to play a vital role in Jewish community life until the Temple's destruction in 70 CE. At that time, the community was faced with the question of whether meat consumption could continue, considering the Temple's essential role. After much debate, it was decided not to require vegetarianism, but instead to implement the kosher rules that make meat available according to traditional requirements. Why not require vegetarianism? Because, it was argued, Judaism was a "religion of life," not of asceticism, and requiring vegetarianism would place an unbearable burden on the community.[87] Why an "unbearable burden"? Here again we confront the question of desire versus need—whether the desire for meat can be easily suppressed, or whether it represents something deeper.

The notion of the vegetarian ideal was kept alive throughout the Middle Ages into modern times by various rabbis who put the sanction to eat meat into an evolutionary or even a critical context.[88] Rabbi Yosef Albo (1380–1444) granted that animals may serve human needs during evolution until the lower nature is overcome; yet meat consumption betrays a lack of enlightenment; and, cognizant of the many laws, the wise refrain from it. Rabbi Yitzchak Arama (1430–1494) was less judgmental: meat is appropriate for those at an intermediate stage of evolution; the advanced, however, are adversely affected and have always refrained. Rabbi Shlomo Ephraim Lunschitz (d. 1619) was openly critical: the Torah's grudging tone conveys "tacit disapproval," and meat represents a "debased craving"; the complexity of the laws is a deterrent, and indulgence should be infrequent.

We have already spoken of Rabbi Kook's contributions at the beginning of the twentieth century and mentioned Rabbi Dresner (1923–2000) as well. Their views display a dynamic understanding of the sanction as a transformative, future-oriented force. Dresner's view that kashrut offers a "middle way" between indulgence and asceticism is worth repeating. Meat is allowed, but the laws cultivate reverence for the life that is taken, refining and educating conscience, and working to discourage consumption.[89]

The distinction between desire and need is useful to apply to the attitudes of the several rabbis cited above. Rabbis Kook and Dresner are the least judgmental. Kook views meat as both a desire and a need; Dresner is more equivocal, speaking of desire and perhaps a need. Rabbi Arama's affirmation that meat is appropriate for an intermediate stage of evolution suggests that it is a need, at least to some extent. Rabbi Lunschitz's critical tone suggests that meat is a desire, which is likely the case for Rabbi Albo as well. All the rabbis, however, as representatives of a tradition that de facto sanctions meat consumption, accept it, if only as a way station on the road back to the vegetarianism that characterized the Garden before the Fall.

Modern Jewish vegetarian societies continue to emphasize the tradition's vegan–vegetarian roots while also raising important, yet nonetheless controversial, issues.

The Jewish Vegetarian Society (JVS)[90] founded in the United Kingdom in the 1960s aspires to a human society without cruelty to humans or animals, in line with the teachings of the Torah and the Talmud. In the very first issue of the society's magazine, however, a rabbi states, "As long as man is prepared to kill a creature in order to satisfy his bodily desires, he will also, if need be, kill his neighbor to satisfy his lusts."[91]

According to this logic, ceasing to kill animals for food will lead to better human relations; vegetarianism in this sense represents a contribution to world peace (Will Tuttle advances this same argument in his book *The World Peace Diet*[92]). This, however, is not the logic of Rabbi Kook, who makes clear that ordering human relationships is first necessary before considering animals. Moreover, and perhaps more importantly, it is not Torah logic, or the logic of the Book of

Genesis, that is the basis for Rabbi Kook's assertions. As previously indicated, the verses that follow the meat-eating sanction (Gen. 9:4) expressly prohibit the shedding of human blood (Gen. 9:5–6), which is to say that shedding animal blood is allowed but not human blood. Furthermore, the traditional rabbinical understanding of the sanction states that it elevates human relationships above animals in order to provide an acceptable flesh source for food. One can object, as do some vegetarians, that this amounts to "speciesism," or elevating the rights of humans over animals. Nevertheless, this is the Torah's view, which is understood as divinely inspired. There may be sound reasons for advocating vegetarianism from a Jewish point of view (as the rabbis above articulate), but asserting that righteousness toward animals leads to righteousness toward humans is not one of them.

It is important to interject, however, that there is logic and justification to Rabbi Rosenfeld's argument cited above, but of a half-truth nature. We have heard from many authors—spiritual ones as well as Weston Price and Dr. D'Adamo—of the link between animal foods and aggression, yet the important counterbalancing argument is that just this very kind of aggressive stimulation is important to human evolutionary development. Here we confront the paradox and even the tragedy of human nature. Chapter 8 will have more to say about the human evolutionary process.

In arguing for vegetarianism, the Jewish Vegetarian Society (JVS) highlights the conflict between Jewish teaching and animal abuse as practiced in current animal food production. Yet to its credit, the JVS avoids dismissing the use of animal foods completely by providing information about sourcing ethically sound eggs.

The US branch of the JVS—the Jewish Vegetarians of North America (JVNA)[93]—cites Rabbi Kook and his views: the meat-eating sanction elevated humans over animals, it guarded against cannibalism, it put the focus on improving human relations, and it also provided meat to satisfy the lust for flesh as a "transitional tax" until the dawn of a "brighter era." The JVNA then asks whether now, after three thousand years, that "brighter era" has dawned, and whether the temporary dispensation should not have expired long ago.[94]

Approximately one hundred years ago, Rabbi Kook judged that the brighter era had not dawned, nor had the dispensation expired. His point of reference was the ordering of human relations, which first had to occur. Has any significant progress truly been made since then? Nevertheless, the JVNA's questions are important and appropriate to the vanguard—whose mission it is to provoke the discrimination between desire and need, discouraging desire while allowing for need, and thereby keeping alive the vitality of the vegetarian impulse.

The JVNA especially advocates plant-based diets and veganism, citing meat consumption as an act of lust and stating succinctly that "consumption . . . is not necessary."[95] But as we have endeavored to show, claiming meat to be a need is supported by reputable witnesses as well as the meat-eating sanction itself. Would God allow killing animals and their consumption merely to satisfy desire? The question is a crucial one—for one's own health and that of others.

Like the JVS, the JVNA also emphasizes animal treatment and notes that abusive practices have been found even at kosher slaughtering houses in the United States and Israel.[96] Richard Schwartz, JVNA's president emeritus, however, argues that shechita slaughtering practices have been unfairly singled out for criticism; and he calls for better regulation and inspection (even though he emphasizes JVNA's vegan and nonslaughter preferences).[97] We can only affirm the call for better regulation and inspection, because shechita offers an important and preferred religious alternative to conventional slaughtering practices and should be encouraged.

Last to mention in the modern-day Jewish vegetarian tradition are the Amirim village in Israel and the Shamayim V'Aretz Institute. Located in Galilee, Amirim was begun in 1959 to pursue vegetarian, vegan, and organic lifestyles. It comprises over 100 households and about 450 people. Tourism is a primary income source, and besides guesthouses, vegan and vegetarian cuisine is offered.[98] The Shamayim V'Aretz Institute was founded by the charismatic American Rabbi Shmuly Yanklowitz. *Shamayim V'Aretz* means "Heaven and Earth," signifying the goal of incarnating heaven on earth "to sanctify the world through all of our just and holy endeavors."[99] The primary focus is protecting animals, who are considered to be the most vulnerable and abused of sentient creatures. The institute promotes animal-welfare activism, kosher veganism, and Jewish spirituality. Both the institute and the Amirim village are important parts of the Jewish vegetarian vanguard.

In summary, the paradisal vegan–vegetarian ideal of the Jewish tradition in the Book of Genesis is soon replaced by the meat-eating sanction occurring after the Fall and the Flood, yet the heartbeat of the impulse remains clearly discernible in the tradition down to modern times. The time for re-realizing the ideal may be debated, but not fulfillment itself.

Christianity and the Vegetarian Undercurrent

The vegetarian undercurrent inherited from Judaism experiences both a high and a low in the Christian tradition—perhaps the highest high and lowest low within the Abrahamic tradition as a whole. The high is the communion meal of Jesus, which one Christian tradition refers to as "the medicine that makes whole."[100] The significance of this communion meal remains to be fully fathomed. The low is the slackening of the vegetarian undercurrent, and then its complete, or seemingly complete, stagnation. What is the cause? There seem to be at least two reasons, one legitimate and the other illegitimate. The legitimate one accommodates the reality of an incipient universal church open to those unused to, and unable to cope with, the rigors of the Mosaic laws. The illegitimate reason misinterprets key aspects of this wider and universal movement. The net sum is a loss of vitality in Christianity for the vegetarian undercurrent (albeit hope for renewal ever springs eternal).

The Communion Meal of Jesus

Some claim that the Temple cleansing depicted in the Christian Gospels[101] indicates that Jesus rejected temple sacrifice and that he himself was a vegetarian. The support for such assertions, however, is unconvincing.[102] Moreover, the Christian rejection of insistent vegetarian sects such as the Ebionites is a consistent theme.

Far more significant for the vegetarian ideal is the communion meal of Jesus itself. Considering its significance and that Jesus was a Jew, and considering also Judaism's travails for the vegetarian cause and Western Christianity's recalcitrance (read on), Judaism deserves the credit. Be that as it may, it is the Christian tradition that has preserved the memory and practice of Jesus's communion meal.

Christians usually understand its institution as consummating an important motivation for temple sacrifice, namely, atonement for sin. By sacrificing his own body and blood (in the form of bread and wine), Jesus atones for the Fall and human sin and obviates the need for further atonement. Yet his communion meal accomplishes much more: it acknowledges the desire or need for flesh and then satisfies it—but with vegetal substances. *The Christian host— the sacrificial meal of the body and blood of Jesus in the form of bread and wine—provides flesh nutrition through the vegetal substances of the fruitarian/vegetarian ideal.*

There are some materialists who think that consciousness is a trick of the brain. If that were so, then the brain deserves to be worshipped as a god for conjuring forth such a rich and happy image.

Consuming what is understood as divine essence through the use of vegetal substances is not unique to Christianity. We previously heard of sacrificial practices also using grain effigies, such as in the Hindu tradition, and other cultures did so as well (see appendix A). Yet the special significance of Jesus's communion meal is its enduring universal practice. The chapter ahead will have more to say about the relationship of this communion to mythological archetypes.

The Undercurrent Slackens

The communion meal of Jesus is an important and profound symbol of the vegetarian ideal. Before its institution, some remarks are attributed to Jesus that are interpreted as loosening the Jewish kashrut laws intended to limit and suppress meat consumption. Jesus says to a crowd:

> "Listen to me, all of you and understand: there is nothing out-side of a person that by going in can defile, but the things that come out are what defile."
>
> (Mark 7:14–15)

The passage continues with the interpretation Jesus gives to his disciples:

> "Do you not see that whatever goes into a person from outside cannot defile since it enters, not the heart but the stomach, and goes out into the sewer?" (Thus he declared all foods clean.) . . . And he said, "It is what comes out of a person that defiles . . . from the human heart . . . fornication, theft, murder, adultery, avarice, wickedness, deceit, licentiousness, envy, slander, pride, folly. All these evil things . . . defile a person."
>
> (Mark 7:18–22)

The context for his remarks is the Pharisees' criticism of Jesus's disciples for not observing the tradition of hand washing before a meal, and in turn Jesus's criticism of the Pharisees for observing human traditions while ignoring the commandments of God that relate to evils of the heart (recall the similarity to the Buddhist Amaghanda Sutra cited earlier in the chapter).

The problem in the passage, however, is the parenthetical comment "(Thus he declared all foods clean)." Many English translations add this comment, but it is not found in the King James Bible or in the interlinear Greek–English Bible.[103] It is generally agreed that the remark is an interpretation, not part of the original biblical text. One commentator notes that the parallel verses in Matthew (15:10–20), and verse 15:20 in particular ("but to eat with unwashed hands does not defile"), clarify that the focus is what a person ingests through unclean hands, not foods.[104] Perhaps, however, the supposition that the passage also applies to foods results from the subsequent events described below that do directly relate to loosening the kashrut laws.

The Book of Acts, which takes place after Jesus's resurrection and ascension into heaven, records a vision of the apostle Peter. While waiting for the preparation of a meal, Peter falls into a trance in which he sees the heavens open and a sheet descending with many kinds of creatures and birds. Then a voice says:

> "Get up, Peter; kill and eat." But Peter said, "By no means, Lord; for I have never eaten anything that is profane or unclean." The voice said to him again, a second time, "What God has made clean, you must not call profane."
>
> (Acts 10:13–15)

This sequence happens three times before the sheet disappears back into the heavens. Immediately thereafter, messengers from the Roman centurion Cornelius appear requesting Peter's visit, and the spirit instructs Peter to go with them. What results is his dawning realization of God's acceptance of righteous Gentiles, the baptism of Cornelius's household, and the beginning of the mission to the Gentiles (Acts 10:17–48). It has, however, been pointed out that Peter interprets his vision, not to mean that he should eat unclean foods, but instead that he should not shun association with Gentiles (in Acts 10:28, Peter says, "God has shown me that I should not call anyone profane or unclean").[105] Nevertheless, the Council of Jerusalem that occurs later in Acts decides indeed to loosen the traditional kashrut laws, at least for Gentile Christians.

The Council was called to deal with controversy about the applicability of Jewish laws to Gentile converts. It decided to require them to abstain only from four things: fornication, foods sacrificed to idols, strangled or unbled animals, and blood (Acts 15:20; some texts lack the prohibition against strangled animals, which is assumed to be covered by the blood prohibition). As a commentary to the Act's text indicates, "The rabbis taught that these, and *fornication*, had been forbidden to Noah's sons, therefore to the righteous of all nations."[106]

The reference to Noah and his sons is important, for it signifies that henceforth Gentile converts will be subject not to Mosaic laws but to Noahide ones, the laws given to Noah and his sons after the Flood, when human history began anew. The first such law was the blood prohibition (Gen. 9:4) that accompanied the meat-eating sanction (Gen. 9:3). Noahide laws were understood to apply to all of humanity, and they preceded the much stricter Mosaic laws coming afterward that only applied to Jews. Hence, the Council of Jerusalem repeats the universal Noahide blood prohibition as a condition for Gentile Christians to eat meat.

The Council's requirements, however, represent a significant slackening compared with the rigorous kashrut laws of the Jews. Notably lacking are the prohibitions against unclean animals and fat. As we have seen, the prohibition against unclean animals was understood as a protection against harmful moral effects (see chapter 2), and the fat prohibition was understood to curb enjoyment (yet in chapter 2 we heard a more significant spiritual rationale from Rudolf Steiner). The blood prohibition remains intact, and its fundamental importance can be understood as emphasizing the sacredness of life (blood symbolizes life) and pricking conscience to recognize that shedding blood for food is not the ideal. Nevertheless, it seems reasonable to assert that the Council's pared-down requirements represent a net loss for the strength of the vegetarian impulse as it subsequently applies to Christianity.

The letters of the apostle Paul also reflect the controversy that leads to the Council's decrees. The primary diet-related issue involves meat sacrificed to idols (vegetarianism also plays a role, but secondarily). Some refuse to eat this meat, which is largely what is available in local markets of the time, and eat only vegetal foods instead. Paul accuses them of being weak in faith and conscience (Rom. 14; 1 Cor. 8) because he is convinced that all foods are clean, including those sacrificed to idols, and he urges buying what the markets sell without scruples (1 Cor. 10:25). Yet he also asserts that brotherly and sisterly charity and community harmony, too, are the ultimate concerns. Therefore, he says that it is better to abstain if others are thereby offended, for this reason:

151

"All things are lawful," but not all things are beneficial. "All
things are lawful," but not all things build up.

(1 Cor. 10:23)

What he does reject firmly is any demand for abstinence from meat,
which he associates with Gnostic teaching (1 Tim. 4:3).[107]

We see through Paul the tension that surrounded a new orientation to diet outside of Temple sacrifice and the kashrut system. As in
Judaism, vegetarianism is not a major concern in Christian communities; the concern instead is with procuring acceptable meat.

Yet as an undercurrent, the vegetarian impulse has become weaker. Allowable and forbidden (harmful) creatures are no longer differentiated; there is no fat prohibition; and Temple sacrifice, which put
the procurement of meat into a sacred context, has also disappeared.
The Council's Noahide requirements that include prohibiting blood
do provide a measure of support to the vegetarian undercurrent. Yet
in succeeding centuries, even they begin to fall away.

The Undercurrent Stagnates

It is understandable that the concern with food sacrificed to idols
would lessen in Christian communities as they grew to exert their
own economic influence and then disappear altogether when Christianity became, first tolerated, and then the official state religion of
the Roman Empire. Less understandable, however, is the erosion
that took place regarding the blood prohibitions.

That erosion did take place was undoubtedly due partly to the
lax standards of Gentile converts who were unused to the discipline developed by Jews through observing the Mosaic laws over
the course of generations.[108] Yet the Noahide blood prohibition
that preceded the Mosaic laws somehow became viewed merely as
a temporal requirement to keep peace between Jews and Gentiles in
the first Christian communities. Writing about 400 CE, Augustine
acknowledges the relationship of the blood prohibition to Noah, at

least metaphorically, by saying that it united different nations into one ark. Then he adds:

> Now that the Church has become so entirely Gentile that none who are outwardly Israelites are to be found in it, no Christian feels bound to abstain from thrushes or small birds because their blood has not been poured out, or from hares because they are killed by a stroke on the neck without shedding their blood. Any who still are afraid to touch these things are laughed at by the rest: so general is the conviction of the truth, that "not what enters into the mouth defiles you, but what comes out of it" [Matt. 15:11]; that evil lies in the commission of sin, and not in the nature of any food in ordinary use.[109]

Here we see that Augustine's justification for disregarding the blood prohibition is twofold: the lack of a need to worry about offending Jews, and the verse from Matthew 15 (see also Mark 7) that he interprets to apply to foods and to blood specifically. As noted above, the corollary passage in Mark 7 contains the parenthetical comment "(Thus he declared all foods clean)," but this comment is acknowledged as an interpretation, not part of the biblical text. Similarly, we can question Augustine's application of the passage to blood. Regardless, we can say that his assertion about "nothing defiling" harmonizes to some extent with Peter's vision in Acts (all animals are clean) and Paul's attitude in his letters (all things are lawful, including food sacrificed to idols). Yet the important counterpoint to reemphasize is that the blood prohibitions were not just Mosaic laws applicable to Jews, but Noahide laws applicable to all of humanity.

Writing at about the same time as Augustine, Cyril of Jerusalem (died 387 CE) expresses a very different view in his baptism instructions:

> And the Apostles and Elders write a Catholic epistle to all the Gentiles, that they should *abstain* first *from things offered to idols, and* then *from blood* also *and from things strangled.* For many men being of savage nature, and living like dogs, both lap up blood, in imitation of the manner of the fiercest beasts, and

greedily devour things strangled. But do thou, the servant of Christ, in eating observe to eat with reverence.[110]

That Augustine's attitude became widespread, yet was still seen as problematic, is suggested by the repeated renewal of the blood prohibitions in the first twelve centuries through various councils and popes: the Council of Gangrene in 325 CE; the Council of Orleans in 536 CE; the Council of Constance in 692 CE; the Council of Trullo in 695 CE; Pope Gregory III in 731 CE; Pope Leo VI in 886 CE.; and Pope Calixtus II in 1120 CE. After the proclamation by Calixtus, however, the prohibitions were discussed by the German scholastic Robert Pulleyn (*Pullen* in English, died 1146) who rejected them, and thereafter they became neglected. The French cleric Stephen of Tournay (Étienne de Tournay, 1132–1203) wondered how this could come about, considering the clear prohibitions of both the Old and New Testaments and Church canons. In places like Geneva, however, the prohibitions stayed in force until around the time of Calvin (the sixteenth century!).[111]

Writing in 2008, the Pontifical Biblical Commission of the Catholic Church stated that the New Testament had imposed the blood prohibition on Gentiles for a symbolic, not a theological reason—"the life (nephes) of all flesh is in the blood" (Lev. 17:11, 14; Deut. 12:23). The Commission then continued:

> After the apostolic era the Church did not feel obliged to make this a basis for formulating precise rules for the butcher and the kitchen. . . . The trans-cultural value underlying the particular decision of the Church in Acts 15 was a desire to foster the harmonious integration of the various groups, albeit at the price of a provisional compromise.[112]

As the restatements of the prohibitions by various councils and popes over the course of twelve centuries seem precise enough, perhaps the commission's declaration can be attributed partly to historical amnesia, yet certainly also to the views of Augustine and Paul, along with the interpretation of the Matthew and Mark passages that "nothing defiles" and all foods have been made clean.

On the other side, the Eastern and Orthodox Churches have always observed the blood prohibitions,[113] as affirmed by the following recent response on an Orthodox website to a question about blood consumption:

> Deliberately eating blood (unbled or strangled) animals is actually condemned by the Scriptures (notably Acts 15) and Holy Canons. Of course, Orthodox Christians may eat meat, but that meat should be bled (as it the normal practice). If informed that meat is not bled or that a dish intentionally contains blood (blood sausage, blood sauce), an Orthodox Christian should abstain.[114]

The response then quotes Canon LXIII (63) of the Canons of the Holy Apostles specifying that ordained persons who eat flesh with blood are to be deposed because the law forbids it, and those of the laity who do so are to be excommunicated. Canon 67 of the Council of Trullo is cited to the same effect if such persons "eat in any way the blood of an animal."

Today, the majority of the Evangelical, Liberal Protestant, and Catholic Churches view blood prohibitions as a temporal compromise and as such no longer binding, although opposing views do exist. The Orthodox Churches, however, are united in the view that the prohibitions remain in force, and nonobservance in the West has even been cited as a reason for schism.[115]

The blood prohibition of Genesis 9:4 is the conditional requirement for the meat-eating sanction of Genesis 9:3. The prohibition emphasizes reverence for life, but it also allows meat for need, not desire or pleasure. In addition, it serves as the prick to conscience cited by Jewish commentators that inexorably leads to the realization of the vegetarian ideal. To ignore the blood prohibition is to hamper this process. Adherents of "temporal compromise" and "nothing defiles" are asked to reconsider their view in the light of all relevant indications. There will be more to say about the blood prohibition in the section on Islam ahead.

CHAPTER 5

Subsequent Christian Vegetarian Threads to Modern Times

The lapse of the blood prohibition in the Christian West may have weakened the vegetarian undercurrent, but the vegetarian impulse did not disappear completely. Augustine cites Christians who abstain from meat as being "without number," even though eschewing vegetarianism himself and denying its necessity.[116] St. Francis of Paola (1416–1507) was a vegan and made veganism the "fourth vow" (next to the traditional religious vows of poverty, chastity, and obedience) of the Order of Minims that he founded; the concerns were compassion for animals, nonviolence, and the absence of cruelty (we hear the echo of *ahimsa*, or nonviolence, in Eastern traditions).[117] The Benedictine, Carmelite, Carthusian, Cistercian, and Trappist monastic orders all have a history of vegetarianism. William Cowherd, the founder of the Bible Christian Church in 1809,[118] Ellen G. White, one of the founders of the Seventh-Day Adventist Church (see chapter 2), and Catherine and Bramwell Booth, the founders of the Salvation Army, and especially their son Bramwell Booth, the second general,[119] have all advocated vegetarianism.

The Mormon Church claims a limited divine sanction for eating meat that includes a dispensation related to cold weather and famine:

> Yea, flesh also of beasts and of the fowls of the air, I, the Lord, have ordained for the use of man with thanksgiving; nevertheless they are to be used sparingly;
>
> And it is pleasing unto me that they should not be used, only in times of winter, or of cold, or famine.[120]

We have otherwise heard of the link between cold weather and meat consumption with Tibetan yogis in chapter 1 and Michio Kushi in chapter 2. A commentary to the above verses indicates that, while Mormon teaching does not stress vegetarianism, sparing use of animal foods is the key.[121] A Mormon association for vegetarians and vegans also exists.[122]

The Christian Vegetarian Association, with independent branches in the United States and the United Kingdom, is an important part of the Christian vegetarian impulse.[123]

To its credit, the US association does not dispute (as do some) that Jesus ate fish after the resurrection (Luke 24:43). To its discredit, it suggests that the primary reason for the meat-eating sanction of Genesis 9:3 was a lack of vegetal food after the Flood. Limited freedom to express violence is the second possible reason.[124] Richard Alan Young, a member of the board of directors, acknowledges in his book *Is God a Vegetarian?* the argument of a lack of vegetal food, yet himself rejoins that Noah doesn't disembark from the ark until a dove appears with an olive branch, signifying the growth of vegetation.[125] In his book Young also refers to Rabbi Kook's work, which clearly emphasizes the sanction's purpose of giving humans limited freedom to express violence by killing animals and eating them.

Also to the discredit of the US branch of the Christian Vegetarian Association is its outdated criticism of the Atkins Diet, which it labels as a fad diet that usually leads to regaining weight, while citing the Ornish low-fat diet as healthy.[126] (Dr. Ornish acknowledges that weight-loss diets generally lead to recidivism, and some would undoubtedly consider the Ornish diet a fad diet—see chapter 7).

Regarding the UK branch of the Christian Vegetarian Association, one cannot find fault with the stated mission of supporting and encouraging the move toward vegetarianism, or with sharing vegetarianism's biblical and theological basis, or even with raising awareness of the relationships between vegetarianism world hunger, animal suffering, human health, and natural resource sustainability. Yet what must be challenged are simplistic assertions linking meat eating with disease, global injustice, and even the deadly sin of gluttony.[127]

Both Christian associations emphasize the health benefits of plant-based diets yet fail to acknowledge the health benefits of animal foods. Even with respect to bodily health, we have seen that such a perspective is one-sided and open to criticism. It is understandable that the full range of benefits from animal foods are not generally known or accepted, and it certainly a purpose of this study to illuminate both sides of the picture—the advantages and disadvantages of both vegetal and animal foods.

What is especially important to highlight and criticize on the part of both Christian associations, however, is the persistent emphasis on animal cruelty as a primary motivation for vegetarianism: "We do not object to meat because it is from God but because man-made factory farming is so harmful."[128]

Is this not the "weak moral voice" cited by Rabbi Kook of ethical vegetarianism, which takes flight into vegetarianism but thereby avoids confronting problems the overcoming of which would build strength? Are not the horrors of factory farming first and foremost economic, political, and social problems to be resolved among humans? Impotence and even despair at the seeming impossibility of systemic change is understandable, but it does not justify a retreat into vegetarianism, especially from a perspective that asserts animal food as a need. Vegetarian associations may well dispute the perspective recognizing that need. Yet by emphasizing the *distinction* between desire and need, they can nevertheless contribute to bringing the vegetarian cause forward.

Islam: Revitalizing the Vegetarian Undercurrent

The notion that Christianity's historical succession to Judaism brought new religious developments of universal benefit and concern is standard to Christian thinking. To suggest, however, that something similar in turn is true for Islam would be greeted with indignation by many Christians. Nevertheless, with respect to diet and the vegetarian impulse, Islam has much to offer "those who have ears to hear" through revitalizing the vegetarian undercurrent and strengthening the claim that the blood prohibition was meant never to lapse, but to endure.

The Qur'an Prohibitions and Amendments

Like other Near and Far Eastern sacred texts, the Qur'an also sanctions the consumption of flesh foods from animals, birds, and fish:

> And the grazing livestock He has created for you; in them is warmth and [numerous] benefits, and from them you eat.
>
> (Qur'an 16.5)

> And not alike are the two bodies of water. One is fresh and sweet, palatable for drinking, and one is salty and bitter. And from each you eat tender meat.
>
> (Qur'an 35.12)

> And the meat of fowl, from whatever they desire.
>
> (Qur'an 56.21)[129]

The list of what the Qur'an forbids also includes familiar themes:

> He has only forbidden to you dead animals, blood, the flesh of swine, and that which has been dedicated to other than Allah. But whoever is forced [by necessity], neither desiring [it] nor transgressing [its limit], there is no sin upon him. Indeed, Allah is Forgiving and Merciful.
>
> (Qur'an 2.173, 16.115)

> Forbidden for you are . . . one killed by strangling, and one killed with blunt weapons, and one which died by falling, and that which was gored by the horns of some animal, and one eaten by a wild beast, except those whom you slaughter.
>
> (Qur'an 5.3)

The foods that are allowed—animals, birds, and fish in general—are straightforward and unremarkable. Yet there is much to say about the prohibitions that can be summed up as follows:

159

- Blood

- Strangled or unbled animals

- Foods sacrificed to idols

- Pork

First of all, these prohibitions repeat the prohibitions of the Council of Jerusalem and the Noahide laws given to Noah and his sons after the Flood (with the exception of pork). In this sense, Yahweh in Genesis 9, the Holy Spirit in Acts 15, and Allah in the Qur'an are in complete agreement with one another, which is not surprising, considering that they are the three faces of the Divine in one tradition, namely, the Abrahamic.

Secondly, repeating the blood prohibition is particularly striking considering the controversy about it that developed in Christianity involving the notion that "nothing defiles." Allah, the Holy Spirit, and Yahweh, in contrast, seem to agree that indeed *blood does defile*. The reasoning, to repeat, is that blood symbolizes life, and life is sacred; killing for food is not the ideal; draining blood is an act of respect and a prick to conscience, leading back gradually to the vegetarian ideal.

Also noteworthy about the prohibitions is the flexibility that Allah shows. The following Qur'an verse seems to apply:

> We do not abrogate a verse or cause it to be forgotten except that We bring forth [one] better than it or similar to it. Do you not know that Allah is over all things competent?

> (Qur'an 2.106)

The implication in the case of the prohibitions above is that they can be excused under duress. To what does this apply? In addition to however it may have applied to Muslims in the seventh century, it seems tailor made regarding the dispute about foods sacrificed to idols in the letters of Paul, which was one of the impetuses for the Council of Jerusalem's decisions. Does it apply equally as well to Augustine's thrushes, small birds, and hares—i.e., to the prohibition against the consumption of blood? It seems reasonable, at least to me, to conclude that flexibility in the face of duress may well apply to meat sacrificed to idols, which is what was available in the markets of Paul's time, but that it does not apply to the inconvenience of draining blood from small animals taken in the hunt. In fact, here is what the Book of Leviticus says about hunting:

> And anyone of the people of Israel, or of the aliens who reside among them, who hunts down an animal or bird that may be eaten shall pour out its blood and cover it with earth.
>
> (Lev. 17:13)

Moreover, here is what Rabbi Kook says about the need to cover blood: it signifies God's protest against the meat-eating sanction, which is based on human corruption and moral weakness, and covering the blood stimulates the process of moral development that will become fully actualized in time.[130]

One may well object that the Levitical laws are Mosaic laws applying to Jews, not to everyone, which is arguably true for the injunction to cover the blood. But the objection does not apply to draining and not consuming the blood—because this prohibition belongs to the Qur'anic, Council of Jerusalem, Mosaic, and Noahide laws, which is to say that *the blood prohibition always has been, and apparently is always meant to be, a fundamental part of the sanction that allows eating meat; and by implication it is an important part of the Abrahamic tradition's vegetarian undercurrent.*

Implications of Repeating the Blood Prohibition

The Qur'an's repetition of the blood prohibition reinforces the notion that it was meant to be universally and permanently binding. It is important to emphasize this and to take a fresh look at what happened in Christianity. There are several interconnected issues to discriminate from one another:

161

- The blood prohibition as part of the Noahide laws, the Mosaic laws, the Council of Jerusalem's decrees, and the Qur'an prohibitions

- The prohibition against food sacrificed to idols as part of the Noahide laws, the Mosaic laws, the Council of Jerusalem decrees, and the Qur'an prohibitions

- Food sacrificed to idols as a temporal issue at the time of the first Christians for two reasons:

  1. Markets sold this kind of meat (arguing for having the flexibility to eat it).

  2. Communities were composed of both Gentiles and Jews, and Jews would be especially opposed to such foods because of their prohibition in the Mosaic laws (arguing for abstention in deference to Jewish Christians).

- The prohibition against unclean creatures in the Mosaic laws

- Peter's vision in Acts 10 portraying all creatures as clean

- The passages in Mark, chapter 7, and Matthew, chapter 15, about eating with unclean hands ("nothing that goes into a person defiles") that are interpreted to mean that all foods have been made clean

- The flexibility shown by Allah in the Qur'an about the food prohibitions in times of duress

Of these various points, readers should take note that Peter's vision is about the unclean creatures of the Mosaic laws being made clean, nothing else, and that all traditions prohibit food sacrificed to idols, which, however, was also a temporal issue for Christians for two different reasons.

The above points result in the following questions:

- Was the Council of Jerusalem *right* in prohibiting food sacrificed to idols because the prohibition was a universal one going back to Noah and his sons, yet nevertheless *wrong* in not allowing for flexibility, considering conditions as they were?

- Was Paul *right* to argue for flexibility about eating food sacrificed to idols because that is what the markets sold, and equally *right* to argue for abstention because of the mix of Gentiles and Jews in the communities; yet nevertheless *wrong* to suggest that all things had become lawful—similar to the interpretation of the Mark 7 and Matthew 15 passages? (That the council upholds the prohibition suggests that Paul's notion was rejected.)

- Was Augustine *wrong* to interpret the blood prohibition as a temporal issue (it was not) and also *wrong* to apply to it the notion of "nothing defiles"—similar to Paul?

- Has the Christian West been in the past, and is it now in the present, equally *wrong* to interpret the blood prohibition as a temporal issue and to invoke the "nothing defiles" statement as the justification for dismissing it?

These are the questions provoked by the Qur'an commands in which *Allah repeats once again the prohibitions against consuming blood and food sacrificed to idols.* The Qur'an lends weight to these things being considered as prohibited—then, now, and always. The notion of the Qur'an as the arbiter in matters doctrinal will undoubtedly strike terror into the hearts of many Christians. Yet we are confronted with evidence of a clear harmony among the different divine voices of the same tradition, namely, the Abrahamic Trinity of Yahweh, the Holy Spirit, and Allah.

Nevertheless, from our perspective there is a sense in which to affirm the notion that "nothing defiles." Readers will recall from chapter 2 that Rudolf Steiner talks about the undesirable effects of tea, then notes that they can be overridden by strength of character. Similarly, Michio Kushi talks about stages of eating that culminate in the freedom to eat what one chooses, knowing about effects and how to counterbalance them. Yet these caveats involve inner strength that cannot be assumed. Prohibitions like the blood prohibition repeated by the Qur'an were meant to provide beneficial, educative guidance for universal populations.

Moreover, the fewness of the Qur'an prohibitions, like those of the Christian and Noahide traditions, demarcates the significance of the numerous and more stringent Mosaic laws. The Jewish laws were limited, not universal, in scope. They applied to a people called to holiness in a special way for a special purpose (to prepare the way of the Messiah). The prohibition against unclean animals, in fact, otherwise only applied in antiquity to priests and holy ones. The fat prohibition similarly demanded a special kind of rigor and religious practice in order to safeguard the effect (see chapter 2). The lack of such prohibitions in the Noahide, Christian, and Islamic decrees suggests decreased expectations. In repeating the Noahide and council prohibitions, the Qur'an suggests that, for general populations, "nothing defiles"—except blood (including unbled animals) and food sacrificed to idols. Paul, Augustine, and the Christian West are right to assert that the Mosaic laws (regarding unclean creatures and fat) no longer apply to Christians, but they are wrong concerning blood and food sacrificed to idols (idols are still a relevant issue, to which we shall return). These prohibitions applied to everyone, beginning in Noah's time, and they still apply today.

Yet let's consider what is at stake by not observing them. Here is what Jesus says about breaking the law:

> Not one letter, not one stroke of a letter, will pass from the law until all is accomplished. Therefore, whoever breaks one of the least of these commandments, and teaches others to do the same, will be called least in the kingdom of heaven; but whoever does them and teaches them will be called great in the kingdom of heaven.
>
> (Matt 5:18–19)

At stake then, apparently, is one's reputation in heaven and not getting kicked out. Jesus is referring, however, to the more numerous and stringent Mosaic laws. Do his comments apply to the fewer and less strict Noahide, Council of Jerusalem, and Islamic laws? For the sake of Christians in the West, we hope so.

Yet in the interest of preserving the integrity of the Abrahamic tradition as a whole, let's try one more argument that is especially relevant to Christians. Jesus summarizes the law with the twofold (or threefold) great commandment of loving God and neighbor as oneself. Does loving God mean observing the unanimous decrees of Yahweh, the Holy Spirit, and Allah? Jews and Muslims say yes. What do Christians say?

Judaism and Islam have much to offer Christianity about understanding and cultivating the vegetarian impulse. On the other hand, the communion meal of Jesus is of profound significance for Jews and Muslims, too. It is so significant that it ought to be universally available, yet it is amazing how miserly attitudes about such things can be. It would be Good News indeed if Jews, Christians, and Muslims could sit down together and have a long chat about all these things. One can only look forward with hope to the time when the combined influence of Judaism and Islam might help to make the blood prohibition something vital again in Christianity, just as one can only look forward with hope to the time when the communion meal of Jesus is available in every temple and mosque (not to mention every corner store).

Prohibiting Pork and Dhabihah Slaughter

Regarding the Qur'an's dietary laws, the addition of pork to the list of forbidden foods, repeating the Mosaic Law's prohibition, is of special interest. Rudolf Steiner indicates that at issue with the Mosaic prohibition is the Jewish difficulty in assimilating sugar, and as a result, the tendency toward diabetes. Pork hinders the utilization of sugar, hence the ban. Steiner continues that the scope of this commandment is racial in nature and that the modern tendency toward nonobservance among Jews has harmful effects.[131] Is it any wonder, then, that the prohibition would be repeated in Islam, as Jews and

Muslims are blood brothers and sisters? The Blood-Type Diet also has something to say about pork—it is the only "avoid" meat for all four blood types. Consistent issues are blood serum flocculation, or causing substances suspended in the blood to drop out as flakes, and modifying disease susceptibility.[132] Allah, not to forget Yahweh, seems to have known something about pork that human beings are just beginning to discover!

Islam's revitalization of the vegetarian undercurrent in the Abrahamic tradition is further enhanced by reinstituting ritual slaughter, or *dhabihah*. That ritual sacrifice disappeared in Christianity is understandable, considering the ideology about the significance of Jesus's sacrifice along with the confusion in the West about "nothing defiles." The horrors of modern-day animal slaughter are arguably one result. Dhabihah returns slaughter to a sacred context while cultivating the distinction between the desire and the need for meat. The following description captures the spirit of dhabihah:

> The act of slaughtering itself is preceded by mentioning the name of God. Invoking the name of God at the moment of slaughtering is sometimes interpreted as acknowledgment of God's right over all things, and thanking God for the sustenance He provides: it is a sign the food is taken not in sin or in gluttony, but to survive and praise Allah, as the most common blessing is "Bismillah," or "In the name of God."

> Thus the slaughter itself is preceded by the words "In the name of Allah (Bismillah)." It is not regarded appropriate to use the phrase "Bismillah al Rahmān Al Rahīm" (In the name of God the Beneficent the Merciful) in this situation, because slaughtering is an act of subdual rather than mercy.[133]

In short, procuring meat through ritual slaughter is about not gluttony or desire, but survival or need. Moreover, although God allows this act of animal subdual, it is regrettable.

The word *slaughter* literally means to kill by "exsanguination," or by bleeding. Its purpose is to remove as much blood as possible, in line with the blood prohibition, as humanely as possible. While there is much debate about the humaneness of ritual slaughter, there is also much evidence that the result when it is skillfully done is a quick and painless death. Proponents of ritual slaughter object to the various forms of stunning that are common in slaughtering houses today for a variety of reasons, including making the animal unconscious, which is not allowed, and inhibiting exsanguination.[134] The debate continues to go back and forth.[135] At its root is often a fundamental difference in values that is perhaps unresolvable—on the part of religious proponents, a meat-eating sanction according to strict slaughtering guidelines; and on the part of animal rights activists, a rejection of meat eating. As long as humane animal treatment remains the focus of debate, however, perhaps it can be considered beneficial.

Muslims have debated the acceptability of Jewish meat but have rejected Christian meat.[136] (Christians everywhere should be voicing a collective "Ouch!") For the reasons indicated above, Christianity lost touch with the meaning of religious slaughter and prohibiting blood. As if in compensation, Islam has reenlivened both. It can only be hoped that Christians reawaken to the cultural significance.

Subsequent Islamic Vegetarian Threads to Modern Times

Steven Rosen notes that Mohammed was reportedly a lover of animals and preferred a vegetarian diet. In his birthplace, Mecca, slaughter is not allowed (Qur'an 5.1 and 5.95), and pilgrims approaching Mecca are enjoined to refrain from killing even insects. The intention of these measures is to exemplify the ideal harmony that should exist among all creatures.[137]

Rosen also notes that although the Qur'an sanctions animal food, other verses emphasize the importance of the fruits of the earth, such as grains, reeds, palms, milk, and bee's honey. He suggests that Islam's meat-eating concession reflects the Torah's notion of "gradualism": compassion for animals and abstinence from flesh are ideals, yet extending "universal compassion" beyond human beings can come only gradually. In this we hear echoed Rabbi Kook's understanding of a necessary human evolutionary development.

One version of the story of Mohammed's death suggests that he was thereby teaching about meat's harmfulness—he deliberately eats poisoned meat that is offered to him deceptively while instructing others to abstain.

The Sufi mystical tradition considers vegetarianism a high ideal. A parable by the Sufi master Muhammed Rahim Baiwa Muhaiyaddeen ("The Hunter Learns Compassion from the Fawn") questions any notion of God's providing animals for food, recommending instead the cultivation of compassion and the resolve not to kill. For Sufis, the inner meaning of the *qurban* slaughtering rituals during the Eid al-Adha Festival is slaying the beasts of the heart through devotion and sacrifice to God. Similarly, the *kalimah* prayer, which is ostensibly recited to purify "the baser qualities of the animal," is understood as purifying the human desire to slaughter. Moreover, qurban's myriad slaughtering details are understood to lessen the number of animals killed. One tradition states that Allah told Mohammed directly that qurban was instituted to reduce unnecessary killing.[138]

Islam also has a vegetarian association—Islamic Concern.[139] A closer look at its website, however, reveals little more than an informational focus with no membership or activities. The site is sponsored by People for the Ethical Treatment for Animals (PETA), and many links go to PETA, which responds to email inquiries. This is not necessarily unusual. Jewish vegetarians have also collaborated with PETA, and Jewish and Christian vegetarian groups also have websites hosted or sponsored by other groups. Yet Islam deserves to have its own independent and fully functioning vegetarian association.

Most of the articles on Islamic Concern are written by Muslims and deal with topics such as vegetarianism's relationship to Islam, animal treatment, the debate about slaughter, and abuses of *halal* standards (i.e., meat that is acceptable to Muslims according to dietary laws). The following quotation summarizes the Islamic association's philosophy:

> The information provided on this Web site demonstrates how factory-farmed meat from industrialized countries and even

meat advertised as "halal" from India, a country in which the second most popular religion after Hinduism is Islam, violates Islamic reverence for life. It is evident that adopting a vegetarian diet is the simplest and healthiest way in which people can guarantee adherence to the gentle teachings of their faith.[140]

At the risk of repetition, adopting a vegetarian diet may seem like the simplest solution, but questions about the health effects and the process of human moral development remain. We will return to these themes, too.

To RECAPITULATE the discussion about the Abrahamic traditions of Judaism, Christianity, and Islam, none embraces vegetarianism as in the Far East, yet points of contact with the ideal exist. Vegetarianism is alive and visible in the lives of individuals and groups. As an undercurrent, it appeared in Judaism through the rigors of kashrut, yet the strength of the impulse today has undoubtedly become much weaker: about one-sixth of Jews in the United States are estimated to follow kashrut fully, and a much greater number to avoid some foods like pork.[141] Islam's vegetarian undercurrent is modest compared with Judaism's, and yet its overall vibrancy and strength is undoubtedly greater through more disciplined observance. Christianity's vegetarian undercurrent has stagnated and is in need of renewal. A good start would be a new understanding of and appreciation for the blood prohibitions of its own tradition as well as the slaughtering rituals of others. All the Abrahamic traditions, however, share alike in the legacy of the Genesis vegan command and the promise of a vegetarian future through the prophecies of Isaiah.

CONSENSUS ON VEGETARIANISM: AN UNEQUIVOCAL YES AND NO

As mentioned at the chapter's beginning, the sum of the world's major religious traditions on the question of vegetarianism reveals ambiguity, or both support and nonsupport at the same time. In the Far East there are a tendency toward qualified support in Hinduism, a split within Buddhism, Jainism's advocacy, and Sikhism's rejection; in the Abrahamic traditions of the Near East, an underlying vegetarian ideal and an undercurrent of varying degrees and strength, with outright support here and there, but, on the whole, acceptance of meat consumption.

I have suggested that the root of this ambiguity lies with the question of desire or need. The question arose in chapter 1 with the mention of Tibetan yogis eating meat for warmth. In chapter 2, a host of voices labeled meat as a despicable desire, lust, or craving; and the Lankavatara Sutra noted that indulgence reinforces desire. Yet we also heard comments by macrobiotic authors and Rudolf Steiner suggesting that the desire can amount to the intuition of a need that is crucial to health. Individual considerations became the all-important criteria. Weston Price similarly suggested in chapter 4 that full health depends on animal food.

In the present chapter, however, we heard from the Anusasana Parva that meat promotes development and strength, that it is superior to all other foods, that it benefits the weak, the sick, and the exhausted, but that the taste can become addictive. In addition, we heard Rabbi Kook's comprehensive vision of the role of meat in human evolutionary development, which is understood as the rationale for the biblical meat-eating sanction. In this vision, animals pay the price, but not for all time.

In short, the question of whether meat is a desire or a need is not easy to answer, but consumption seems to span a spectrum from "desire" at one end to "need" at the other, and this spectrum of possibility itself appears to lie at the root of the ambiguity surrounding this issue.

Our foundation stone for spiritual dietary teachings, the Bhagavad Gita, seems equally ambiguous in that it names no foods, offering instead the criterion of choosing a sattvic-type diet that is holistically nourishing. Yet earlier this chapter quoted the Gita as allowing meat only if it has been properly sacrificed. Thus its support for vegetarianism, like other Hindu teachings, would also be qualified.

The witness of the Bhagavad Gita is worth considering in more detail: As mentioned, the Gita appeared when Hinduism was consolidating its own identity; the sacred text tried to resolve the tension between the Vedic and Brahmanic legacies of the past and the new morality of the times that involved nonviolence. Its solution was to affirm that the different yogic paths of action, knowledge, and devotion were part of one another and led to the same liberation goal. Thus, the Gita was able to give people of different characters and responsibilities a common sense of purpose.[142]

Its story, as previously indicated, involves a crisis in the life of Arjuna, a warrior of the Kshatriya class, for whom "there is no greater good ... than righteous battle" (Bhagavad Gita, 2:31).[143] Despite his warrior duty, Arjuna shrinks before the horror of civil war and battling against his own kinsmen.[144] His lament about the sinfulness of doing this reflects his conflict about the call to compassion. Krishna, the image of the Supreme Divine, appears as his charioteer to instruct him on the path leading to freedom from fear and ignorance.

True liberation, Krishna says, consists of uniting action (*karma-yoga*), knowledge (*jnana-yoga*), and devotion (*bhakti-yoga*). He argues that works cannot be renounced (as they are for the Vedic path of knowledge), for if the Divine ceased incessant activity, the world would soon end. Works are necessary for "the holding together of the peoples" (Bhagavad Gita 3:20), and, performed in imitation of the Divine, they are the surest way to union and to liberation. In this view, full engagement according to the demand of external circumstances is the ideal, seeking neither what is agreeable nor shunning what is disagreeable, and without attachment to the result (Bhagavad Gita, 18:9–10).

Krishna continues that the present battle involves a confrontation with immorality, and engaging in this battle is vitally important. Revealing himself as the Supreme Divine, the *Purushottama*, who transcends but embraces creation and destruction, Krishna commands Arjuna to fight—because this battle and destruction have a place in the divine will and divine purpose, however inscrutable they may seem to be. Krishna desires Arjuna's understanding (knowledge, or *jnana*), his devotion and faith (*bhakti*), and lastly his participation (action, or *karma*) by fighting, but without attachment to the result.

Needless to say, Krishna succeeds. Arjuna accepts his warrior duty and resolves to fight, putting his trust completely in Krishna. He accepts Krishna's words: "Abandon all *dharmas* [righteous behaviors] and take refuge in Me alone. I will deliver thee from all sin and evil, do not grieve" (Bhagavad Gita, 18:66).[145] As Sri Aurobindo writes:

> We must acknowledge Kurukshetra [the field of battle]; we must submit to the Law of Life by Death before we can find our way to the life immortal; we must open our eyes, with less appalled gaze than Arjuna's, to the vision of our Lord of Time and Death [Krishna] and cease to deny, hate or recoil from the universal Destroyer.[146]

We have heard of this "Law of Life by Death" before, at this chapter's beginning, as the archetypal foundation of creation mythology. We also heard of this notion in the Laws of Manu in the form of a divine ordinance for creatures to eat one another in order to sustain life (as a justification for eating meat).

This notion of "life by death" is related to the "context-sensitive" nature of Hindu ethics (which is arguably true for other ethical systems, including the Bible's).[147] *Ahimsa*, or nonviolence, is an ethical ideal but not an absolute, and implementation depends on one's social class (Arjuna is a warrior) and stage of life (ahimsa applies mostly to the hermit and wandering-ascetic stages of later life). Just as ahimsa cannot be Arjuna's standard regarding human life because he is a warrior, so too can ahimsa not be the standard regarding animal life because of the social importance of sacrifice as well as the importance of sanctioned meat eating for human health.

In short, the Bhagavad Gita teaches pursuing a sattvic-type diet, and this suggests eating vegetal foods, whose tendency is sattvic. Yet the action essential to "the holding together of the peoples" is also vitally important; and, in Hindu culture, this meant animal sacrifice and sanctioned meat eating, especially for warriors like Arjuna, who needed the rajasic stimulation provided by meat. Thus we see more clearly that the support of the Bhagavad Gita for vegetarianism would indeed be qualified.

Qualified support from a different perspective is provided by the Mother, Mirra Alfassa, the coworker of Sri Aurobindo, who was considered a manifestation of the Feminine Divine. Diet, the Mother writes, depends on individual consciousness and life. For the ordinary person leading an ordinary life, meat nutrition is optional as long as the effect is helpful, useful, and good. But when a person aspires to higher life, food takes on new importance because some foods support refinement while others inhibit it. She then cautions:

> Before you come to that point, you have a lot of other things to do. It is certainly better to purify your mind, purify your vital before you think of purifying your body. For even if you take all possible precautions and live physically with every care to eat only the things that help to refine the body, but the mind and the vital remain full of desire and inconscience and obscurity and all the rest, your care will serve no purpose. Your body will become perhaps weak, disharmonious with your inner life and drop off one day.[148]

We hear in this caution an echo of Rudolf Steiner and Rabbi Kook about the possible negative effects of vegetarianism.

In light of the Mother's remarks, and in light of the synthesis of all voices and opinions so far in this book,[149] the answer to the question of vegetarianism from a religious and spiritual point of view is an unequivocal Yes and No:

- Yes—in the biblical tradition, vegetarianism is the legacy of an ideal past and the direction of an idealized future, and many spiritual teachings recommend it because of beneficial effects. "Yes" acknowledges the "desire" side of the urge for meat and admonishes to suppress unnecessary desire. This is the reason for all meat eaters, especially the religious and spiritually minded, to reconsider consumption habits, yet with the caveat that vegetarianism presupposes spiritual activity in order to utilize the inner forces that are released in the correct way (see the section on Rudolf Steiner in chapter 2).

- No—important considerations that include but go beyond physical health preclude making vegetarianism a general and habitual recommendation for everyone. "No" acknowledges the "need" side of the urge for meat and is the reason for cautioning vegetarians and especially vegans about excluding animal foods from the diet. (Even for those on a spiritual path, individual considerations may preclude a fully vegetarian diet.)

Negotiating the balance between the Yes and the No, of course, is an individual challenge requiring discernment. Yet considering the ambiguity among religious traditions as a whole and that Jainism, the strictest among them, is lacto-vegetarian and includes dairy; considering also that Weston Price highlights the importance of animal fats for nutrient assimilation and asserts the lesser health of those who exclude animal foods; and considering as well the traditional dietary practice of including small amounts of animal food with meals and research indicating that as little as 2 percent significantly boosts vegetal protein assimilation[150]—in the light of all these considerations, it seems advisable to include some form of animal food in the diet (meat, poultry, fish, eggs, or dairy) *unless one knows that one has transcended such a need.*[151]

This is what can be said about individual choice for or against vegetarianism. But relevant issues go beyond individual choice. Weston Price has documented the effect of parental nutrition on offspring and the traditional special diets for parents before and after conception, highlighting animal foods (high-quality dairy and green vegetables; animal organ meats; fish and fish oil; and fish eggs for women and fish sperm for men—see chapter 4). In this light, Sally Fallon Morell, president of the Weston A. Price Foundation, asserts that "to promote veganism or vegetarianism to young men and women before and during child-bearing age is completely irresponsible."[152] Nothing about spiritual teachings contradicts this view, and much arguably supports it, albeit indirectly. First, there are the ambiguity of spiritual teachings as a whole on the question of vegetarianism and the lack of overt support in the Abrahamic traditions. Second, the Hindu tradition distinguishes between the religious practice for householders and the practice for emancipation seekers (see the

Anusasana Parva in this chapter). This distinction involves the division of life into four stages (students, householders, hermits, and ascetics—outlined previously in the Hinduism section) and the association of vegetarianism with the hermit and ascetic stages of later life. The householder stage presumes participation in rituals like animal sacrifice and meat consumption as well. As for the pro-and-con debate about vegetarianism within Buddhism, it largely, if not exclusively, has involved monks, or celibates. The Jaina requirement for vegetarianism includes dairy, yet the small number of Jains relative to other Indian sects demonstrates the unattractiveness of Jaina rigors, including dietary ones. And Sikhism does not require vegetarianism at all. In short, the consumption of animal foods among child-bearing parents can be expected within most religious traditions as the habitual norm.

Morell further asserts that rearing children as vegans or vegetarians is comparable to child abuse.[153] Rudolf Steiner, for his part, recommends paying close attention to and honoring the dietary instincts of young children. He even indicates, for example, that a child in a meat-eating environment may reject meat because of poisonous effects on the intestines. Steiner argues that such instincts can be trusted and should be promoted, while also acknowledging the need for intervention in the case of bad habits. After puberty, when healthy instincts have begun to wane, he recommends health and nutrition education to reinforce forming good habits.[154] Considering the health ramifications, Weston Price's work certainly deserves to be part of such a curriculum.

Regardless of personal dietary preferences, parents should bear the above considerations in mind. The distinction between personal choice and responsibility for children's health is an important one to make.

IMPLICATIONS: PROMOTING VEGETARIANISM AND ETHICAL ANIMAL-FOOD SOURCES

The first implication of the yes-and-no answer relates to the "yes"—that religious teachings do encourage vegetarianism. This does not mean eliminating animal foods completely. The fundamental issue is one of discerning and controlling desire, which belongs to the discipline of spiritual development with regard to all human desires. In the case of meat, there may be some or even much desire that is not need. This is the difficult distinction to make. From a spiritual point of view, consuming animal foods and especially meat should not be automatic but deliberate. Undoubtedly, consumption could be lessened if such distinctions were made. The final criterion, however, is limiting consumption in a healthy way, as health is the ultimate consideration.

The second implication relates to the "no"—that there is value in animal foods and even a need. The issue that arises is satisfying the need with ethical sources.

Awareness in recent times of ethical problems associated with animal foods goes back to Peter Singer's seminal work *Animal Liberation*, which helped expose the horrors of factory farming and conventional animal slaughter.[155] Singer revealed the confluence of science, technology, and business interests geared to maximizing profits at the expense of ethical treatment (unless exempting farm animals from animal cruelty laws can be considered ethical).

Religious voices such as the vegetarian associations referred to above have decried the modern-day system yet feel helpless in the face of effecting meaningful reform. Although religious practices would seem to offer an alternative, Jewish vegetarian author Richard Schwartz has argued that Judaism's shechita guidelines could not cope with the animal numbers slaughtered daily—the slaughterer, or *shochtim*, would find it impossible to maintain the requisite spirit of holiness that requires, for example, a prayer for each individual animal.[156] As a result, Schwartz advocates vegetarianism or even veganism to minimize the harm done. We have heard this same argument from all religious vegetarian associations, yet the issue remains that it overlooks or denies the issue of need. The viewpoint of this book is the absolute necessity of providing ethical sources of animal foods because of those who need meat, despite any controversy that continues to attach to such an idea.

The necessity for providing animal-food sources that are ethical is easy to assert, but the realization of that goal is difficult to imagine, just as Richard Schwartz suggests. Yet it is precisely here that the crux of the paradox becomes manifest. A solution requires cultural transformation, which presupposes human transformation, and meat consumption is understood to play an important role in the development of human inner strength. Human transformation is first necessary, according to Rabbi Kook, before righteousness can be genuinely vouchsafed to animals—not out of the moral impotence that resigns in the face of an unethical cultural system, but with the fullness of the moral voice strengthened through personal transformation. Systemic reform may seem daunting and even impossible, but it is a necessary part of the process of both human and cultural evolution. In terms of the Bhagavad Gita, the struggle for reform represents a modern-day battlefield of *Kurukshetra*, the place where Arjuna himself hesitated to become engaged but was encouraged to do so.

Kurukshetra was a place of confrontation with immorality, a term that is easily applied to the present system of animal food production. A further especially relevant characterization identifies this system's products as *foods sacrificed to idols*—to the idols of money and profit, or *Mammon* (Matt. 6:24; Luke 16:13). This is the true spiritual nature of the current secular system, and foods sacrificed to idols are forbidden to all of humanity through the Noahide prohibitions and the Mosaic, Christian, and Muslim prohibitions as well. *Foods sacrificed to idols are forbidden to everyone.*

Thus, if the need for animal foods can be accepted, then there is also a need to provide ethical sources. Does this mean waging jihad against the present system? Perhaps the most appropriate answer once again is yes and no—no, not directly; but yes, indirectly. Religious alternatives exist, and, were they supported on a wider scale, pressure would be exerted on the conventional system to follow suit. The shechita practices of Jews, the dhabihah practices of Muslims, and the jhakta practices of Sikhs are religious-based ethical approaches, and it is they that must all be supported. This is where religious and spiritually minded people can turn. If Christians were to lend their collective weight to the effort, the resulting impact could be tremendous; yet for Christians this would mean accepting that some things such as blood, indeed, do defile.

The costs of building an alternative system—cost in terms of effort and money, also—cannot be avoided. One can only respond with Sufi faith in the necessity of troublesome effort exerting downward pressure on consumption. Certainly such effort would reinvigorate the vegetarian impulse.

The yes-and-no answer to the question of vegetarianism comprises a simultaneous awareness of the importance of vegetarianism from a spiritual point of view and the importance of meat, as well as the need for ethical animal husbandry practices. Cultivating this awareness and striving for necessary personal and cultural transformation represent the "work" called for by the Bhagavad Gita for "the holding together of the peoples."

This religious and spiritual answer to the question of vegetarianism, however, is preliminary and incomplete. It remains to grapple with carbohydrates and grains, which are important foods for vegetarian diets, and to outline a deeper understanding of the Genesis call to veganism and its realization. The chapter ahead takes up both topics.

6

GRAINS, CIVILIZATION, AND THE PALEOLITHIC REVIVAL

We pivot now to grains, the second major theme of our study next to spiritual teachings about vegetarianism. Grains, of course, would be a major, if not the most important, component of a vegetarian diet.

There is good news and bad news about grains. In chapter 1 we heard that grains are sattvic foods supreme, but also that the sattva-tending effect can become rajasic or tamasic depending on preparation. (Again, *sattva* is the quality associated with equilibrium, harmony, and balance; *rajas* with energy, motion, and passion; and *tamas* with inertia, inconscience, and ignorance.) This spectrum of possible effects is an indication of potentially good and bad sides. Chapter 2 discussed that some consider grains the principle or most important food, and many teachings recommend them, undoubtedly reflecting the sattvic potential. Chapter 3 discussed negative mental effects related to refining. Chapter 4 cited two ancient teachings about the primary importance of grains, and we saw them at the base of food pyramids. Yet with the carbohydrate hypothesis of disease, the shadow side appeared again—refined grains that are quickly digested easily lead to metabolic problems. The vegan paradigm of the Physician's Committee for Responsible Medicine in chapter 4 asserted that vegan foods including grains are sufficient for health, yet this view was challenged by Weston Price.

The debate continues in the present chapter and involves twists that both elevate grains higher and degrade them lower. On the positive side, we hear about beneficial effects of grains for body, soul, and spirit and their important role for civilization at the dawn of

179

the agricultural revolution. On the negative side, we paradoxically hear about the adverse health effects of grains when civilization began and more, including a critique of grains in the whole form. This negative aspect is given as the justification for returning to the meat-centered diets of the Paleolithic era. We have heard hints of this kind of attitude before within the debate between the carbohydrate and fat hypotheses of disease, but now the objections to carbohydrates will be given full voice and presented in more detail. Before turning to them, as well as to a full acknowledgment of the health benefits of Paleo-style diets, we turn to the good news about grains from the time when they first began to be cultivated. There is important information to reap here that eventually leads to a more comprehensive understanding of the idealized vegan diet.

GRAINS AND CIVILIZATION

Grains are defined as the edible seeds and fruits of grass plants. Examples include amaranth, barley, buckwheat, corn, millet, oats, quinoa, rice, rye, sorghum, and teff. Amaranth, buckwheat, and quinoa are not edible seeds of grasses, yet they are usually counted as grains because of nutritional use.

In the history of food and mythology, two themes recur about grains: their importance for the body and for the soul.[1] The importance for the body appears self-evident, yet the range of health-related associations may seem surprising. Importance for the soul is less well known or clear. There are two aspects to this soul dimension—a quickening effect on the intellect and on the life of spirit.

Grains and the Body

The bodily benefits of grain begin with ensuring survival and providing a source of medicine and strength. The development of farming provided a more dependable and voluminous food source, and cereal grains were the most important crop. Different types were peculiar to different parts of the world. Corn was predominant in the

Americas, barley and wheat in the Near East, and millet and rice in the Far East.[2] The myths of all cultures testify to the association of grains with the gods and to their cultural importance.

A Native American Ojibwa corn myth emphasizes the relationship to survival. When the shaman Wunzh seeks spirit guidance because his people are starving, a spirit-man appears and wrestles with him. When Wunzh defeats him, the man instructs Wunzh to bury his body, and the result is that corn springs forth. Subsequently, the people no longer have to rely on hunting and fishing alone for food.[3] In a similar Chinese rice myth, the ears of the rice stalks are empty, and people live solely by hunting and fishing but are starving. The goddess Kwan Yin then enters the rice fields in compassion and squeezes her breast milk into the empty ears. Some become white while others turn red, because in the end, she has to squeeze very hard and the milk becomes mixed with blood.[4] Millet myths in China and quinoa myths in South America also emphasize survival and the assurance of life.[5] In Mayan culture, amaranth was a staple and the key to survival because it provided energy and protein when other sources were unavailable.[6]

The theme of grains as an important source of life and strength is a familiar one today because they are recognized as the most important source of bodily fuel. Slow-burning, complex-carbohydrate energy in the form of grains is civilization's most common and least expensive fuel.[7] In myth and tradition, various grains are praised for providing endurance, energy, growth, health, strength, and vitality. In one Buddhist myth, rice revives Siddhartha, the future Buddha, when he is near death.[8] For Incas and Aztecs, corn was a sacred symbol of the sun and the plant with the greatest life energy.[9] For the Indians of central Mexico, eating amaranth was a guarantee of "health and life for all."[10] According to a legend of Togo's Bassavi tribe, the god Unumbatte gave the gift of sorghum and millet (and yams) to provide sustenance.[11]

One reason for the association between grains and medicine is their relationship to herbs. As with herbs, the growth cycle of grains is annual. When herbs are prescribed in traditional medicine, the diet is restricted to grains, and for this reason they are considered the soul of herbal medicine and the most precious of the healing herbs.[12]

181

The traditional use of sorghum and amaranth also attests to a medicinal quality. The Yoruba-Dahomey of Nigeria use sorghum for medicine because of its association with Osanyin, the god of medicinal crops.[13] Wherever amaranth has been grown—in the Americas, Europe, or Asia—it has always been considered divine and medicinal. In Honduras, people carry the seeds close to the chest to prevent as well as to cure colds.[14]

Grains and the Intellect

The relationship of grains to the intellect involves the transformation of human life as well as of nature. Erich Neumann invokes both themes in discussing the archetype of the Great Mother, whose guises include the ancient Earth Mothers or goddesses responsible for agriculture and grains.

Transforming nature is an integral part of human culture, and using fire to improve foods through methods such as frying, roasting, and boiling has been part of the process. Bread baking is an example.[15] Yet in carrying out such processes and learning to apply fire, human consciousness also becomes transformed.

This reciprocal process began at the dawn of the agricultural era. Humans modified wild grasses by selecting seeds based on observable and desirable plant traits. Corn seed was selected for size, taste, and the speed of maturation in order to promote an abundant, simultaneous harvest, leading to the ability to live from harvests. Human intelligence was responsible, but plants provided the stimulation. Myths describe grains as gifts of the gods and agriculture as being "taught" to humans *by* the gods; science describes a gradual process of learning taking place over time. In both views, the result is the same: agriculture and civilization develop side by side through stages of learning and applying intelligence.[16]

In the words of Maguelonne Toussaint-Samat, rice growing and Chinese ingenuity are so tightly interwoven that it is impossible to say which determined the other. Admiring a seventeenth-century irrigation pump whose principles are still in use, she muses about the relationship between cultivating rice and the development of social structures:

> Rice was the making of Chinese civilization, which owed it, besides a meticulous cast of mind, that vast administrative apparatus that neither time nor revolution have changed. . . . All communal irrigation systems depend on riverside dwellers cooperating, and on firm social rules. In Provence, for instance . . . the man with the job of opening and closing the . . . small irrigation channels is one of the most important people in rural life.[17]

Dawn E. Bastian and Judy K. Mitchell sound similar themes about the significance of corn cultivation for civilizational development:

> Agriculture is more labor intensive than hunting and gathering. Fields must be guarded, watered, and weeded. Crops must be planted and harvested. Storage containers must be created. Both the work and the workers must be organized and supervised.[18]

This activity, they continue, led to hunting-and-gathering bands evolving into villages, which resulted in the need for even more crops. One can imagine such a process slowly building societies and civilizations over time: as more crops are raised, more people can be fed, and more labor is freed up for diverse purposes; societies become more complex, evolving political systems, universities, medicine, arts, and sciences. Toussaint-Samat sums up this interweaving process between agriculture and the intellect succinctly: "Not for nothing does the same word, culture, apply to both intellectual development and the tilling of the soil."[19]

Grains and the Spirit

Beyond the effect of agriculture and grains on the intellect is their effect on the human spirit. In its simplest form, mythology documents how the appearance of agriculture and grains coincided with a turn from barbarism.

In Egypt, people lived as cannibals before the cultivation of barley and wheat. By introducing the cultivation of grain, the god Osiris saved people from savagery, and he traveled the world over to distribute the blessings of grain.[20] Inca creation mythology speaks of people living like wild animals until the son and daughter of the sun god are sent to teach agriculture and maize—or corn—cultivation, which becomes a sacred crop.[21] There are many strikingly similar myths about goddesses and gods giving the gift of grain, followed by civilization and an end to barbarism.[22]

The highest expression of grain's effect on the human spirit, however, involves awakening to the idea of life after death. Understanding life as a cycle that comprises birth, death, and rebirth goes back to the eighth millennium BCE and Old Europe's Neolithic society. Living with natural cycles like those of the moon and agriculture stimulated basic faith in the continuity of human life. The belief took different forms in different times and places—regeneration, transmigration, resurrection in heaven, reincarnation on earth, cosmic renewal through cycles of time, and resurrection on earth and final cosmic renewal at the end of time.[23] Grains were a special symbol of the faith in rebirth in association with mythological stories of gods and goddesses dying yet continuing to live (echoing the creation mythology discussed in chapter 5).

In the Greek myth, wheat is the gift of Demeter, goddess of grain. One day Hades, god of the Underworld, abducts Demeter's daughter Persephone, carrying her off to his realm of the dead. While Demeter grieves Persephone's loss, all vegetation dies, threatening to extinguish life itself on earth.

Eventually Zeus, the king of the gods, grants Demeter's plea for Persephone's release, and Persephone is allowed to return to earth, but only to spend part of her time there. For some months of each year, she must return to the Underworld.

The grain harvest, which represents the "death" of grain and the onset of winter, is associated with Persephone's descent to the Underworld, the realm of the dead, just as the sprouting anew of grain in springtime is associated with her coming back to life and returning to the earth. In this way, the life cycle of grain becomes a symbol of the story of Persephone, who descends to the realm of the dead, but returns to life.

The worship of Demeter with agricultural rituals throughout the year guaranteed the harvest's productivity, but there was another dimension as well:

> Demeter, and the other grain goddesses like her, nurtured not only the body but the soul. For the initiates in Demeter's cult, the Eleusian Mysteries, worshipping the grain goddess guaranteed their own life after death.[24]

Just as the story of Persephone involved a symbolic death and return to life in imitation of grain's cycle, Demeter's devotees hoped for rebirth by worshipping her.

The story of the Egyptian grain god Osiris, who dies but continues to live, provides another example. Drawing on the myth, Egyptians placed Osiris effigies stuffed with grain into their tombs and addressed deceased ones with the name of Osiris in expectation of attaining new life through him.[25] In addition, they put funerary beds of sprouted barley on mummies[26] to imitate an Osiris image showing sprouted barley.[27]

Other mythological stories of gods dying and becoming reborn also used grain as the symbol—Aphrodite and Adonis in Syria; Cybele and Attis in Phrygia; and Tammuz and Ishtar in Babylonia (the story of Dionysus in Greece used grapes).[28] Christianity, too, used grain to symbolize rebirth. As Paul says:

> Fool! What you sow does not come to life unless it dies.... You do not sow the body ... but a bare seed, perhaps of wheat or of some other grain. But God gives it a body.... So it is with the resurrection of the dead.
>
> (1 Cor. 15:36–38, 42–44)[29]

In addition, Jesus uses wheat in a passage understood as a prophecy of his death and resurrection:

> Very truly, I tell you, unless a grain of wheat falls into the earth and dies, it remains just a single grain; but if it dies, it bears much fruit.

(John 12:24)

The rapid spread of Christianity in Asia Minor in antiquity is attributed to the similarity of the Christian story to various grain mythologies involving death and rebirth.[30] Yet the grain myths themselves were a reflection of a deeper and more comprehensive myth, namely, the myth of creation cited in chapter 5. It was Christianity's deep similarity to key elements of this myth that undoubtedly provoked the recognition that allowed its rapid growth. A comparison of key points is revealing (see table 3 on page 187).

The diverse elements of creation mythology and the story of Jesus interweave in a remarkable way. Jesus is understood as the source of life ("In the beginning was the *Word*"), and then he reappears to sacrifice himself for a higher form of life—resurrected life. Blood sacrifice by crucifixion leads to this new form of life, and bloodless sacrifice takes place with the communion meal he institutes using bread and wine (combining grain mythology and Dionysian grape mythology). Both the bloody crucifixion and the bloodless communion sacrifice obviate the need for further blood sacrifice to commemorate the creation myth, at a time when human sacrifices were still being practiced. In an astonishing way, the need for further blood sacrifice becomes sublimated.

Readers may recall the mention in chapter 5 of the Avestan people holding the evil spirit, Angra Mainyu, responsible for instituting the practice of blood sacrifice, whose domain was solely the province of the gods. In this sense traditional blood sacrifice inappropriately recreated a divine–mythical reality. Jesus's bloody sacrifice on the cross invoked the creation myth but then redirected its memorialization to bloodless sacrifice with bread and wine, both sublimating and ennobling it. Critics point to the repulsiveness of a Father

TABLE 3. COMPARISON OF THE CONCEPTS OF CREATION MYTHOLOGY WITH THE STORY OF JESUS		
CONCEPT	CREATION MYTHOLOGY	STORY OF JESUS
Life Originated in Divine Sacrifice	The universe and all of life come into being through the body and blood of a deity, sacrificed by itself or by other gods; "death becomes life."	Jesus is the source of life ("In the beginning was the Word. . . . All things came into being through him, and without him not one thing came into being" (John 1:1, 3). The new life of resurrection comes into being through Jesus's sacrificial death on the cross.
Sacrifice Honors the Deity and Renews Life	Sacrifice honors the act of the deity's death and helps to sustain universal life; blood sacrifices are made using humans and animals; grain effigies and fruits of the field are also used.	For the sake of renewing life, Jesus offers the bloody sacrifice of his death on the cross to the Father.
Sacrifices Represent the Deity, Consumed in Communion	All sacrifices—human, animal, grain effigies, and "first fruits" of the field—represent the deity and are consumed as communion with the deity.	Before his death, in the Last Supper Jesus institutes a sacrificial communion meal of bread and wine, mystically impregnated with his body and blood, commanding that this communion be continued in his memory.
Communion Signifies Life after Death	Just as the sacrificed deity survives death, communion with the deity guarantees eternal life.	The communion meal of Jesus signifies eternal life: "I am the living bread that came down from heaven. Whoever eats of this bread will live forever; and the bread I will give for the life of the world is my flesh" (John 6:51).

God demanding the bloody sacrifice of the Son. Yet this sacrifice stilled once and for all a deeply imbedded archetype within human consciousness, and therein lie its divine justification and its divine-human tragedy as well.

The relationship of Jesus's sacrifice to Jewish sacrifices is also worth considering. Jewish sacrifices were of different types (see Leviticus 11): sin sacrifices; "offerings of well-being" preceding the consumption of meat; and offerings of praise and thanksgiving. The third type, offerings of praise and thanksgiving, corresponds to the blood sacrifices made to memorialize the creation myth. Sacrifice on the cross fulfilled this kind of sacrifice, and the bloodless communion meal became its substitute and replacement (as with creation mythology above). Bloody sacrifice on the cross also fulfilled sin sacrifices—"the Lamb of God who takes away the sins of the world"—and bloodless communion fulfills "offerings of well-being" that were made before the consumption of meat (body and blood are provided as food, but in the form of bread and wine, in a kind of "homeopathic" way). No one will argue that the communion meal of Jesus replaces any human nutritional need for flesh. Nevertheless, it speaks to this existential dilemma and points to the fulfillment of the vegetarian ideal by using mystically impregnated vegetal substances.

The story of Jesus certainly evoked recognition based on the grain mythologies of the times, but it is the blood themes of his story that would have evoked a deeper response, consciously in those cultures still practicing blood sacrifice and unconsciously in those that had evolved to the use of vegetal sacrifices. Appendix A of this book lists some of the astonishing number of correspondences between Jesus's story and those of other cultures. The way in which people recognized in his death and resurrection the fulfillment of various ancient mythologies still in vogue at the time is surely one factor in the remarkable spread of Christianity throughout the ancient Near East and then the entire world.

After this long digression, let's return to Christianity's use of grain to symbolize rebirth, just as it was used in other cultural contexts. As previously noted, the idea of rebirth took different forms in different cultures and times—regeneration, reincarnation, resurrection, transmigration, and cosmic renewal. In the Near East, the dominant form became resurrection and a final cosmic renewal taking place at the end of time. In the Far East, the dominant form became reincarnation throughout recurring cycles of time (with rice as a symbol[31]). Despite the outward contrast, both beliefs are inwardly complementary, and together they provide the key to a deeper understanding of the biblical vegan ideal. These relationships will be taken up in chapter 8.

The association of grains to rebirth and renewed life represents its highest spiritual fruit. This spiritual benefit, next to those for the body and the intellect, is worth keeping in mind as we turn to the critique of grains expressed through the Paleolithic revival, a revival harkening back to the meat-centered diets that preceded the agricultural revolution.

THE PALEOLITHIC REVIVAL

The Paleolithic diet, alternately called the Paleo, caveman, Stone Age, or hunter-gatherer diet, focuses on the food use of animal protein. This kind of diet is understood to have been the predominant diet of the Paleolithic era that lasted about 2.3 million years and ended with the agriculture revolution ten thousand years ago. Curiously, interest in the revival of this diet coincides with the appearance of Peter Singer's *Animal Liberation*, which heralded widespread interest in vegetarianism.[32] Before publishing *Animal Liberation*, Singer characterized eating meat as catering to palate and taste, as it is unnecessary for fulfilling nutritional requirements.[33] Almost as if in rejoinder, the interest in Paleo-style diets began to surge.

The premise behind the Paleo-style diet is that our genes remain adapted to animal foods and are still maladapted to relatively new foods such as grains, beans, and dairy. The diet has been receiving increasing attention for decades because research does show that Paleolithic forebears were healthier in important ways than the agriculturalists who followed, just as contemporary hunter-gatherer tribes are healthier than modern populations.[34]

Paleopathology, or the analysis of ancient skeletal remains, reveals the decline in health occurring during the agricultural revolution. Numerous health issues have been revealed:

- Increased bone and bone membrane inflammation

- Bacterial infection and tuberculosis

- Smaller teeth and teeth defects

- Reductions in jaw size and strength

- Iron-deficiency anemia

- Hookworm, shorter stature, and probable decreasing longevity

Numerous factors have undoubtedly contributed to this overall health decline, including population concentration, sedentism or lack of exercise (at least compared to hunter-gatherers), feces accumulation, increased parasites, susceptibility to animal-borne disease, and stress. Yet declining food quality and variety are also considered vitally important factors.[35]

"Foraging theory," which describes the succession of feeding patterns within a particular environment, illustrates the decrease in food quality. The first food resources to be used are high-quality ones such as readily available plants and large, nutrient-rich game animals that provide the best energy return for expended effort. Then smaller game, fish and shellfish, and lower-quality starchy seeds become utilized as the environment and resources are more intensively exploited. Finally, the landscape is modified through tilling and planting, and low-priority, but calorie-rich, starches are emphasized that can be produced in large quantities and easily stored. In the process, marginal foods disappear, resulting in a loss of nutrients and variety. Staple foods (grains, potatoes, manioc, and taro) develop and are increasingly relied upon. Yet nutritional deficiencies can result and even worsen because of nutrient loss while foods are being stored.[36] In such a scenario, foods such as grains that are lower in rank because of quality and taste become primary only because higher-ranking resources have been depleted.

The decrease in variety is dramatically illustrated by relevant figures for contemporary hunter-gatherer groups. The !Kung tribe of southern Africa utilize 105 plants and 144 different types of animals for food; Australian Aborigines, 240 types of plants and 120 different animals; and the Dogrib of subarctic Canada, 10 different plants and 33 animals. Agriculturalists, in contrast, generally eat 4 plant species (wheat, corn, potatoes, and rice) and 2 animals (beef cattle and pigs).[37] The relatively better health of contemporary hunter-gatherers and Paleolithic ancestors is attributed to many more food varieties as well as quality (chapter 4, however, cites Vilhjalmur Stefansson and Weston Price as suggesting that quality is the more important key).

A closer comparison of the Paleolithic with the modern diet shows the following distinctive features of the Paleolithic:

- Less caloric energy per unit of food weight (signifying a decreased tendency toward weight gain compared with highly processed and refined carbohydrate foods that easily lead to gaining weight, as outlined in chapter 4)

- More nutrients because of fruits and vegetables rich in vitamins, minerals, fiber, and phytochemicals

- Less fat and less saturated fatty acids, due to the consumption of lean game meat

- A more balanced ratio between essential polyunsaturated omega-3 and omega-6 fatty acids (we heard this in chapter 4; omega-6 fatty acids are linked with heart disease and are overabundantly found in meat from grain-fed animals compared with grass-fed ones)[38]

Other disadvantages for modern diets are the presence of separated oils or fats, a dramatic increase in sodium (only 10 percent of ingested sodium is inherent to foods), and artificial additions such as pesticides, hormones, fertilizers, antibiotics, dyes, and food additives.[39] In fact, the Paleolithic diet could be characterized as a "natural, whole, and organic" plant and animal diet—but without grains, dairy, processed oils, refined sugars, and alcohol, which together make up approximately 70 percent of the modern diet.[40]

To be sure, however, Paleolithic diets were not uniform in content. Contributions from hunting and gathering varied, and food and nutrient ratios depended on geographical location and other factors such as latitude and rainfall.[41] Among the fifty-eight known hunter-gatherer societies extant today, twenty-nine live predominantly from gathering, eighteen from fishing, and eleven from hunting.[42] Recent estimates for Paleolithic food ratios are 56–65 percent animal and 36–45 percent plant foods; and for macronutrients, 19–35 percent protein, 20–40 percent carbohydrate, and 25–58 percent fat.[43]

Such estimates contrast with official recommendations today as well as with typical consumption habits. Food pyramids typically group plant foods at the bottom and animal foods toward the top. The approximate macronutrient recommendations are 15 percent protein, 55 percent carbohydrates, and 30 percent fat (while typical consumption habits are 15 percent protein, 48 percent carbohydrate, and 34 percent fat).[44]

Paleo proponents make the following points about Paleo-era consumption:

- *Protein*: Levels were high, but not necessarily unhealthy. High protein has adverse kidney effects only if a disturbance already exists. The Eskimo high-protein diet does not show an unusual incidence of kidney disease. Colon cancer and elevated cholesterol result from a high concentration of saturated fat, not protein. A high-protein/low saturated-fat diet actually lowers cholesterol.

- *Carbohydrates*: Most Paleo carbohydrates were complex and came from vegetables and fruit (which raise blood sugar levels at a slower and healthier rate). Paleo ancestors ate virtually no grain. Contemporary carbohydrates come mostly from grains and refined grains.

- *Fats*: Paleolithic ancestors ate more fat, but mostly from game meat, the fat of which is primarily monounsaturated, to a lesser extent polyunsaturated, and to an even lesser extent saturated. They ate little to no trans-fatty acids (which today come mostly from hydrogenated vegetable oils). The omega-3 to omega-6 fatty acid ratio was mostly balanced, and heart disease was virtually unknown.

- *Micronutrients*: Intake was 1.5 to 5 times higher than current recommendations. Fruit and vegetable phytochemicals appear to be more important than grain phytochemicals. In the past, potassium intake was higher than sodium intake; today the reverse has become true.

- *Fiber*: Current recommendations stress the importance of fiber and suggest eating about 20 grams daily. Paleo intakes varied. In high latitudes, the intake was less than contemporary levels. Of the two types of fiber—soluble, which is good for cholesterol absorption; and insoluble, which is good for the intestines—a modern refined-grains diet has higher proportions of insoluble fiber. Paleo fiber from fruits and vegetables contains a more beneficial soluble/insoluble ratio.

All the above differences, and the better health of Paleolithic ancestors (reflected by the comparably better health of contemporary hunter-gatherers), support the claims that human genes remain adapted to the Paleo diet and are maladapted to the modern diet, and that current recommendations are wrong.[45]

Yet criticisms of Paleo-style diets also exist. One notes that dietary assumptions are based on analogy with known hunter-gatherer groups, which, however, exhibit a wide variety of diets. The argument continues that ancestral diets may well have been nutrient-rich compared with modern diets, yet specific plant-to-animal food ratios or macronutrient distributions did not exist (we shall hear that this argument has been acknowledged and estimates revised).[46] Another criticism notes the genetic adaptations to new foods that have occurred, such as developing a tolerance to lactose, or milk sugar, to a high degree within a few thousand years, and recent increases of the amylase enzyme to digest starch. A related argument asserts that present-day problematic foods such as refined grains and sugars are not "new" foods of the agricultural revolution but instead high-energy, devitalized foods widely available only in the past few hundred years. Yet another criticism emphasizes that a high protein Paleo-style diet from animals fed on grass (to assure a healthy fatty acid ratio) is unfeasible for most of the world.[47]

Despite the criticisms, a recent reevaluation by early proponents S. Boyd Eaton and Melvin Konner emphasizes the continued relevance and importance of Paleo diets.[48] While making adjustments for variety among ancestral diets, they nevertheless assert that the claims about protein, fat, fiber, and cholesterol levels have held up remarkably well. Moreover, scientific studies have confirmed positive health effects. The reevaluation by Eaton and Konner makes the following points:

- The expansion of protein ratios to 35–65 percent reflects the new understanding about fish's importance as a Paleo food. The high consumption of lean meat high in omega-3 fatty acids (from animals fed on grass rather than on grain) has no adverse health effects.

- The primary difference between Paleo and modern carbohydrate consumption is not total calories but carbohydrate type (Paleo diets have more vegetables and fruit; the modern diet has more grains). The hunter-gatherer diet is more effective than the Mediterranean diet (see chapter 4) for controlling insulin resistance and the risk of heart disease for type 2 diabetics (grains and especially refined grains are implicated in all these conditions).

- The previous estimates of 20 percent total fat and 6 percent saturated fat have been revised to 20–35 percent total fat, closer to the official recommendations of the 1980s (30 percent total fat, with advice to reduce saturated fat). Yet the proper relationship between omega-3 and omega-6 levels is now clearer. Hunter-gatherers show a 1-to-2 ratio, but present-day recommendations range between 1-to-8 and 1-to-10. The differences argue that official recommendations should drop further.

- Hunter-gatherer cholesterol intake (approximately 480 milligrams daily) is higher than the typical American diet and current recommendations (200 milligrams daily). Yet research shows that fatty-acid ratios and refined carbohydrate consumption are more important health factors. Hunter-gatherer cholesterol levels are safe because of the protein and fatty-acid quality.

- The range of hunter-gatherer fiber levels is significantly higher than present recommendations and potentially more beneficial. Vegetable and fruit fiber ferments more completely than grain fiber and has a soluble-to-insoluble ratio of approximately 1-to-1. Grain phytates (phosphorus compounds that bind nutrients, making them unavailable) negatively affect mineral absorption. Modern recommendations focus too much on quantity instead of quality.

- The sodium level and sodium-to-potassium ratio of hunter-gatherer diets are both extremely low compared with modern diets. Research shows that reductions have benefits.

- Fruits and vegetables create alkalinity in the body. The modern grain-oriented diet produces acidity that can cause problems.

Eaton and Konner add the results of several studies in favor of a hunter-gatherer diet:

- More effective than the Mediterranean diet for improving diabetes symptoms

- Better results in a comparison study with the Diabetes Diet for fatty-acid, diastolic blood pressure, and body-weight measures

- Beneficial decrease in measures such as blood pressure and insulin levels after Australian hunter-gatherers change back to their traditional diet

The researchers also reflect on a Paleo-style food pyramid—vegetables and fruit on the bottommost tier; meat, fish, and low-fat dairy on the second tier; whole grains as a possible next tier; and refined carbohydrates, fats, and oils on the highest and smallest tier. They also, however, acknowledge the health benefits of alcohol (a product of the agricultural revolution) while conceding that the Paleo model is not definitive.

THE CHARACTERISTICS AND the benefits of Paleo-style diets and their animal-foods focus should come as no surprise after hearing about the low-carbohydrate movement and the work of Vilhjalmur Stefansson and Weston Price in chapter 4. Paleo diets are a type of low-carbohydrate diet focusing on lean animal protein. Certainly, one of their important contributions is greater attention to meat and fat quality: fat from lean game meat and grass-fed animals has healthier fat ratios (saturated to monounsaturated to polyunsaturated), and healthier fatty-acid ratios (omega-3 to omega-6).

Emphasizing a lower saturated fat level, however, is questionable because saturated fat's health effects have been vindicated (chapter 4). Yet the emphasis on omega-3 to omega-6 ratios does highlight the importance of animal feed. The criticism that a grass-fed meat diet is unavailable to most people remains, yet at least awareness about the importance of animal feed has increased.

Besides offering a general critique of the agricultural revolution and defense of Paleo-style diets, the Paleo movement has additional criticism to level against carbohydrates and grains. With grains, the issues go beyond refining's adverse effects to problems with whole grains themselves. Although Konner and Eaton's proposed pyramid considers including both whole and refined grains, other Paleo proponents are more adamant about rejecting both.[49]

CRITIQUE OF CARBOHYDRATES AND GRAINS

Besides the adverse health effects of grains in the refined form, they, along with milk—another food that has become more prevalent since the agricultural revolution—are primary sources of allergies and other problems as well.

In the case of milk, the protein casein is difficult to digest, and many people also have difficulty creating the enzyme lactase that is necessary to digest milk sugar (lactose). The amino acid tyramine found in cheddar cheeses is also cited as a cause of problems.[50]

In the case of grains, the gluten, phytates, and lectins they contain are all problematic. Gluten is also a protein that is very difficult to digest. US wheat is a hybrid that has been bred to increase the gluten content, and the flour made from it has been called "the most indigestible flour in the world." It is also claimed that the gluten content of wheat has increased five hundred times compared with wheat from the time of our forefathers, and coeliac disease, which is caused by the inability to digest gluten, has at least quadrupled in the past thirty years. Sensitivity to gluten is steadily increasing, and those who are sensitive or allergic must avoid barley, rye, and wheat completely (and some people, oats and corn, too). Gluten intolerance has also been linked to alcoholism, arthritis, dementia, Down syndrome, schizophrenia, and vitamin B_6 deficiency.[51]

Phytates are phosphorus compounds in the hulls of grains as well as in legumes, nuts, and seeds.[52] They can bind minerals, which makes them unavailable for absorption, and also vitamins such as niacin (B_3), which causes the deficiency disease pellagra. Native American cultures prevented the phytate-binding action of corn by soaking it in acid solutions such as lime or mixing wood ash into the cooking pot, which releases niacin, and makes it nutritionally available (a process called "nixtamalization"). Native cultures also complemented corn with beans, thereby adding more of the amino-acid tryptophan that the body can use to synthesize niacin.[53] No native cultures are known to have developed a niacin deficiency. Yet after colonization, when corn was imported to Europe, pellagra became rampant. US milling practices after 1910 produced the same result: milling removed the phytates by removing the corn germ, but in doing so, the tryptophan content was cut in half. Subsequently mixing the corn meal with white flour increased the tryptophan level, but not enough, and pellagra ensued. Modern-day flours prevent this problem by enriching corn meal with niacin.[54] The contrast with native practices demonstrates the primitive wisdom of which Weston Price spoke.

Yet the claim is also made that phytates bind minerals only if the diet relies too heavily on grains or if there is an excess of bran; balanced eating should provide sufficient minerals.[55] The problems with phytic acid are claimed to be temporary, and yet adaptation may depend on overall nutrition and health.[56] In such comments we again encounter the individual considerations that make diet such a complex issue.

Phytates are also said to have a positive side: they keep minerals such as iron at safe levels by removing them from the body; they prevent the absorption of toxic heavy metals; they regulate blood glucose absorption; and they enhance the immune system by increasing the activity of cells that attack cancerous cells. They also protect against diabetes, heart disease, kidney stones, and osteoporosis. Moreover, a phytic acid compound has been developed to treat Parkinson's disease because of the potential benefits for the brain—removing toxic iron, mediating the supply of glucose, and controlling the calcium that leads to cell death. (We hear here an echo of the positive psychological effects attributed to whole grains by orthomolecular proponents and Weston Price in chapter 3 and the negative effects attributed to refined grains.) Even a Paleo perspective now acknowledges that the benefits of phytates may outweigh the risks![57] In short, phytates may indeed cause problems, but the problems are potentially resolvable, and phytates may also have benefits.

Another problematic carbohydrate issue is lectin proteins found in high concentrations in grains, beans, seeds, and nuts. As with phytates, lectins have disadvantages as well as advantages. On the negative side, they can lead to nutritional deficiencies, trigger allergic and immune-system reactions, and cause chronic diseases as well. Readers will recall from chapter 4 that the problem of lectin sensitivity is a focus of the Blood-Type Diet; blood-type tolerance for lectins in different foods varies, resulting in diverse dietary recommendations for different blood types. Yet whether lectins become harmful also depends on the quality of the gut bacteria, which itself is affected by factors such as increased hygiene and antibiotic overuse (individual considerations yet again!). Some lectins, however, are beneficial; one example is providing protection from cancer.[58]

The carbohydrate problem with phytates and lectins leads us back to the motivation for refining grains in the first place. In Western culture, the history of refining goes back to biblical times and the practice of sifting. Sifted flour was a prerequisite for prayer offerings and foods prepared for special guests. In the past, sifting was considered the "prerogative of the privileged,"[59] and the desire for sifted flour continued throughout history. Not until the Industrial Revolution, however, did milling techniques finally make refined flour cheaply and easily available to everyone.

Why was sifted or refined flour so desirable? The reasons are complex and include factors such as digestibility, taste, nourishment, and preservation. By removing part of the bran, sifting produced a flour that was tastier, lighter, and even more digestible according to physicians. In Roman times and throughout history, sifted meal was considered more nourishing, and even more so the more it was refined.[60] This idea seems counterintuitive today, but in fact refined flour compared with whole wheat flour allows the assimilation of more protein and energy (95 to 85 percent), yet at the expense of removing half or more nutrients.[61] The same is true for rice. The usual rationales for refining are taste and color, yet removing the rice bran through polishing makes protein more available and reduces digestive gas—again by removing important vitamins and nutrients.[62] Moreover, refined flour can be stored longer because germ oils that cause rancidity and attract pests have been removed. As we can see, there are many motivations to refining, but the net result is a mix of benefits and disadvantages. Carbohydrates are, indeed, complex as well as problematic foods.

Yet perhaps the ultimate and most revealing argument against the new carbohydrate foods of the agricultural revolution is that they are absolutely unnecessary. In contrast to proteins and fats, *there are no essential carbohydrates that the body needs*. Essential protein amino acids and essential fatty acids, yes; essential carbohydrates, none whatsoever. The primary function of carbohydrate is to provide bodily fuel in the form of glucose, or blood sugar; yet protein and fat can fulfill all fuel needs as well as synthesize glucose, which some cells do require. In the absence of carbohydrates, bodily functions will not be impaired at all.[63] In the words of carbohydrate-critic Gary Taubes, excluding them from the diet will allow the body to return to "biologic normalcy."[64]

In sum, although carbohydrates have benefits, they are absolutely unnecessary foods. In the past they have caused, and in the present they continue to cause, many problems. Carbohydrates contributed to a decline in health at the dawn of civilization, and grain carbohydrates are particularly troublesome, both in the refined and whole forms.

These criticisms are important to take seriously. They put the recommendations we have heard for whole grains into a different light, and ultimately they challenge the sattvic status of grains (and dairy as well). We will attempt to confront and resolve these issues in the final chapter. Yet before doing so, in the chapter ahead it is important to refocus attention on the benefits and detriments of each of the three major dietary types: low-carbohydrate (including Paleo-style diets), low-fat, and low-calorie diets.

7

WEIGHT LOSS VS. LIFESTYLE: LOW-CARBOHYDRATE, LOW-FAT, AND LOW-CALORIE DIETS

In the previous chapter, we heard that Paleo-style diets are effective for weight loss and that they alleviate obesity and other disease conditions as well. Yet proponents usually consider the Paleo to be first and foremost a lifestyle diet, or the food normally eaten for daily nourishment. Weight loss is an added bonus.

The word *diet* does have the dual meanings of habitual daily food on the one hand and food eaten to lose weight on the other. An ideal diet aspires to be both, according to the famous Hippocratic dictum, "Let your food be your medicine and your medicine your food." This book's focus has been the sattvic lifestyle diet that nourishes all dimensions of the human being simultaneously. The sum of considerations so far suggests that a mixed diet of animal and vegetal foods is appropriate for most people, because both types of food have advantages for complete health.

A mixed diet may be the best choice of lifestyle, yet it is not the most effective for losing weight. This is because the inclusion of all macronutrient food groups—proteins, fats, and carbohydrates— more easily leads to fat storage (see chapter 4). Low-carbohydrate- and low-fat diets are both more effective for losing weight.

Readers will recall from chapter 4 that low-carbohydrate diets were used for treating obesity and diabetes in the nineteenth century and continued to be used to treat obesity until the 1950s, but then the ascendency of the fat hypothesis of disease made low-fat diets the preferred choice. The paradox is that both worked, which can be explained by the metabolic principles peculiar to each. Both are very effective for weight loss. Yet from a spiritual point of view, both have disadvantages as lifestyle diets: low-carbohydrate diets because of an overabundance of animal foods, and low-fat diets because of too little. This chapter reviews the three major dietary types—low-carbohydrate, low-fat, and low-calorie[1]—in more depth to clarify advantages and disadvantages from a spiritual perspective.

LOW-CARBOHYDRATE DIETS

There are different types of low-carbohydrate diets, and all are effective for losing and controlling weight. Yet each depends on different physiological principles, and each as a lifestyle diet raises particular spiritual concerns.

The Atkins Diet

The Atkins Diet promulgated by Dr. Robert Atkins is the best known and perhaps the most popular low-carbohydrate diet. It is divided into four phases: In the initial phase, carbohydrates are limited to 20 grams net. *Net* signifies total carbohydrate grams minus total fiber grams. Fiber is subtracted because, being indigestible, it does not add calories. In succeeding phases, more carbohydrate can be added as long as weight balance is maintained. If weight is gained, or if it stabilizes at an undesirable level, the carbohydrate level is lowered again.

The quality of carbohydrate foods is vitally important. Refined carbohydrates are not recommended because of the link to gaining weight[2] (just as low-carbohydrate diets were used to treat obesity until the mid-twentieth century).

The amount of protein in the Atkins Diet is flexible. The daily recommended level of 13–22 ounces is higher than USDA government recommendations, but it is nevertheless considered optimal. Common fears about kidney damage and calcium loss due to high protein content are considered misconceptions. Protein's satiating nature (and that of fat as well) is one of the keys to weight loss on a low-carbohydrate diet.[3] Yet eating a lot of protein does not necessarily mean eating animal protein. The "new-look" Atkins includes vegetarian and even vegan options.[4]

Fat is the primary key to the Atkins Diet's success. Trimming or avoiding fatty meats is considered unnecessary if carbohydrates are restricted. The diet's philosophy considers fat to provide more consistent energy than carbohydrates, in addition to having a satiating quality. The importance of fat for assimilating the fat-soluble vitamins A, D, E, K and beta-carotene is also stressed (as we have heard from Weston Price). Dr. Atkins adds that if fat is trimmed, olive oil should be added for nutrient absorption.[5] Fat is the key to weight loss by providing *ketones* (substances resulting from the breakdown of fat) that the body uses for fuel.

In addition to the emphasis on fat, the metabolism of ketones through the process known as *ketosis* is another reason why the Atkins Diet has been considered controversial. In modern times, carbohydrates have been the primary source for bodily fuel in Western nations.[6] Yet when carbohydrates are absent but fats sufficient, the liver can create ketones from fatty acids to meet fuel needs. Another reason for controversy is confusion with *ketoacidosis*, a dangerous buildup of blood ketones that can occur in type 1 juvenile diabetes. The level in ketoacidosis, however, is much greater than that normally attained through ketosis.[7]

Stimulating ketosis has long been criticized with low-carbohydrate diets, and yet periodic ketosis is now seen as normal. It occurs to some degree through overnight fasting, and it even has benefits such as protecting against cellular injury.[8] Ketosis, in fact, has a long therapeutic history. Beginning in 1921, ketogenic diets were used to treat epilepsy, a practice that continued until the advent of antiseizure drugs in the 1950s. In the 1990s, ketogenic diets were actually revived to treat epileptic children unresponsive to drugs. Many clinics use such diets today with seizure patients, and researchers are exploring the application to Alzheimer's disease, autism, brain tumors, Lou Gehrig's disease (ALS), and other conditions.[9]

In short, ketosis remains an important, and now more reputable, principle of the Atkins Diet. Yet other aspects have changed, partly in response to criticisms:

- Fiber's importance is acknowledged with a correspondingly greater emphasis on carbohydrate vegetable greens in early dietary stages.

- Vegetarian and vegan options challenge the Atkins Diet's traditional image as a high-protein and -fat diet. Tips to decrease meat costs are also provided.[10]

- Consumption of unlimited red meat and fat—especially saturated fat—is discouraged, despite the insistence that dietary fat is not harmful if carbohydrate levels are kept low. Atkins proponents emphasize that carbohydrate levels have always been the most important factor, not fat.[11]

Research indicates that the Atkins Diet does not increase heart-disease risk. Numerous studies show that such a diet is effective for weight loss, and in some cases more effective than other diets for reducing disease measures.[12] Although major health organizations and professionals opposed the Atkins Diet in the past, the American Heart Association and the American Dietetic Association have changed their positions and now acknowledge the potential benefits.[13]

An important weight-loss factor is the satiating effect of this type of diet. Satiety may relate to the longer digestive time required for proteins and fats, which effectively stills hunger.[14] Yet here's another explanation for why more people stick with the Atkins Diet longer than with other diets: "There are some meat lovers, and on this diet you can eat a lot of meat."[15] (Again we must ask: Is the choice of meat from desire or need?)

One criticism, however, relates the high-fat content of the Atkins Diet to low energy, fatigue, and lethargy, and another adds that ketogenic diets lead to impaired cognitive functioning.[16] Both criticisms are understandable from a spiritual perspective and are important to review.

Chapter 2 cited Rudolf Steiner saying that when the diet lacks fat, the body can create its own, and the activity that is stimulated has spiritual significance. The logical converse is that dietary fat results in less activity, just as the above criticism about low energy, fatigue, and lethargy suggests. This decreased activity as it relates to fat digestion can be explained by the *thermic effect* and the *basal metabolic rate*, names for metabolic functions.

The *thermic effect* is defined as the energy cost for converting nutrients into forms the body can use. Protein metabolism has the highest thermic effect. Between 20 and 30 percent of ingested protein calories are required just to metabolize the protein. Carbohydrate metabolism costs less—between 3 and 20 percent—depending on whether it is refined and the fiber content. Fat metabolism costs the least—between 2 and 3 percent.[17] The significance is quicker and easier conversion and less physiological activity.

The *basal metabolic rate* (BMR) is defined as the rate at which calories are burned when the body is at rest. A diet high in fat significantly lowers the BMR compared with a diet high in carbohydrate,[18] once again signifying less activity. The issue, however, is not effectiveness for weight loss or even for improving physical health—diets high in fat do lead to these results—but decreased activity resulting from the ease with which fat is metabolized.

In referring to the guna-quality terms of the Bhagavad Gita, the effect of this decreased activity is tamasic, the quality associated with inertia, lethargy, and even sleep.[19] We can say that tamas correlates with fat, just as rajas correlates with protein (protein has the highest thermic effects) and sattva with carbohydrate (carbohydrate has an intermediate effect between the values for fat and protein).[20] These associations, however, are meant to be not judgmental but merely descriptive. Most foods, in fact, are combinations of protein, fat, and carbohydrate in different proportions,[21] and we have already emphasized that there are essential fats and proteins that must be supplied through diet, in contrast with carbohydrates.[22] The effect of decreased activity through eating a high-fat diet, however, becomes a concern over prolonged use.

The reputation of high-fat diets such as the Atkins for weight loss has been rehabilitated in recent years, and rightly so. Yet a spiritual perspective raises concerns about possible effects such as lethargy and impaired cognitive functioning that logically relate to the tamasic effects of dietary fat.

Contrary indications about such effects, however, do exist. Atkins's literature states that any perceived loss of energy passes once the body has adjusted to ketosis, and the physician's report on Vilhjalmur Stefansson's one-year-long, high-fat diet stated "no subjective or objective evidence of any loss of physical or mental vigor."[23] Nevertheless, the facts about thermic effects stated above, as well as Rudolf Steiner's remarks about fat in chapter 2, are worth noting.

Dr. Atkins himself notes that, in his diet's later stages, more healthy carbohydrate foods (whole and unprocessed ones) can be added if the protein and fat levels are reduced.[24] In this way, there is flexibility that does not require adhering to high fat levels. If one chooses to use the Atkins Diet to lose weight, the health benefits can be realized and then adverse effects mitigated by gradually decreasing protein and fat and increasing carbohydrate.

Paleo-Style Diets

Paleo-style, low-carbohydrate diets[25] emphasize lean animal protein. Fruit and vegetable carbohydrates also play an important role. The reasons for these particular emphases are both ideological and biological.

In Paleolithic times, dietary protein levels were high, but the source was meat from animals feeding on grass, which produces a leaner meat that is high in monounsaturated fat. Today's farm animals that eat grain produce meat with a higher saturated fat level (and higher omega-6 fatty-acid levels).[26] Monounsaturated fat lowers blood cholesterol, and hunter-gatherers had low cholesterol levels and little heart disease.[27] Saturated fat, in contrast, increases cholesterol levels. A diet high in fat together with refined carbohydrates leads to metabolic syndrome (see chapter 4), one symptom of which is a high cholesterol level (and yet saturated fat leads to high cholesterol levels only if excess calories result in fat storage; the Atkins high-saturated-fat diet has been proven healthy). These are reasons why Paleo proponents prefer lean protein.

Paleo-style diets rely on animal protein for losing and stabilizing weight. The thermic effect of protein (the caloric cost of metabolizing ingested protein) is between 20 and 30 percent, and lean protein has the highest rate—almost 30 percent.[28] As a result, more calories are expended just through protein metabolism, resulting in efficient weight loss. Some studies indicate that a high-protein diet is more effective for weight loss than high-carbohydrate diets. Others show that a high-protein diet is more satiating than a high carbohydrate or even a high-fat diet, leading Loren Cordain, the author of *The Paleo Diet*, to assert that "lean protein should be the starting point for all weight-loss diets."[29]

Cordain acknowledges, however, the danger of a high-protein diet leading to toxicity. Too heavily relying on animal protein creates toxic byproducts that stress the liver, the kidneys, and eventually all cells.[30] The inclusion of either fat or carbohydrate mitigates the effect, and Cordain's Paleo-style diet emphasizes fruit and vegetable carbohydrates. Fruits and vegetables also provide fiber and bulk that contribute to satiety. The combination of fruits, vegetables, and lean meat easily leads to weight loss until optimal levels are reached.[31]

Thus the Paleo approach to weight loss relies on protein's thermic effect and the satiating effects of lean meat, fruit, and vegetables. Not only are Paleo-style diets proven to be effective for weight loss, but they benefit other biological health measures as well (see chapter 6).

Yet as a lifestyle diet, the concern with Paleo-type diets is the cumulative effect of rajasic animal influences. In chapter 2, Rudolf Steiner talks about the human task of manifesting qualities such as "stamina, courage, and even aggressiveness" through the strength of individual astral effort, saying that animal influences inhibit this process.[32] The effect can be potentially beneficial because we must live effectively in the world, but it can also be potentially harmful due to narrowing the horizon to material reality. This ability for living effectively through animal influences, yet with a narrowed focus, correlates with protein's high thermic effect and the rajasic quality of impelling toward external activity, but in an overstimulating way.[33] The concern here is with the degree of such effects over time.

DESPITE THE CAUTIONS about the Atkins and Paleo-style, low-carbohydrate diets, each can an effective tool for losing weight and restoring health. Both add variety to weight-loss options and can be chosen according to taste and need. Once health has been restored, however, spiritual points of view are also important to consider.

LOW-FAT DIETS

Low-fat diets focus on carbohydrate foods. They also satiate and lead to weight loss (like low-carbohydrate diets), but through the peculiarities of carbohydrate-oriented metabolism.

The diet of Dr. Dean Ornish has a very low fat content (about 10 percent) and is basically, though not strictly, vegetarian.[34] The primary aim is treating heart disease, and because saturated animal fat and cholesterol are associated with heart disease, they are excluded (yet we can ask whether the cause is saturated animal fat and cholesterol or excess calories; see chapter 4's discussion about the cause of disease). The Ornish diet stabilizes and reverses heart disease and has earned Dr. Ornish accolades for achieving the "implausible."[35] Medicare covers the Ornish lifestyle program.[36] Weight loss is considered an extra benefit, but if it is the primary concern instead of heart disease, then the fat in the diet can be increased.[37]

The low-fat Hawaii Diet of Dr. Terry Shintani is a model for traditional ethnic diets (such as the Mediterranean Diet cited in chapter 4). Like the Ornish Diet, Shintani's also contains about 10 percent fat (with 78 percent carbohydrate and 12 percent protein).[38] The animal-food content is also low, yet the diet is meant not to be strictly vegetarian but to illustrate international traditional practices.[39]

Martin Katahn's T-Factor Diet offers more flexibility with fat. To lose weight, fat is limited to 20–40 grams for women (about 7–14 percent of total calories) and 30–60 grams for men (about

11–22 percent).[40] Katahn emphasizes, however, that stable food habits are the key to dieting. Many people lose weight only to re-gain it, which can damage health. Bodily adaptation to repeated dieting can also make losing weight more difficult. After weight loss has been achieved, Katahn suggests a maintenance diet with 24 percent fat.[41]

Despite any differences, all the above low-fat diets achieve weight-loss effectiveness by relying on caloric density along with the other metabolic functions previously mentioned, but in ways that favor carbohydrate metabolism.

Caloric density is defined by the number of calories per gram con-tained in different foods. Fat's caloric density is generally considered to be 9 calories per gram, and carbohydrate and protein are both considered to contain about 4 calories each per gram. The figure for carbohydrate, however, applies to refined carbohydrates like flour and sugar; complex whole carbohydrates contain significantly less calories—between 0.6 and 1 per gram.[42] This means that whole car-bohydrates satiate more effectively by providing greater bulk with fewer calories.

The principle of providing greater bulk is illustrated by compar-ison food plates. A plate of complex carbohydrates such as vegeta-bles and grain weighs 1,885 grams and contains 1,125 calories. A contrasting plate with a cheeseburger, French fries, and milkshake weighs 636 grams and contains 1,195 calories. Both calorie amounts are similar, but the plate of grains and vegetables weighs almost three times as much, providing more stomach bulk and leading to satiety over a longer time.[43]

The principle of providing fewer calories is illustrated by a study comparing a "low energy density" (LED) group and a Standard American Diet (SAD) group. The LED subjects ate a complex-carbohydrate diet containing about 15 percent fat; SAD subjects ate a diet with about 42 percent fat. The LED group needed about 1,570 calories per day to achieve satiety, but the SAD group needed ap-proximately 3,000 calories.[44]

The carbohydrate thermic effect and basal metabolic rate are also advantageous for controlling weight. Although the thermic effect for

209

refined carbohydrate is about 3 percent (similar to fat), for whole carbohydrates it is between 6 and 20 percent, depending on the fiber content (see note 17). This means that metabolizing complex carbohydrate expends more energy. The basal metabolic rate for a high-carbohydrate diet is also significantly higher than that for a high-fat diet and amounts to burning as much as 200 to 300 additional calories daily (comparative diets: 75 percent carbohydrate, 10 percent fat, and 15 percent protein vs. 45 percent carbohydrate, 40 percent fat, and 15 percent protein).[45] Both metabolic functions for carbohydrates expend many calories and lead to weight loss.

A further weight-control advantage relates to the body's preference for metabolizing carbohydrates (and proteins too) before fats, utilizing the carbohydrate for immediate fuel needs or converting it for later use. On a daily basis, only 4 percent of carbohydrate calories are normally converted to fat and stored. When this happens, the thermic effect increases to about 25 percent, which expends even more calories just for the conversion process. In addition, instead of converting carbohydrate to fat, the body prefers to speed up the metabolic rate to burn up any excess.[46]

The difference in metabolic rates for whole and refined carbohydrates, however, is important to reemphasize: the caloric density for whole carbohydrates is significantly lower (0.6–1.0 vs. 4 calories per gram) and the thermic effect is greater (6–20 percent vs. 3 percent). The result is cumulative beneficial effects for whole carbohydrates—providing more bulk and creating greater satiety, adding fewer total calories, and burning off a higher percentage of calories just through metabolism.

Carbohydrate diets usually contain foods such as grains, beans, vegetables, and fruits, and these are the foods associated with the sattvic guna (chapter 1) and generally recommended by spiritual teachings (chapter 2). This kind of diet increases bodily activity through the operation of the various metabolic functions indicated above. Yet the effect is more moderate compared with the high-protein diet, the effect of which is increased activity but in a rajasic, overstimulating way.

A spiritual perspective, however, also has concern with low-fat diets, which tend to be vegetarian. As mentioned above, comparison studies show a better dieter retention rate for the Atkins Diet, and Dr. Ornish himself acknowledges the high recidivism rate attaching to dieting in general (66 percent regain weight within a year and 97 percent within five years).[47] The concern with low-fat diets, especially if the fat content is very low, is the ability to stick to them and to find the transition to a healthy lifestyle diet. In addition, we heard in chapter 2 that animal foods can lead to balancing earthly and spiritual life and that vegetarian diets themselves can lead to imbalance. We also heard that vegetarian diets can be outright harmful if the inner activity they generate is not properly channeled. The madness of Adolf Hitler, a notorious vegetarian,[48] is a possible demonstration of the dangers of vegetarianism divorced from spiritual grounding. These are reasons for caution with low-fat diets as well.

THE BLOOD-TYPE DIET

The four blood-type diets are lifestyle diets and not about losing weight, yet Dr. Peter D'Adamo indicates that they are effective for losing weight by helping to restore metabolic balance. This makes sense, especially for types O and A, the diets for which are respectively low carbohydrate and low fat. According to the metabolic principles outlined above, each of these types of diet works to stabilize weight and to support overall health. The diets for types B and AB mix carbohydrates and fats to a greater degree. As indicated in chapter 4, the key consideration for mixed diets is total calories and food quality, i.e., the use of unrefined carbohydrates and even whole-fat products as much as possible.

As discussed in chapter 4, the Blood-Type Diet is noteworthy for several reasons, including the focus on individual considerations and the personality characteristics associated with each type. Yet questions arise about perpetuating the blood-type diets as lifestyle diets. This is particularly the case with type O's animal-food focus, the intention of which is to support a more active and aggressive personality, and with type A's vegetarian diet to support a more cerebral and placid nature. As emphasized, the balance between worldly and spiritual pursuits is the ideal from a spiritual point of view, which means cultivating the total personality. Diet does have an effect on personality, as Dr. D'Adamo's associations corroborate, but the point is movement toward balance. The question then becomes the extent to which the various types can develop tolerance for foods normally considered outside their respective comfort zones. That, of course, is an individual question, but the ideal of balancing between extremes is important to keep in mind. The next chapter will have more to say about Blood-Type Diet issues.

LOW-CALORIE DIETS

Low-calorie diets are the third major category and make up the majority of weight-loss diets. No macronutrient food group (carbohydrate, fat, or protein) is deemphasized, and so these diets can be characterized as mixed diets. As we heard in chapter 4, mixed diets disadvantage fat metabolism, and so total calories become a concern. Hence these diets are characterized as "low calorie." Calories, indeed, are controlled very closely—food portions are limited and calories are counted. In addition, exercise is also very important for burning up extra calories.

Low-calorie diets claim to focus more intently on both sides of the "healthy living equation"—sensible eating and exercise.[49] Sensible eating means including all macronutrient food groups and not avoiding preferred foods. Low-calorie diets embrace official recommendations such as those of the USDA, which similarly advocate sensible eating and can be considered mixed in that they take an "excess-calories" view of disease (the problem is not carbohydrates or fats, but total calories).

In the low-calorie philosophy, exercise is important because, in order to lose weight and maintain weight balance, "calories in" (i.e., ingested) must equal "calories out" (metabolized).[50] If the ingested calorie amount exceeds immediate bodily needs, then more must be expended through exercise to restore balance.

Weight Watchers exemplifies low-calorie diets. Unrestricted food choices include hot-fudge sundaes (although healthier choices are recommended). This still qualifies as sound dieting because calorie restriction and exercise are emphasized, which is what most experts recommend.[51]

The low-calorie view states that dieting can be effective only to the extent that total calories are restricted; if low-carbohydrate and low-fat diets work (which they do), it is because calories are being limited, not carbohydrates or fats. Yet we must object that this is a half-truth, for we have seen that low-carbohydrate and low-fat diets are effective by limiting either carbohydrate or fat and satiating hunger by means of specific metabolic principles favorable to fat, protein, or carbohydrate metabolism.

The low-calorie view, however, has further points to make against low-carbohydrate and -fat diets:

- Low-carbohydrate diets (with a high-fat content) easily lead to overeating because fat's caloric density is high (on the average, nine calories per gram).

- Low-carbohydrate diets (with a high-protein content) stress the liver and kidneys.

- Low-fat diets are boring ("fat is one of life's pleasures"). Insufficient fat affects hair, nails, and skin adversely. In the absence of exercise, a low-fat diet elevates blood triglycerides (blood fats) and leads to health risks.[52]

As may be apparent, such criticisms ignore the fact that each type of diet anticipates and avoids such problems through unique guidelines (except perhaps in the case of boredom).

Dr. Ornish, in turn, points to the weaknesses of low-calorie diets: they base themselves on deprivation (counting calories, restricting portions, eating less) and so lead to hunger, cheating, regaining weight, and ultimately self-recrimination.[53] Of course, low-fat and low-carbohydrate diets also may have such problems—with the exception of hunger.

Thus as each type of diet does, low-calorie diets also present a conundrum: they appear to be more balanced by including all macronutrient food groups; yet by relying on limited calories, they easily lead to hunger and can become ineffective for losing weight. Low-carbohydrate diets, on the other hand, effectively lead to weight loss by satiating hunger with ample calories of protein or fat—but they may lead to craving carbohydrates. Low-fat diets lead to weight loss by satiating hunger with lots of carbohydrate calories—but may lead to craving fats. Low-calorie diets allow all food groups, but lead to craving calories of any kind. Such is life in the material world.

Yet despite the difficulty with losing weight, low-calorie diets are the clear choice as lifestyle diets from multiple points of view— those of conventional paradigms, of most people as evidenced by their habits, and of spiritual considerations as well. In the spiritual view, balancing the new carbohydrate foods of the agricultural revolution with fat and animal foods is an economic necessity as well as a necessity relating to physical, psychic, and spiritual health for most people to one degree or another. Nevertheless, the potential for health problems that results from mixing carbohydrates and fats remains as an area of concern regarding low-calorie mixed diets.

THE SATTVIC LIFESTYLE DIET

Each of the major dietary types has distinct advantages and disadvantages:

- Low-carbohydrate and low-fat diets are most effective for weight loss, but each is disadvantageous as a lifestyle diet due to an excess or a lack of animal foods.

- Low-calorie or mixed-foods diets may be least effective for weight loss, but they are the best choice as lifestyle diets because of the inclusion of all food groups.

As chapter 4 discusses, the potential for consuming excess calories with mixed diets seems best resolved by emphasizing food quality and whole foods—whole carbohydrates as well as whole fats. Food quality—optimum levels of vitamins, minerals, and other nutrients—is undoubtedly as important to the sense of satiety and well-being as are adequate numbers of calories. The importance of quality is easy to assert but difficult to control, dependent as it is on factors such as agricultural practices, soil quality, and animal husbandry practices. Nevertheless, it is an important variable to highlight. The recommendation for whole fats in addition to whole grains goes against conventional wisdom. Yet fats in the whole form have always been a part of traditional diets, and their satiating quality argues against overconsumption in limited amounts, which also has been the traditional practice. The satiating effect of whole carbohydrates further argues against the overconsumption that leads to excess calories and disease.

Reemphasizing whole carbohydrates, however, leads us back again to the critique of grains, even in their whole form. This problem and the enigma of the biblical vegan ideal that promotes carbohydrate foods remain as subjects for the next and final chapter.

8

DIET AND TRANSFORMATION

The time has finally arrived to deal forthrightly and fully with the much praised and much maligned new carbohydrate foods of the agricultural revolution in all their glory and balefulness. They are, on the one hand:

- The Gift of the Gods—as we hear in Genesis 1.29, "See, I give you every herb bearing seed and to you it shall be for meat." The new carbohydrates are the sattvic food supreme; *the* principle food; the basis of civilization; the foundation of food pyramids; the harborer of a wealth of vitamins, minerals, enzymes, phytochemicals, trace elements, and yet-to-be-discovered nutrients; and an effective basis for losing weight and controlling disease.

And on the other hand, the new carbohydrates are:

- The Curse of the Gods—the basis of declining health at the turn to the agricultural revolution; the least-valued food in any environment, according to foraging theory; harborer of dangerous glutens, lectins, and phytates; the underlying cause of caries, obesity, metabolic syndrome, and other diseases; and of the three macronutrients (proteins, fats, and carbohydrates), the only one that is absolutely unnecessary.

If there is any way to reconcile these two faces of carbohydrates, it undoubtedly leads through transformation—the transformation of foods and transformation of the human being.

TRANSFORMATION AND FOOD

The agricultural revolution is synonymous with the beginning of civilization and culture. We heard in chapter 6 of Erich Neumann characterizing the essence of culture as transforming nature.[1] Applied to the agricultural revolution, this meant not only the transformation of wild grass into a staple crop but also transformations that made the new staple food both edible and palatable: "Food begins to be improved by frying, roasting, and boiling. A later development is the bake oven, intimately bound up with the mysteries of agriculture: grain and bread."[2]

Neumann develops the idea of improvement further by relating the transformation of grain to the "mystery of spiritual transformation," from grass, to grain, to bread, and then to the Host, the communion meal of Jesus. Communion with the human-divine Jesus is linked to human transformation or divinization.[3] Yet before turning to food's relationship to this dimension, it is important to dwell on transformational processes involving foods and grain.

As Neumann indicates, the purpose of transformation is to improve the natural state. The rationale for refining grains was the same—to limit the effects of bran, cellulose, fiber, lectins, and phytates in the outer cover that inhibit digestibility and nutrient assimilation.

Typically, though, refining removes too many nutrients, making the breakdown of ingested grain into glucose or blood sugar too easy and leading to metabolic syndrome and the diseases associated with it. Rudolph Ballentine notes that US refining practices have typically removed 28 percent of the grain (known as a 72 percent extraction rate), resulting in the loss of half or even more of nutrients. In contrast, India's practice developed over a millennia-long involvement with health and nutrition removes 5–10 percent of the grain (a 95–90 percent extraction rate), preserving most nutrients, but removing indigestible portions and phytates as well. The flour that results is not "whole" in the absolute sense, yet represents a beneficial compromise. Regarding European practices, Maguelonne Toussaint-Samat points approvingly to Germany's 85 percent extraction rate.[4]

Rice, like wheat, is also refined or polished to remove the bran, leading also to more protein availability (as with wheat), less digestive gas, and better preservation, yet at the cost again of losing many nutrients. Traditional Indian practice polishes rice grains lightly, and potential nutrient loss is solved by steaming or boiling ("parboiling") before husking, preserving nutrients by pushing them deeper inside the grains. Parboiled rice also becomes harder and less likely to break, and it is insect resistant and safer for storage. In addition, cracks are repaired and foreign matter removed.[5]

Corn milling practices are particularly important, as Betty Fussell notes, because the germ, which contains most of the oil, comprises a larger portion of the kernel compared with wheat (11.5 vs. 2 percent). Removing the germ eliminates not only nutrients but taste. Modern roller milling removes the germ more efficiently and improves shelf life, but it amounts to "genocide of the living germ." Traditional stone-ground milling removed less and was done in small batches to keep the oil from spoiling (recall Weston Price's remark that traditional cultures insisted on using cracked grains quickly). A new generation of corn millers is resurrecting traditional techniques, but keeping the meal cool to preserve freshness is an additional problem. Nevertheless, reviving traditional practices is important to give "new life to a murdered grain."[6] In a similar vein, Rudolf Steiner indicates that stone grinding preserves life forces in the grain that affect nutritional quality.[7]

These examples with wheat, rice, and corn illustrate the advantages of traditional practices that deserve to be deliberately reclaimed. This kind of "deliberate processing" would minimize nutrient loss, check too-rapid assimilation by the body, and also maximize digestibility and nourishment value.

Next to milling, other traditional processing practices involve dynamic changes. One example already mentioned is parboiling, which drives nutrients deeper into the grain to prevent their loss from refining. Baking, fermenting, germinating or sprouting, malting, scalding, soaking, and sour-dough baking are other examples.[8] Sally Fallon emphasizes new insights into the importance of these traditional techniques, next to which modern practices seem like a radical departure or even a "fad."[9]

Sprouting activates enzymes that break down complex protein, starch, fat, and sugar compounds into simpler ones. This facilitates their bodily use and eliminates undesirable antinutrients such as phytic acid and enzyme inhibitors. Sprouting also increases the content of proteins, fats, some essential amino acids, total sugars, B vitamins, and crude fiber (a major constituent of cell walls) while decreasing the starch content and making it more digestible. And sprouting stimulates minerals to chelate, or combine with protein, thereby enhancing mineral functions. Vitamin C is also produced, as well as enzymes that facilitate digestion.[10]

In addition to these benefits, we can ask whether sprouting can help to solve the dilemma with animal feed. Grain feed results in meat that is high in saturated fat and unbalanced in omega-3 to omega-6 fatty-acids. Grass feed produces a healthier result, yet it seems impractical, especially for large-scale operations. Sprouting, however, transforms grain into grass!

Other dynamic traditional techniques are culturing, fermenting, soaking in acidic liquids, and sour leavening. All these methods neutralize phytates, deactivate enzyme inhibitors, increase vitamins, and begin the predigestive process that encourages beneficial enzyme production. Like sprouting, these methods also help to break down proteins such as gluten. Sally Fallon suggests that grains will be better tolerated by those who are allergic to them when they are prepared using such methods. And she cautions that glutinous grains (oats, rye, barley, and wheat) should not be consumed without presoaking. Even whole-meal flour benefits from soaking in acidic milk, becoming softer, rising easier using just baking soda, and resulting in a lighter product. The acids from buttermilk, cultured milk, yogurt, whey, lemon juice, and vinegar activate the phytase enzyme, which breaks down phytic acid in grain bran. Lactic dairy acids also help to break down complex starches and tannins. Baking bread by using sourdough instead of brewer's yeast produces bread that is tastier, more digestible, and less easily spoiled, even though brewer's yeast produces bread with more rapid and regular fermentation and better rising. Sourdough fermentation takes longer, but it destroys almost all of the phytic acid. Fallon adds:

> The nourishing traditions of our ancestors require us to apply more wisdom to the way we produce and process our food and, yes, more time in the kitchen, but they give highly satisfying results—delicious meals, increased vitality, robust children and freedom from the chains of acute and chronic disease.[11]

Neutralizing phytates through acidic treatment is also exemplified by the traditional Native American practice of corn "nixtamalization" mentioned in chapter 6 (mixing lime with corn, or adding wood ash to the cooking pot). Neutralization releases vitamin B_3 (niacin) and prevents scurvy. As previously noted, studies of fifty-one different Native American cultures showed that all were using nixtamalization to release niacin.[12]

Other traditional practices involve deliberate harvesting methods. Lorenz Schaller notes that in the past, rice was allowed to ripen in the sun before reaping. The kernels were then left on the fields for further weathering, developing the cracks and fissures that aid thorough cooking. Typically today, rice is harvested while still immature to prevent cracking and fissuring, which is now considered undesirable.[13] Sally Fallon adds that when grain sheaves are stacked and left on the fields, they begin to sprout, initiating the array of beneficial changes previously discussed. When properly grown, she asserts, wheat produces an oil rich in desirable omega-3 fatty acids.[14] In addition, Weston Price notes the importance of field-curing hay: unless hay has been carefully dried to retain the chlorophyll necessary for developing vitamin A, cows feeding on it cannot synthesize important fat-soluble vitamins.[15] A final harvesting example involves pest control: the Angoumois grain moth—which is, according to the newspaper *The Hindu*, "the most serious pest injurious to rice, both in the field and storage"—is controlled by drying the grain under the sun for three days to reduce moisture.[16]

With legumes such as beans, traditional preparation included presoaking, changing the water, skimming off the cooking foam, and sometimes even replacing the water again. Such methods neutralized phytic acid and enzyme inhibitors, broke down complex and difficult-to-digest sugars, and assured thorough digestion and nutrient assimilation (we nevertheless keep in mind Pythagoras's caution about beans).[17]

Rudolph Ballentine adds that skillful use of legumes is a hallmark of good vegetarian nutrition, and once again traditional Indian practice has much to offer. Coriander, cumin, and turmeric (in ratios of 3 to 2 to 1) are browned in ghee, or clarified butter, and used for foundational flavoring. Many spices are medicinal, yet some have toxic compounds; coriander, cumin, and turmeric are considered the safest and are known for their healthful effects.[18] In addition to soaking beans overnight and changing water to reduce intestinal gas, cooking with onions, garlic, herbs, and spices—and then adding acidic seasonings (such as tomato or lemon juice) and fat or oil at the end—stimulates digestion.[19] (We have to wonder whether the reason Indian culture does not caution about eating beans is because no such caution is necessary, due to these preparation methods.)

Widespread dairy consumption is another hallmark of the agricultural revolution, and dairy also is a focus of criticism because of adverse effects. Yet traditional practices once again have much to recommend them. Sally Fallon makes the startling observation that only the West consumes milk without fermentation. Souring (lacto-fermentation with bacteria) yields many positive changes: restoring helpful enzymes; breaking down milk sugar and protein; and increasing vitamins B and C, friendly intestinal bacteria, and calcium and phosphorus availability. Lactic acid produced by fermentation preserves the milk and inactivates putrefying bacteria.[20] As previously indicated, soaking grains in milk-derived acidic solutions (and lemon juice and vinegar as well) provides the same benefits as does fermentation for milk.

We have heard that the Hindu tradition considers milk to be a sattvic food supreme, yet rawness is an important criterion. Products made from fresh, raw milk are consumed the same day (except clarified butter or ghee, which keeps indefinitely). Atmavadan Reddy, who oversees dairy operations at the Sri Aurobindo Ashram in Pondicherry, India, reports that local villagers like to consume raw milk immediately, but after a few hours, it must be boiled because of rapid bacteria growth. Milk that is not immediately consumed can then be refrigerated for up to two weeks, but it is boiled before consumption. Pasteurized and homogenized milk, and milk produced using pesticides or genetically modified organisms (GMOs), are considered poisonous.[21] Rudolph Ballentine notes that the traditional practice of boiling milk at 212 degrees Fahrenheit (pasteurization heats to 161 degrees) sterilizes it more completely without affecting nutrient value and makes it less mucus forming, leading to improved health, growth, and weight for children.[22] Sally Fallon, on the other hand, acknowledges the better digestibility of boiled milk, yet she claims that boiling destroys enzymes and decreases vitamins. Her recommendation: use clean, certified, raw whole milk and ferment it.[23]

Another traditional dairy practice is using clarified butter, or ghee, for cooking. Ghee is made by boiling butter to remove the water. According to the Ayurvedic tradition, ghee acts as a preservative and has a special capacity for assimilating medicinal effects of herbs and spices and passing them on to the body. Ballentine notes that foods cooked in ghee are noticeably fresher after refrigeration in contrast to those cooked in vegetable oil.[24]

Lorenz Schaller adds a fitting summary to these indications about traditional practices by noting the symbiotic relationship that existed between grain cultivation and human ingenuity: "Grains have developed in unity with humanity's intelligence. They are an *object* produced by human wisdom."[25]

He means that intelligence and wisdom were necessary in the past to transform a wild grass into a staple crop. Both intelligence and wisdom continue to be necessary today to make these staple foods of the agricultural revolution fully nourishing and to inhibit harmful effects. The use of transformative practices, no longer habitual, must become deliberate. Such methods may not solve all modern problems with carbohydrates and grains, but they can undoubtedly help. Nonetheless, the final solution to making the new foods of the agricultural revolution fully nourishing also involves human transformation.

CHAPTER 8

TRANSFORMATION AND THE HUMAN BEING

On a fundamental level, the body is able to respond to the regular consumption of foods such as grains by creating phytase enzymes to break down phytic acid, thereby making minerals like calcium available that otherwise remain bound.[26] This latent ability, however, depends on the state of health that allows such dynamic processes to take place. Differing abilities to create phytase demonstrate that coping successfully with carbohydrates does not rest with food transformations alone.

Biological transmutations represent another more significant bodily potential—the capacity to transmute elements from one to another. The phenomenon was revealed through the work of French scientist Louis Kervran.[27] Kervran was called to investigate the mysterious deaths of metal workers who had died from carbon-monoxide poisoning despite the lack of an apparent carbon-monoxide source. Kervran hypothesized that working with heated metal had caused nitrogen to transmute in workers' lungs, creating carbon monoxide. Such a transmutation could be explained in terms of protons splitting off from nitrogen atoms to create carbon and oxygen atoms, and then both those atoms combining to create carbon monoxide.

Nitrogen (N_2) is composed of two atoms with seven protons in each nucleus ($_7N$), giving a total of fourteen protons ($2_7N = 14$). If one proton jumps from atom to atom, the result is atoms with six and eight protons, the requisite numbers for carbon ($_6C$) and oxygen ($_8O$). If both of these then combine, the result is one molecule of carbon monoxide (CO).

This transmutational theory helped Kervran make sense of other unusual and inexplicable phenomena. As a child, he had witnessed hens picking out and eating bright specks of mica in the sand. Yet when the hens were killed and cut open, no mica was found. Again Kervran hypothesized that a transmutation had taken place, turning potassium into calcium.

Mica is rich in potassium, and potassium atoms contain nineteen protons ($_{19}K$). Adding a hydrogen proton ($_1H$), as could occur from the air or water, would create one atom of calcium ($_{20}$Ca). If indeed such a transmutation was taking place, this would explain why hens could lay eggs with firm, calcified shells despite the lack of a calcium source. A subsequent experiment supported the hypothesis: hens that were denied calcium stopped laying eggs; but when they were given mica, they eagerly ate it up and within a short time produced eggs with strong, hard shells. Kervran further hypothesized that such transmutations were taking place through the action of bodily enzymes working at low levels of energy.

As Drs. Rudolph Ballentine and Gabriel Cousens note, *biological transmutations* contradict the law of the conservation of matter, which states the immutability of elements. The significance for nutrition is profound: if the body can create its own elements, then nutrition is *not* just a matter of ingesting or assimilating food nutrients. Ballentine points, for example, to credible reports of Eastern masters living for years without food, and Gabriel Cousens points to the nun Therese Neumann, reported to have lived solely on the communion host.[28]

Ballentine suggests that the human capacity for transmutation points to the power of consciousness over matter, which has always been a tenet of Eastern philosophy. This power is potentially available to everyone, yet not everyone can make use of it. Both he and Cousens report great diversity among patients in nutritional needs and in the ability to assimilate ingested nutrients. The key appears to be the state of health, which is itself affected by various spiritual practices such as yoga, meditation, and prayer. As we have heard in chapters 2 and 5, religious and spiritual recommendations for vegetarianism are given in the context of spiritual practice; and we also heard that, without such practice, vegetarianism can be dangerous.

Yet beyond the capacity to transmute elements, there is a more profound level to human transformations relating to the rebirth doctrines that resulted from living with the changes in nature (chapter 6). Readers will recall that the cycles of the moon and agriculture led to a cyclical understanding of human life and ideas such as resurrection, reincarnation, and cosmic renewal, and that grains became a special symbol.

On the surface, the rebirth ideas of resurrection and reincarnation stand in opposition to one another. Traditionally, Christianity views each person as having but one earthly life and death,[29] and resurrection with an immortal body occurs at the end of time along with cosmos renewal. The traditional Eastern view sees reincarnation in multiple earthly bodies occurring throughout cycles of time until enlightenment extinguishes the thirst for life. Yet some conceptions of reincarnation and resurrection combine the two. In this view, human evolution proceeds through multiple reincarnations until the climax at the end of time, when resurrection with an immortal body occurs.

Such a synthetic view is represented by the anonymous author of the spiritual classic, *Meditations on the Tarot*. As for the orthodoxy of reincarnation from a Christian point of view, he writes:

> Reincarnation is neither a dogma, i.e. a truth necessary for salvation, nor a heresy, i.e. contrary to a truth necessary for salvation. It is simply a fact of experience, just as sleep and heredity are. As such, it is neutral. Everything depends on its interpretation. One can interpret it in such a way as to make it a blasphemy. When one says: to forgive is to grant the opportunity to begin again; God forgives more than seventy-times-seven times, always granting us opportunities anew—what infinite goodness of God! Here is an interpretation to the glory of God.[30]

The author continues that suggesting that previous lives morally determine subsequent ones without the possibility of divine grace's intervening would be a blasphemous interpretation of reincarnation. He then adds that the church opposed the idea of reincarnation to prevent an undue focus on future earthly lives.[31] Yet he asserts that reincarnation is actually an intermediary principle between heredity and salvation, which together "constitute the cosmic drama of evolution."[32] The resurrection body must become the perfect manifestation of individuality free from heredity's influence and reestablishing God's image and likeness[33] (note the relevance to the Blood-Type Diet's idea of continuing to stimulate a personality type through diet). The resurrection body grows gradually throughout reincarnations and evolution. Theoretically, only one incarnation is necessary to bring it to perfection, but many are necessary in practice.[34]

Hope is the force that moves and directs this process of spiritual evolution.[35] Resurrection finally results through the union of two free wills, one human and one divine:

> Resurrection is not an all-powerful divine act, but rather the effect of the meeting and union of divine love, hope, and faith with human love, hope, and faith. The trumpet sounds from above the whole of divine love, hope, and faith; and not only the human spirit and soul but also all the atoms of the human body respond "yes" in chorus, which is the free expression—a cry from the heart of the whole being and of each particular atom—of the love, hope, and faith of man.[36]

Next to the anonymous author, Rudolf Steiner is another who represents the view of multiple incarnations gradually leading to resurrection, and he provides a wealth of detail about the constitutional changes taking place. In chapter 2 we spoke about Steiner's fourfold human paradigm—the physical body, the etheric body, the astral body, and the ego—that helps to explain nutritional effects on spiritual development. Steiner also has a ninefold conception comprising three bodies, three soul sheaths, and three spiritual sheaths that exist initially only in germinal form.[37]

According to Steiner, the ego, or "I," is a reflection of divine Nature[38] and has the task of transforming the bodily sheaths over the course of evolution in order to manifest the spiritual sheaths. The first focus is transforming the astral body, the body of passion and desire, into the lowest spiritual sheath, called the "spirit self." Concurrently, but at a slower pace (the hour hand of the clock compared with the minute hand), the etheric body of life forces is being transformed into the second spiritual sheath, called the "life spirit." This takes longer because the forces that are involved lie deeper within human nature. The transformation of the physical body into the third spiritual sheath, the "spirit body," represents the actual resurrection body; and this process lasts longest because the forces involved lie deeper still within human nature. All these transformational processes are taking place with everyone in the course of normal earthly life without conscious participation, and yet the work can be taken up directly through conscious spiritual practice and initiation.

The anonymous author adds a fitting coda to this transformational vision: the law of the "struggle for existence" will eventually give way to the law of "cooperation for life":

> The end of the "law" of the struggle for existence and the future triumph of the law of cooperation for life has been foretold by the prophet Isaiah:
>
>> The wolf shall dwell with the lamb,
>> And the leopard shall lie down with the kid,
>> And the calf and the lion and the fatling together,
>> And a little child shall lead them.
>
> (Isaiah 11:6)
>
> This will be, because the new "law"—i.e., a profound change in the psychic and physical structure of beings—will replace the old "law," first in consciousness, then in desires and affections, then lastly in the organic structure of beings.[39]

In this way, transformational changes are occurring slowly over time and culminate in structural changes, which is what Isaiah's vision is understood to represent.

The time of fulfillment in the biblical tradition involves a new heaven and earth and the appearance of the New Jerusalem:

> For I am about to create new heavens and a new earth; the former things shall not be remembered or come to mind. But be glad and rejoice forever in what I am creating; for I am about to create Jerusalem as a joy.
>
> (Isa. 65:17–18)
>
> Then I saw a new heaven and a new earth; for the first heaven and the first earth had passed away. . . . And I saw the holy city, the new Jerusalem, coming down out of heaven from God.
>
> (Rev. 21:1–2)

The descent of the New Jerusalem comes at a time of cosmic renewal and represents a return to Paradise. As biblical scholar Bruce Metzger puts it, "Then a new divine order will be established, when the End will be as the Beginning, and Paradise will be restored."[40]

These juxtapositions—resurrection and a transformed body, the descent of the New Jerusalem and a return to Paradise—put the biblical vegan command at the time of the first Paradise into an illuminating context: just as a vegan-vegetarian diet applied to the Paradise of Genesis (1:29–30), *so too will it apply to the Paradise of New Jerusalem at the end of time, when the resurrection body will have been fully formed.* It is the structural changes inherent to the process of resurrection that finally enable vegan-vegetarian nutrition for both humans *and animals* (Gen. 1:30), suggesting that *bodily needs themselves will have changed.* Readers will recall Erich Neumann relating the communion meal of Jesus to the transformation of human nature. That is what communion signifies and what resurrection signifies as well.

It is a curious fact that the spiritual traditions of the West, which are largely meat eating, have generally passed over the biblical vegan command in silence, while the lacto-vegetarian traditions of the East have never ceased to proclaim their vegetarian ideal. Is this because the biblical vegan ideal held sway in an idealized past and cannot hold sway again until an idealized future, when the changes relating to resurrection have taken place?

It is important to add some points about this evolutionary process. The first is that blood-type O, which the Blood-Type Diet associates with an animal-foods diet, involves a defective gene. This gene is considered defective, inactive, or nonfunctional because it does not build antigens on blood-cell surfaces as the genes of the other types do to distinguish friendly from foreign substances in the blood. When the other types detect foreign substances, they create protective antibodies in response.[41] Lacking such antigen identity markers, type O creates antibodies more indiscriminately and aggressively and as a result has a stronger immune system.

Type O's lack of antigens is important for the debate about which blood type came first. Dr. D'Adamo suggests type O did because it was dominant during the hunter-gatherer era, with type A becoming increasingly prevalent after the agricultural revolution. The counter-argument cites the unlikelihood of seemingly normal genes such as those in types A and B mutating from an abnormal one. In addition, evidence for type A's appearance first also exists. The debate so far is inconclusive. The evidence suggests that either type A or type O appeared first; or that type A appeared first, then disappeared, and subsequently reappeared.[42]

This debate is intriguing to our spiritual perspective for several reasons. The first reason is that the human-related primates who preceded hunter-gatherers and represented the first phase of human history ate a largely vegetarian diet, the one associated with blood-type A.[43] Hence, the appearance of type A first accords with the initial vegetarian diet prescribed in chapter 1 of the Book of Genesis.

The second reason is that the association of meat eating with a defective gene is profoundly significant theologically; that is, meat eating was not the original divine intent and necessitated an abnormal gene that could create the necessary stomach acid for digestion, along with a strong immune system capable of resisting pathogens (both characteristics of blood-type O).

The third reason has to do with why the subsequent appearance of this defective gene happened. The biochemist Lawrence Moran cites the assumed appearance of blood-type O *after* type A as an argument against "Intelligent Design Creationism"—because why would the Creator first create a normal gene and then a defective one?

> Could some of our IDiot friends please explain . . . using their favorite paradigm?
>
> Why would the "designer" make a perfectly good gene like the one encoding the A enzyme and then wreck it by introducing a single base pair deletion to make the O allele?[44]

Here is this IDiot's response: *The divine purpose* was *spiritual evolutionary development—to gain the personality characteristics associated with meat diets that help to develop ego strength* (see the section on the Blood-Type Diet in chapter 4). According to Dr. D'Adamo, blood-type B, which follows types A and O, balances the personality characteristics of each, and the later appearance of type AB adds more of A's influence. D'Adamo also notes that type AB is associated with Jesus Christ via blood samples from the Shroud of Turin, but he doubts the association because type AB first became visible much later. Yet the association to Jesus Christ is intriguing, and the characterization of type AB as an enigma and even "quirky" suggests that whatever evolutionary process may be underway is by no means complete.

In brief, the above relationships suggest that the vegetarian diet associated with blood-type A was the original diet, and that type O's meat-centered diet became a necessary aberration for the sake of ego development. In effect, such a scenario supports the biblical notion of an initial Paradise followed by a Fall and then a subsequent process of evolutionary development—as suggested by the anonymous author, Rudolf Steiner, and, of course, the leader emeritus of the religious vegetarian impulse, Rabbi Abraham Isaac Kook. This developmental process is continuing and will continue until the promise of the vegan ideal is reclaimed, yet from a position of the ego strength that has been gained.

Another important and complementary point about this entire evolutionary process is Rudolf Steiner's assertion that the resurrection body will have no need for food at all (according to Steiner, the need for nutrition resulted from a change in the various bodily sheathes after the Fall).[45] This may seem surprising, yet biblical verses do prophesy a future without hunger or thirst:

> They shall not hunger or thirst.
>
> (Isa. 49:10)
>
> They will hunger no more, and thirst no more.
>
> (Rev. 7:16)

These verses can be variously interpreted to mean a lack of need as well as the presence of abundant food. Yet a Cabalist view also asserts the lack of need: "The World to Come is unlike this world. There, there is no eating or drinking."[46] If indeed the resurrection body will have no need for food, will the time for vegan nutrition precede the resurrection? Considering that structural changes take place incrementally over time, perhaps. The post-resurrection stories about Jesus breaking bread and eating fish and a honeycomb (Luke 24:30, 42), however, suggest that eating will at least be optional (food lovers everywhere will breathe a collective sigh of relief).

A final point about the evolutionary process is that locating its culmination in the distant future runs the risk of justifying the church's opposition to the doctrine of reincarnation—namely, putting off until tomorrow the actions that can and should be done today. As chapter 5 stated, the answer to the question of vegetarianism is yes and no, which in practical terms means distinguishing between the desire and the need for animal foods. The full embrace of the highest ideal may well lie in the future, yet there are many transitional steps along the way—from limiting or even eliminating meat, fowl, fish, and eggs, and then on to lacto-vegetarianism itself. Taking seriously the impulse to vegetarianism in the present is an important part of the transformational work.

As for implementing the call, Rudolph Ballentine offers a balanced perspective. Tracing the origin of the word *vegetarian* to the Latin *vegetare*, which means "to enliven," he additionally relates it to the words for *arouse* (*vegere*) and *flourish* (*vigere*), the English words *vigorous* and *vigil*, and finally to the very ancient root *wag*, which means "lively" or "strong." He then continues:

> The basis of the term "vegetarian," then, is a sense of liveliness, vigor, and alertness, rather than merely an indication of a diet of vegetables. The issue is not whether the diet is or isn't made up exclusively of foods of plant origins (vegetable foods) but whether it is enlivening and health-giving. What is used as a supplemental source of protein and other nutrients, be it milk, eggs, fish, or even fowl or meat, is a less important consideration.[47]

This focus on the health-giving effect, of course, is the Bhagavad Gita's own perspective. Ballentine reinforces the notion of flexibility by emphasizing the importance of moving freely among different phases—including or excluding meat, fowl, fish, etc., as need and circumstances dictate. The culture-wide trend toward less animal food, he says, may seem inevitable, but applying the process to one's own life should never feel constrained.[48]

Yet if, in good conscience, one is unable or unwilling to limit animal foods in the present, the host of important changes in the social and economic spheres remain to be achieved involving the production of animal food. Chapter 5 addressed the importance of providing ethical animal-food sources and the religious practices already in existence that put production into a sacred context and need support. Insisting on strengthening such social frameworks contributes to developing the ego strength that leads to the vegetarian ideal.

Creating the agricultural conditions that produce truly nourishing food is also important to the transformational task. As Gabriel Cousens indicates, today's sattvic diet would undoubtedly be organic because of the concern for deliberate practices that enhance nutritional quality.[49] In this regard, the *biodynamic* form of organic agriculture, which seeks to heal and energize the earth besides replenishing nutrients, is especially noteworthy, because its enhanced transformative practice results in enhanced nutritional quality. One can imagine a food system in which deliberate cultivation and production practices become the standard, but of course this will not happen without effort and struggle.

With the above considerations in mind, we are in position to draw a final conclusion about the relationship of transformation to grains and the new carbohydrate foods of the agricultural revolution: *absolutely unessential carbohydrate foods such as grains, in need of deliberate care and transformation to make them fully nourishing and palatable, are archetypically perfect foods for human beings and human societies, themselves engaged in processes of transformation.*

Individual needs in the present may vary, just as the Blood-Type Diet and many of our authors indicate, and just as individual taste intuitively seems to dictate; but seemingly problematic carbohydrate foods do have the capacity to nourish, and they do represent the direction of an ideal future.

With this conclusion, we come to the end of these reflections on spirituality and diet; and so we turn once again to the Bhagavad Gita and its appropriately unspecific recommendations, keeping in mind everything that has been discussed and also that, in the course of spiritual development, the gunas, too, must be transcended:

> The food...which is dear to each [human] is of triple character. ... Hear... the distinction of these.
>
> The sattvic temperament ... turns naturally to things that increase the inner and outer strength, nourish at once the mental, vital, and physical force and increase the pleasure and satisfaction and happy condition of mind and life and body, all that is succulent and soft and firm and satisfying.
>
> The rajasic temperament prefers naturally food that is violently sour, pungent, hot acrid, rough and strong and burning, the aliments that increase ill-health and the distempers of the mind and body.
>
> The tamasic temperament takes a perverse pleasure in cold, impure, stale, rotten, or tasteless food or even accepts like the animals the remnants half-eaten by others.[50]

Amen.

Epilogue:
Diet and Spiritual Evolution

Of the Bhagavad Gita's seven hundred verses, four are about food. The other 696 largely comprise the rest of what Krishna has to say to set Arjuna's feet firmly on the path leading to salvation. Diet plays a role, but a very modest one. In effect, Krishna says to Arjuna, "Eat in a dignified manner the food that will keep you fully healthy!" One can imagine, however, Arjuna's conflict—wanting to take up the spiritual path, but thinking on the one hand about ahimsa, karma, and the new vegetarian movements of the times, and on the other hand about the dietary practices of himself and his warrior friends, and even his own tastes—and then his objection, "Yes, but *what* should I eat?" One can then also imagine that Krishna, fully aware of Arjuna's conflict and the personal considerations involved, might look Arjuna in the eyes and repeat with firmness and compassion, *"Eat what will keep you, Arjuna, fully healthy!"* (Yes, a call to discernment, but that's life, including spiritual life!)

Chapter 8 concluded with the opinion that carbohydrates, with all their faults, are nevertheless archetypically perfect foods for human beings. This is a spiritual view based on perceived beneficial effects for human and cultural evolution. Yet some caveats resulting from our study that might easily be overlooked or forgotten are important to reiterate. Here's the first one:

The use of carbohydrates for food, and the practice of vegetarianism, too, are matters of choice; health does not depend on them. The agricultural revolution that began some ten thousand years ago introduced the large-scale consumption of carbohydrate foods such as grains, which continues today, and their predominant use is economically advantageous because of abundance and low cost. Yet physical health does not compel the consumption of carbohydrates; they are unessential foods, and health can be maintained or even improved on high animal protein or fat diets. This latter point surprised me, as stated in the introduction, because I grew up in the cultural milieu of the trend toward vegetal foods and away from animal foods, as outlined in chapter 4. This trend has its justification in the context of a predominantly carbohydrate diet that must deemphasize animal foods to remain healthy, yet it is not the only option. The low-carbohydrate movement has generated a plethora of studies to prove that meat diets are healthy, as long as the condition is met of restricting or even eliminating carbohydrates. There is no health benefit to carbohydrates, or even vegetarian diets, unless one accepts and values the paradigm that links body, mind, and spirit and scientifically unproven assertions about holistic dietary effects. For the assertion that one's diet has spiritual effects does favor carbohydrate foods and even vegetarianism. Accepting the paradigm and valuing carbohydrate foods, however, are matters of choice and belief. One is free to choose because health is not at stake here, and that this is so makes sense from a spiritual point of view because human freedom is inviolable. In matters of diet, as in matters of belief, there is no compulsion, only absolute freedom. Carbohydrate foods and vegetarianism may be ideals from a spiritual point of view, but health—whether physical or spiritual—does not depend on them. But now we arrive at the second caveat to the idea that, spiritually speaking, carbohydrates are the ideal food:

Vegetarianism is not synonymous with spiritual life; it can assist spiritual development, but without spiritual practice, it can even be harmful. Rabbi Kook, George Ohsawa, Michio Kushi, and Rudolf Steiner all contribute to the notions making up this statement. Rabbi Kook, in addressing the Jewish interest of his time in vegetarianism as a sign of the coming Messianic Age, put the Torah's meat-eating sanction into a framework that encompassed the Fall and then, through evolution, the return to spiritual heights. Within this process, meat plays a role in helping the human personality develop strength. Rudolf Steiner voices a similar view. Such ideas may seem shocking, but they nevertheless belong to the history of religious ideas about diet and spirituality. In Kook's view, premature vegetarianism out of a "weak moral voice" impedes rather than fosters spiritual development. His insights apply today as a caution to the ethical vegetarianism associated with the animal-rights movement. Ohsawa, Kushi, and Steiner in turn stress the importance of balance—between yin and yang, vegetal and animal foods, and the inner and outer life—and Kushi and Steiner the imbalance resulting from one-sided vegetal and meat diets. Steiner articulates that restricting meat and fat through a vegetarian diet stimulates the inner activity that contributes to spiritual development, but he also asserts that without spiritual practice to channel the force correctly, harm results. He mentions ordinary intellectuals who are vegetarians and suffer possible brain impairment without an active spiritual life, and I have offered Hitler as a possible example. Kook, Ohsawa, Kushi, Steiner—and even Weston Price—all help to clarify the potential harm resulting from vegetarianism. Yet we do not rely on their witness alone. They only articulate more precisely the rationale behind the ambivalence seen in religious traditions as a whole toward the question of vegetarianism, an ambivalence rooted in the multiplicity of factors to be considered and ultimately in vegetarianism's secondary, not primary, role for spiritual development.

FINALLY, WE CALL once more upon the Bhagavad Gita to characterize the proper relationship between diet and spirituality: Diet relates to spiritual development in the same way as the Gita's four verses about diet relate to the seven hundred verses that comprise the fullness of its teaching. Spiritual evolution and the healthy role of diet within that process ultimately depend on treading the path in its fullness.

AFTERWORD

In January of 2013, I spent two weeks in one of the guesthouses of the Sri Aurobindo Ashram in Pondicherry, India. As a guest, I had the opportunity to eat in the ashram's dining hall—called the Mother's Dining Hall—which was about ten minutes away by bicycle. When I first requested coupons from the guesthouse desk clerk for three days, he replied: "Better try just one day, the food there is very plain."

By the time my stay ended, I had eaten almost all of my meals at the dining hall and grew increasingly to look forward to them, even to breakfast, despite the need to get up earlier than usual to finish my morning routine before getting to the dining hall on time.

The meals were indeed simple: breakfast consisted of grain porridge, bread, a banana, and the choice of yogurt or milk with optional sugar; lunch consisted of rice topped with dal and vegetable curry, along with bread, yogurt or milk, and two bananas; and dinner, of porridge, bread, and yogurt or milk. In the course of my two-week stay, there was some variation—sometimes a spoonful of butter, sometimes a ball of cheese, or a sweet dessert, or a dish of sprouts. Helpings dished out by the ashram staff were certainly adequate. At first I didn't realize that I could request more when moving through the line. Some people did, but I never felt the need; nor did I feel the need for snacks between meals.

As the result of eating there, what I first noticed was an improvement in digestion, as evidenced by solid, compact stools light brown in color. In truth, I commonly experience improved digestion during vacations, which undoubtedly relates to lack of stress (and, needless to say, the environment within the ashram surroundings was indeed relaxing). In addition, when I finally returned home, I also noticed that an untreatable cavity between the roots of a back molar had stopped hurting. My unconfirmed suspicion is that a veneer filled it over, just as Weston Price describes can happen when the diet provides all necessary nutrients (a few months later, the cavity's sensitivity had returned).

I wish I could attribute any improvement to the "what" of the foods I ate at the Mother's Dining Hall, because the menu would be relatively easy to duplicate. Yet the real issue is undoubtedly quality and all the other intangibles that go into making the fare there the unique experience it is: mostly organic foods from ashram farms; freshly baked bread from the ashram bakery; fresh milk from ashram dairies and from cows looked after with care, fed wholesome foods and played classical and soothing music that makes them happy (as ashram administrator Devdip Ganguli reports); food preparation and service through ashram members; and the meditative atmosphere itself, including the "food for thought" boards with relevant sayings of Sri Aurobindo and the Mother—such as these words of Aurobindo: "The food given from the dining room has the Mother's force behind it. It contains everything that is necessary to keep you in good health to do the sadhana [the spiritual practice]. Keep that attitude and eat. Everything will go well." And surely, everything did go well.

Granted, sadhana in an ashram is different from that of life in the world, for which a heartier fare may be necessary. But quality, I am convinced, is the ultimate key to heartier fare, too—fresh, organic, unadulterated foods, nutritious and robust to the highest degree.

Evolution is, of course, a process for human beings and societies. The New Jerusalem heralded in Revelation 21:2 is one image of the civilizational goal toward which we head. It may be impossible to know whether there will be cafeterias, kitchens, or restaurants in the New Jerusalem or what they might serve. But if they do exist, I think that in the Mother's Dining Hall I have had a foretaste.

FOR THOSE CAUGHT in the predicament of living east or west of Eden, a few more diet-related words are appropriate. *The Yogi*

Diet was never intended to include recipes, for it is impossible for me to improve on what already exists. But I do have a few tips to pass along, in keeping with the theme of grains as an important sattvic food.

The first is to start the day with a bowl of freshly cooked grains, especially underutilized ones such as amaranth, barley, buckwheat, oats, millet, and quinoa. Choices are barely exhaustible within a week's time. This kind of breakfast is immeasurably preferable to packaged cereals, granolas, or flour products such as muffins, bagels, and breads (depending, as always, on quality).

Deliberate preparation is the key. In *Nourishing Traditions*, Sally Fallon recommends overnight soaking for most grains (with the exception of rice), especially for oats, and lacto-fermentation for flakes and grain meals by adding cultured milk products, the benefits of which my chapter 8 explains.[1] Fallon also advises that cereals such as cornmeal porridge will taste even better if soaked several days before cooking. As for cooking, slow cooking will use about half as much water if you have the time. If you don't, grains cooked the night before can be left on the stove or in the refrigerator for several days without spoiling, according to George Ohsawa, which has also been my experience. Toppings are limitless—yogurts and milks (dairy or nondairy), butter or oil (especially olive oil), honey and other sweeteners, fresh and dried fruits, nuts, seeds, and spices. For a wealth of good recipes and tips, see Fallon's book.

This grains type of breakfast has worked well with me for years, and perhaps it can work well for you, too. As for lunches and dinners, I defer to the experts (such as Sally Fallon) who have written recipe books.

Appendix A

The Communion Meal of Jesus: Mythological and Traditional Parallels

Chapter 6 explored how the communion meal of Jesus synthesizes key elements of the mythological complex about the divine origins of life and sacrifice: a deity is sacrificed to create life; sacrifice is offered back to the deity to renew life; consuming the sacrifice signifies communion with the deity; communion with the deity promises life after death. The words of Jesus succinctly summarize these various elements:

> I am the living bread that came down from heaven. Whoever eats of this bread will live forever; and the bread I will give for the life of the world is my flesh.
>
> (John 6:51)

Below are some relevant points of the mythological complex, along with references to parallels in various traditions:

- *On the divine origins of life and the sacrifice of the deity*: the universe and all of life come into being through the body and blood of a sacrificed deity, either sacrificed by the deity itself or through other gods; "death becomes life."

  - In imitation of the vegetation cycle, vegetation gods die annually and resurrect—Adonis in Babylonia, Syria, and Greece; Attis in Phyrigia and Rome; Osiris in Egypt; and Tammuz in Sumeria.[1] Dionysus, the Greek god of grapes and wine, also dies and resurrects.[2] The Aztec maize goddess Chicome Couatl is responsible for the growth of plants and beans; maize originates from drops of blood or the dead body of the Native American Corn Woman.[3] In the Ojibwa myth, the maize plant originates from the body of a spirit-man.[4] Rice and other crops grow from the body of the slain Japanese food goddess Ogetsu-hime.[5]

- In the myth of the Tree of the Middle Place, the tree emerges from an Aztec goddess (or her representative) and is watered by blood, personifying the fertile earth and representing life resulting from death; the Aztec goddess Tlalteutli is ripped apart, giving birth to the world.[6] The notion of food plants originating from the body of a benign being appears in the Americas and throughout Oceania and Southeast Asia.[7] Consider, for instance, the Papua New Guinean Marind-anim myth of the Dema deity, the mythological figure from whose body life originates,[8] and the Huichol legend of the maize plant understood as the body of divinity.[9]

- The Aztec deity Nanahuatzin sacrifices itself for the sake of universal life, becoming the sun of the present and last age;[10] the Mayan maize god exemplifies divine sacrifice for the sake of food plants (a common worldwide theme), and in Mayan-Toltec-Aztec cultures, divine sacrifice sets the universe in motion.[11]

- Rice grains originate from the breast milk and blood of the Eastern goddess Kuan Yin (although in this example, the goddess does not die).[12]

- The Japanese "food genius" goddess Uke-mochi is slain; from her body spring forth foods, animals, and the silk-worm (the legend is considered of Korean origin because of elements like wordplay).[13]

- In Indonesian mythology, the divine Samyam Sri is killed by gods; from the body, rice and grasses grow for human nourishment.[14]

• *On the sacrifice to the deity renewing life*: sacrifice honors the slain deity and sustains universal life; blood sacrifices take place with humans and animals, but with grain effigies and fruits of the field as well.

- Animals are sacrificed and their blood buried to renew nature's strength and fertility during the Durga festival of the Indian goddess Kali, the source of nourishment.[15] The Aztec earth goddess, torn apart to create the world, craves human hearts and refuses to bear fruit without blood.[16] The Aztec Snake Woman yields nature's fertility through blood sacrifice.[17] The Great Mother is dismembered, becoming the source of life; blood sacrifice, dismemberment, and strewing bodily remains on the fields become part of the fertility ritual;[18] the Great Goddess everywhere demands sacrifice.[19]

- Aztec sacrifice replicates the primal sacrifice, harmonizing social order with "the energies of the tide of life";[20] ceremonials represent the primal divine sacrifice and result in world renewal.[21] Aztecs justify sacrifice as honoring gods sacrificed for the sake of life; Aztecs, Mayans, and others sacrifice to keep the sun in motion and increase nature's fertility.[22]

- The dismembered body of Osiris is strewn over the fields as fertilizer.[23]

- The sun refuses to move without sacrifice; continuing motion requires further sacrifice.[24]

- In Celtic myth, children and animals are sacrificed to obtain corn and milk from the gods;[25] people along the Volga River—and Votiaks, Mordvins, and Baltic Finns—practice sacrifice for the sake of the earth's fertility.[26] In Hopi myth, witches demand the sacrifice of a youth and maiden in exchange for the "seeds of all things."[27]

- Human and animal sacrifices induce rice-field fertility.[28]

- *On sacrifices representing the deity being consumed in communion*: human, animal, grain-effigy, and "first fruits"-of-the-field kinds

245

of sacrifices all represent the deity and are consumed as communion with the deity.

- In the festival of the Aztec war god Huitzilopochtli, an idol made of amaranth is consecrated and eaten as the god's flesh and bones.[29]

- Human and animal sacrifices represent the corn spirit and are eaten sacramentally;[30] eating the "first fruits" is understood as a sacrament of divine communion.[31] Aztecs make and consume a dough god, entering into mystic communion; Aryans do the same with rice cakes.[32] Huichol Indians and the Malas (of southern India) commune with the deity through a divine effigy.[33] "First fruits" are understood as filled with divine spirit or life; later, they are considered created, not animated, and are offered in gratitude and honor.[34] Sacrificial consumption signifies assimilating the god's attributes and powers.[35]

- Mexican sacrificial victims are identified with the gods.[36]

- In the reenactment of the Papua New Guinean Dema deity myth, an *iwag*—a female human sacrifice—represents the ancestral Dema; victims are always understood as the god's incarnation.[37]

- In the Aztec myth of the Tree of the Middle Place, a tree growing from the belly of a human sacrifice represents the primal earth goddess;[38] a sacrificial young woman represents Xclomen, the Aztec goddess of young maize.[39] Sacrifice and consumption of a maiden at the Aztec midsummer corn festival represents the corn goddess Xilonen; a maiden representing the goddess of ripe corn and the Earth Mother Coatlicue is ritually put to death at the harvest festival.[40]

- *On communion signifying life after death*: just as the deity survives death and continues to live, communion with the deity guarantees life after death.

– The Attis resurrection festival signifies the promise of resurrection for worshipers.[41] Osiris's resurrection pledges eternal life to believers; resurrection is conceived bodily, not just spiritually.[42] The sprouting of grain leads to an augury of immortality;[43] the growth-cycle of corn and Demeter's Eleusian mysteries offer the hope of resurrection and eternal life.[44] Divine attributes and powers are assimilated by consuming a sacrificial animal or human.[45]

The above examples about resurrection to a life beyond earthly life have been found only in Near Eastern traditions, suggesting that this idea was confined to them (reincarnation to earthly life was the parallel afterlife teaching in the Far East).

COMMENTATORS HAVE NOTED the parallels between the traditions cited above and Christianity. Sir James Frazer compares the Egyptian hope of resurrection through invoking the name of Osiris to the same hope in Christianity through Christ.[46] He also notes that, despite the Christian air of superiority toward heathen superstitions, the ideology of Christian communion mirrors the notion of gaining divine attributes and powers by eating the sacrificial offering.[47] In addition, he links Christianity's rapid spread throughout Near Eastern cultures to the shared ideologies between them.[48] Frazer has been criticized greatly for lumping together into one category different mythologies about dying and rising gods, including Christianity, while understanding all as psychological projections of the nature cycle. Yet scholars still study him because of the parallels that he demonstrates, and that is the point—that the parallels do exist and that they facilitated being able to relate to Christianity for ancient peoples.[49]

Likewise, Betty Fussell points out the similarity between the New World mythology of the death and resurrection of corn and the Christian cross and mass, and she further notes Western ignorance of the parallel between Christian communion and primitive cannibal practices.[50] Joseph Campbell also points to the cannibal parallel[51] as well as to the sacrificial nature of Mary's self-offering at the Annunciation ("greatly humanized") that evokes Christ's supernatural response.[52]

Yet all these comments fail to recognize the transformation taking place through Christianity: Jesus, the mythical divine origin of life, dies in the historical present to reenact the blood sacrifice understood as necessary for renewing life. Moreover, his sacrifice obviates the need for further sacrifice and institutionalizes the use of bread and wine, not flesh and blood (although mystically impregnated with flesh and blood), as the proper communion form.

Critics express repugnance at the idea of the deity Father demanding the bloody sacrifice of his Son. Yet through this sacrifice, a deeply imbedded archetype within human consciousness that demanded blood sacrifice[53] is stilled once and for all. In addition, the institutionalized use of vegetal substances ennobles communion practice. Christian practice effectively demonstrates divine rejection of expiatory blood sacrifice and cannibalism, while at the same time acknowledging the human desire for consuming flesh but supplying it through vegetal substances. It is no wonder that evoking these mythological and existential themes, but then enacting and ennobling them historically, would call forth such an affirmative response among diverse peoples in the world.

APPENDIX B
ALCOHOL

Next to vegetarianism, the question of using alcohol is also of vital concern to spiritual seekers.

All the spiritual teachings in this book that mention alcohol characterize it negatively: chapter 1 recounts that Bhagavad Gita commentators Jayadayol Goyandka, Swami Prabhupada, and Dr. Rudolph Ballentine list alcohol as tamasic; chapter 2 recounts that Pythagoras and the Pythagoreans are generally said to avoid wine. For the Lankavatara Sutra as well as Seventh-Day Adventist founder Ellen White, alcohol is undesirable. Misogi-harai, the Japanese Shinto purification practice, requires abstention; macrobiotics teacher Michio Kushi characterizes alcohol as excessively yin and leading to violent and warlike-behavior; and esoteric philosopher Rudolf Steiner says that, substituting for ego activity, alcohol creates a state of subservience. On the secular side, the health organization Oldways's paradigms recommend moderate consumption, as does the Harvard School of Public Health if alcohol is consumed at all; and the Paleo retrospective of Melvin Konner and S. Boyd Eaton acknowledges alcohol's potential health benefits (even though its use originated with the agricultural revolution, whose products the Paleo movement otherwise generally eschews).

A brief review of the history of alcohol consumption reveals a general cultural and religious ambivalence that acknowledges the benefits of moderate consumption on the one hand while warning against misuse and the "sin" of drunkenness on the other. Trends toward abstention and prohibition extend into modern times. A few voices distinguish between the moderate use that is appropriate in general versus the abstention more appropriate to spiritual seekers.

As with vegetarianism, Rudolf Steiner provides many details about alcohol's effects as well as an evolutionary framework for understanding its significance, which, however, questions appropriateness for modern times.

Hindu Ayurvedic, Sumerian, and Egyptian texts, as well as the Bible, variously speak of alcohol's beneficial effects, which include medicinal ones, but also of disease-related effects. In Greece and Rome, wine was generally consumed by everyone, but in diluted form. In the Middle Ages in Europe, the beer that was generally consumed had a small alcoholic content. The discovery of the Americas revealed that the Aztecs used wine (*pulque*) only for religious purposes, but it was freely available to the elderly. In ancient China, alcohol played an important role in religious and spiritual life, but warnings cautioned against abuse. In Egypt, beer was considered to be a gift of the god Osiris and a life necessity, but moderate use was also stressed. In Greece, the cult of Dionysus exempted the use of wine from the moderation otherwise characterizing behavior (see Pythagoras and the Pythagoreans in chapter 2). Intoxication was encouraged and led to communion with the god and liberation from care and worry. In Hindu Ayurvedic medicine, fermented juices and herbs are used but not recommended for everyone without proper diagnosis. Jainism does not allow alcohol. Buddhists avoid it. In Sikhism, initiates are not allowed intoxicants, including alcohol.[1]

Within the Abrahamic tradition, the Bible characterizes alcohol both positively and negatively. For the Hebrews, wine was part of the created world and something largely positive and good despite the possibility of abuse, which was recognized and condemned. Kings and priests, however, were required to abstain at particular times. Being a Nazarite, John the Baptist was forbidden wine. The letters of the apostle Paul exhort against drinking wine (or eating meat) if it is offensive to others. Christian ethics incorporated the Greek notion of temperance as a virtue and applied it to wine; drunkenness was considered a form of gluttony and deadly sin. In his monastic rule, Benedict (died c. 547 CE) intended to exclude the daily use of wine, but he relented in the face of opposition while still believing that abstinence was best to curb bodily appetites. Islam's dietary rules consider the consumption of fermented drinks sinful. Thomas Aquinas (died 1274) allowed for moderate use, which did not hinder salvation, yet he linked abstinence to perfection as something for individual concern. A range of views existed within Protestantism and the Reformation. Luther, Calvin, and Zwingli all considered wine a blessing. Drunkenness, however, was considered a sin and inconsistent with the prevailing notion of self-mastery. John Wesley, the founder of Methodism, called alcohol a poison. For Methodist preachers, wine was recommended only in a sacramental context or as a medicine. Views about alcohol became more heated and controversial in the wake of the increasing drunkenness associated with the Industrial Revolution and urbanization. It was at this time that the temperance movement began, culminating in 1919 with Prohibition in the United States through the Eighteenth Amendment to the Constitution. Today's Christians are split among positions of moderation, abstention, and prohibition. Prohibitionists think that God ordinarily requires abstention. Abstentionists consider voluntary abstention a matter of prudence. Roman Catholics, Eastern Orthodox members, Anglicans, Lutherans, members of the Reformed churches, and Jehovah's Witnesses all generally adhere to moderate use. This viewpoint stresses the importance of temperance in all behaviors and that abuse originates with the abuser, not the substance abused. The Mormon Church dissuades against using alcohol outside of communion, which is considered binding on all church members. Presently the Mormon rite uses water.[2]

As we can see, religious attitudes toward alcohol are overall as diverse and ambiguous as attitudes toward vegetarianism and meat, yet the sentiment for opposition and prohibition appears to be prevalent.

Rudolf Steiner stresses the potentially harmful and negative effects. As chapter 2 indicates, he criticizes alcohol for usurping ego functions, which he also sees as a potentially negative effect of meat and fat consumption. Yet whereas meat and fat also have benefits (outlined in chapter 2), in the case of alcohol Steiner finds no mitigating benefit in the present, even though there was one in the past (outlined below).

Steiner expressly states that alcohol is more harmful than meat.[3] Under its negative effects, emotions are strengthened but reason's influence is weakened. Abstaining from alcohol is the best means for developing ego forces.[4] Steiner characterizes alcohol as a "veritable opposing power," creating a kind of "anti-ego" that hinders the spiritual ego and makes it powerless; alcohol's interference stifles true spiritual development.[5]

He reveals that the body naturally produces alcohol as a preservative, especially to preserve dissolved protein. Yet the preserving action of alcohol affects the blood by hindering the production of new cells and contributing to general weakening. Too much alcohol in the system enlarges the liver and begins to impair metabolic functions.[6] Alcohol heats the blood and accelerates the circulation, causing much energy to be expended. The overall effect weakens the body and results in the deposit of waste products in the head, leading to hangovers.

Steiner also details alcohol's destructive effects on human offspring: Female red blood corpuscles become heavy, carrying over to the developing fetus and leading to improperly formed organs and conditions such as hydrocephalus. Male white corpuscles are also affected, leading to abnormally mobile sperm and damage to the fetal nervous system (we are reminded that Weston Price attributed negative fetal effects to parental nutrition; see chapters 3 and 4). Steiner asserts that the negative effects on offspring also affect succeeding generations (we are reminded of the proverbial iniquity of the fathers affecting children unto the third and fourth generations [Exod. 34:7; Deut. 5:9; Num. 14:18]).

Steiner emphasizes that explaining such negative effects works in a beneficially educative way by affecting the feelings, in contrast to laws working through the intellect. Outlining effects clearly and letting individuals decide on appropriate action achieves more and preserves human freedom. This, he says, is the true path to social reform.[7] Regarding the time of Prohibition in the United States, Steiner laments using laws to control behavior rather than providing rational explanations about effects (which, of course, he is uniquely able to do).

Steiner continues that alcohol works like arsenic on the astral body and ego and that the astral effect on children is particularly harmful.[8] The earliest of his lectures touching on alcohol puts its development and use into an evolutionary framework. In the course of evolution spanning eons and different planetary conditions, human nourishment took on various forms. The first was a kind of milk that was sucked directly out of the earth as it existed at that time. The second was nourishment from the upper parts of plants, such as blossoms and fruits exposed to the warmth of the sun. Both forms continued to exist side by side and had to do with life forces. The third and first "dead" form of nourishment was obtained by killing animals. Though lifeless, this form of food allowed for the important transition to ego-hood and independence (we have touched on this theme before, both in Steiner's dietary indications recounted in chapter 2 and in the Blood-Type Diet's personality characteristics recounted in chapter 4). A subsequent phase began to include vegetables from below the earth (root vegetables), which were similarly "dead" in the sense of not exposed directly to the life principle of the sun. (In chapter 2, we heard of negative effects associated with foods like potatoes that grow under the earth.) A later phase introduced purely mineral substances (such as salt), similarly coming from below the earth. The latter three phases represented nourishment from the kingdoms of minerals, plants, and animals. The next phase involved chemical processes applied to fruits and plants, namely, the fermentation that produces alcohol. A sacred character was ascribed to wine (e.g., in the cult of Dionysus), and paradoxically Steiner explains the religious significance as cutting human beings off from the direct experience of spiritual reality. This, however, represented a further and necessary evolutionary step down to the physical plane of material reality. Spiritual initiates had previously used water in rituals to cultivate the direct experience of spiritual reality, yet wine cut off direct contact in order to complete the descent to the lowest point. According to Steiner, the Wedding of Cana in the Gospel of John, where Jesus changes water into wine, reflects this change in emphasis. Now that the process of descent has been completed, however, the next evolutionary phase begins to ascend and involves transitioning from dead to living nourishment. The communion of Jesus (flesh and blood in the form of bread and wine: see chapters 5 and 6) symbolizes the transition from nourishment with dead animals to nourishment with dead plants (wheat dies through harvesting and baking, grapes through fermentation). Eventually the stage will be reached when humans no longer need natural nourishment but will instead create their own mineral source of food.[9]

As we have seen, ego development is an important part of this nutritional evolutionary understanding. The transition to dead food involved the development of ego-hood, and the use of wine signified full descent to the physical-material plane. Reascending evolution now relies on continuing to develop and exert ego strength. Within this context, it is understandable that alcohol's negative ego effects are counter-evolutionary.

As we saw in chapter 2 regarding vegetarianism, Steiner puts pro-and-con assessments about alcohol into an evolutionary framework. Steiner is, of course, not the only or ultimate authority, but one among many voices. What remains is a broad consensus among religious and spiritual traditions recommending at best moderate alcohol consumption and perhaps none at all, especially for spiritual seekers. Arguably the best rationale for abstention is not divine prohibition or the desire to exercise virtue but knowledge of the effects.

Appendix C
Raw Foods

Raw foods are a dietary issue of current interest for many spiritually minded people. Dr. Gabriel Cousens, who has been cited a few times in this work, emphasizes in his book *Spiritual Nutrition* the importance of live foods for feeding and energizing the Kundalini vortex, the focus of his spiritual path. Cousens acknowledges that the Indian Ayurvedic tradition does not stress raw foods and that his emphasis on their use represents a new nutritional paradigm.[1] He justifies this emphasis on the basis of his own experience, both personal and with patients, and on Essene teachings such as those found in *The Essene Gospel of Peace*, translated by Edmond Bordeaux Szekely, which assert that the Essenes and Jesus himself recommended raw foods:

> But I do say to you: Kill ... [not] the food which goes into your mouth. For if you eat living food, the same will quicken you, but if you kill your food, the dead food will kill you also. For life comes only from life, and from death comes always death. For everything which kills your foods, kills your bodies also. And everything which kills your bodies kills your souls also.[2]

Next to these witnesses, Cousens cites scientific evidence suggesting that unheated, intact enzymes and nutrients are more nourishing for the body.[3]

In classifying the nutritional value of different kinds of food, Cousens uses Edmond Bordeaux Szekely's fourfold system:

- Biogenic: life renewing; includes germinated cereal seeds, nuts, and sprouted baby greens

- Bioactive: life sustaining; includes organic, natural vegetables and fruit

- Biostatic: life slowing; includes cooked, stale foods (but legumes must be cooked after sprouting them first)

- Biocidic: life destroying; includes processed, irradiated foods and drinks[4]

Based on this system, Cousens recommends a diet composed of 80 percent biogenic and bioactive foods and 20 percent biostatic,[5] which is close to Szekely's own recommendations (biocidic foods, of course, should be avoided). These, however, are general recommendations. Cousens allows for individual considerations and also emphasizes that diet is but one of his six foundations for spiritual life, all of which work together. Nevertheless, live foods are the focus of dietary recommendations.

An opposing voice from the authors cited in this book is Rudolf Steiner's. He criticizes any emphasis on raw foods in asserting that cooking aids nutrition. Applying heat is necessary to transform carbohydrates into starch and sugar, allowing the body to conserve energy. Applying heat also helps the body to get the full benefit from foods such as potatoes, which nourish the head but get stuck in the intestines if they are ingested raw. Steiner continues that raw foods seem to boost the body's energy at first due to increased digestive effort, but harm later results. Cooking is especially important for foods not directly exposed to warmth during growth (such as potatoes) and foods without leaf and foliage (i.e., grains).[6] Bodily constitution, Steiner continues, is another factor. People with strong constitutions may benefit from a raw foods diet, but not those with weak ones.[7]

Cousens, for his part, acknowledges that some people may not have the digestive power necessary for a vegetarian diet and allows for individual variation. (To arguments in favor of raw foods, we can add the beneficial effect of sprouting seeds, which greatly enhances nutritional contents and digestibility.)

Perhaps the most controversial among Cousens's arguments for raw foods is the authority of *The Essene Gospel of Peace* and Jesus himself. Edmond Bordeaux Szekely, the translator and publisher of *The Essene Gospel of Peace*, claims to have found the different manuscripts used for compiling it in various languages and in different places (the Vatican Library, the Royal Archives of the Hapsburgs in Vienna, and the monastery of Monte Casino in Italy). Yet no one other than Szekely claims to have seen these manuscripts, nor did Szekely ever provide documentary proof. The Vatican Library denies the existence of a manuscript and also denies Szekely's visit. The Royal Archives in Vienna similarly denies the existence of a manuscript, and the monastery in Monte Casino was destroyed during World War II. Most critics and scholars agree that Szekely himself authored *The Essene Gospel of Peace*, which is to say that Szekely's claims are fraudulent. Alleging his own authorship accords with what is known about the history of raw foods as a subject of interest. Sylvester Graham is cited as the first proponent in the 1830s, and interest in the early twentieth century is seen as a reflection of the natural health movements and spiritualities that became popular after World War I, the period when *The Essene Gospel of Peace* first appeared.[8]

The lack of original manuscripts undermines the authority of *The Essene Gospel of Peace* and of Jesus for justifying a raw-foods diet. Proponents may well cry conspiracy and cover-up: Jesus's advocacy for raw foods would seem so controversial and threatening to mainstream understanding today that the evidence must be suppressed. One can only reply that in popular culture, standards exist for truth, and documented evidence for novel claims is one such standard.

The authenticity of *The Essene Gospel of Peace* and its raw-foods message versus the contrary view of Rudolf Steiner has personal relevance and significance for me. In the late 1970s, I encountered *The Essene Gospel of Peace* and Dr. Szekely's other works and attended his last seminar, held in Costa Rica in the winter of 1979, a few months before his untimely death (I appear in the photographs of Szekely's book *The First Essene*, which documents this seminar). After a personal interview with Dr. Szekely in which I attested to having studied particular books among his works, I was granted the certificate of "Teacher of Biogenic Living." When I mentioned that I had recently become interested in the work of Rudolf Steiner, Dr. Szekely replied, "You don't need all of that, you just need the Essene teachings."

During the seminar a protrusion was visible above Szekely's waist on the front of his body. When he died a few months later, it was reported that this sac had burst, killing him. I was left wondering how this healer of thousands through means such as raw foods had been unable to heal himself. When anthroposophy and Steiner's work subsequently became the major focus of my spiritual path in the decade ahead, superseding interest in Szekely's own work, I wished I had asked Szekely what he had meant in saying, "You don't need all of that."

Spirituality can be succinctly defined as the pursuit of the Beautiful, the Good, and the True (otherwise known as God, understood as a real person in whose image and likeness human beings are created, but also as an impersonal and universal principle or force). As for anthroposophical spirituality, I have in the past and would still characterize it today as an "Alaska" experience. One of my deepest and most lasting impressions from having lived in Alaska for two and a half years has been the feeling of awe before the grandeur and majesty of nature, something I've experienced nowhere else and difficult to adequately convey in words or through pictures. This was an experience of nature qualifying as a peak experience and a spiritual experience—of the beautiful, the good, and the true with regard to the natural world. Anthroposophy represents a similar kind of experience for me with regard to spirituality. It has not been the end point. Rudolf Steiner himself emphasized that the spiritual world is continuously speaking to human beings, and the Eastern notion of Sanatana Dharma similarly speaks of the eternal unfolding of truth. Two significant manifestations of the spiritually Beautiful, Good, and True in the twentieth century since the time of Steiner are the Integral Yoga of Sri Aurobindo and the Christian Hermeticism of the anonymous author cited in chapter 8. Nevertheless, anthroposophy remains for me a standard by which to judge other spiritual conceptions; and, by this standard, the Essene works of Edmond Bordeaux Szekely occupy lesser status.

Yet this is not to say that Szekely's work has no spiritual value, even if it is alleged to be wholly or partly a creation of his own mind. The widespread availability of Essene or manna breads today, the roots of which are easily traceable to *The Essene Gospel of Peace*, is reason enough to celebrate Szekely's memory as the bequeather or renewer of this nourishing gift of food. (The manna bread made by Manna Organics quotes *The Essene Gospel of Peace* on the back of the package, and readers will recall that the Blood-Type Diet recommends Essene or manna bread for all blood types despite an otherwise general caution about wheat products.) In addition, poetry from the Essene Gospels is listed among the world's sacred poetry, even though it is attributed to Szekely himself due to the controversy about authenticity.[9] His memory deserves to be honored, but not in terms of authoritative claims for a raw foods diet that invoke the name of Jesus.

As has been pointed out several times, this book seeks the harmony between different points of view. In this sense, the debate about raw foods is not resolved by Rudolf Steiner's view or the questionable authenticity of *The Essene Gospel of Peace*. The question remains as to how raw foods otherwise measure up to the witness of cultural traditions. The record suggests that the therapeutic use of raw foods, and especially their recommendation as a lifestyle diet, are relatively recent phenomena and therefore to be approached with caution.[10]

Sally Fallon, on the other hand, can be recommended as someone who takes a balanced approach to raw foods. In favor of cooking, she makes the following points:

- Cellulose in vegetables must be broken down by humans and herbivorous animals.

- Animals use stomach fermentation; humans apply external heat.

- No traditional culture has ever eaten only raw foods, even in the tropics.

- Cooking makes some nutrients more available while also neutralizing toxins.[11]

Fallon recommends cooking grains, legumes, and some vegetables. Yet she also notes that the traditional diets Weston Price cites all include some raw animal and vegetable foods.[12] In their favor, raw vegetables keep the intestines moist and provide bulk and roughage, which helps to eliminate wastes and keep muscles strong, yet they can also cause irritation if the intestines are inflamed.[13] For those who are unable to tolerate them or disinclined to eat them, Fallon recommends including enzyme-rich condiments with meals in emulation of Asian cultures.[14]

Some final comparative remarks are appropriate about the link Cousens makes between raw foods and energizing the Kundalini vortex—the focus of his spiritual practice, involving the ascent of the Kundalini through the chakra system. Steiner indicates that the chakras have been evolving and that spiritual development for modern times focuses on a top-down movement, not a bottom-up one.[15] In Steiner's understanding, the illuminating influence of the Holy Spirit is involved, similar to the Christian understanding of the Holy Spirit's descent at Pentecost. This is yet another issue for reader consideration and discrimination.

NOTES

Foreword

1. Salynn Boyles, "Tomatoes Don't Prevent Prostate Cancer," *WebMD*, May 17, 2007, accessed September 28, 2016, http://www.webmd.com/prostate-cancer/news/20070517/tomatoes-dont-prevent-prostate-cancer.

2. Helen Briggs, "Tomatoes 'Important in Prostate Cancer Prevention,'" *BBC News*, August 27, 2014, accessed September 28, 2016, http://www.bbc.com/news/health-28950093.

3. Diogenes Laertius 8.19; trans. C. D. Yonge, accessed September 28, 2016, http://www.classicpersuasion.org/pw/diogenes/dlpythagoras.htm.

4. Richard Smoley, *Forbidden Faith: The Secret History of Gnosticism* (San Francisco: Harper San Francisco, 2006), 36. The quoted passage is from Herodotus 2.37.

5. "Favism," *G6PD Deficiency*, accessed September 28, 2016, http://g6pd-deficiency.org/wp/g6pd-deficiency-home/favism-2/#.V-wfWySoeVs.

6. Robert S. Lynd and Helen Merrell Lynd, *Middletown: A Study in American Culture* (New York: Harcourt, Brace & Co., 1929), 156–57. The "Middletown" in this famous study is not named in the book, but it is known to have been Muncie, Indiana.

7. Anahad O'Connor, "Why Your Granola Is Really a Dessert," *The New York Times*, August 30, 2016, accessed September 29, 2016, http://www.nytimes.com/2016/08/30/well/eat/why-your-granola-is-really-a-dessert.html?_r=0.

8. W. K. C. Guthrie, *A History of Greek Philosophy*, vol. 1, *The Earlier Presocratics and the Pythagoreans* (Cambridge, UK: Cambridge University Press, 1962), 251.

9. Philostratus, *Life of Apollonius of Tyana*, 1.32; in Christopher P. Jones, ed. and trans., *Philostratus: Apollonius of Tyana, Books 1–4* (Cambridge, MA: Loeb Classical Library, 2005), 111.

10. Nate Jenkins, "More Horses Sent Abroad for Slaughter," *USA Today*, November 26, 2008, accessed September 30, 2016, http://usatoday30.usatoday.com/news/nation/2008-11-26-2714067585_x.htm.

Chapter 1

1. "Hinduism," *Wikipedia*, accessed March 3, 2016, http://en.wikipedia.org/wiki/Hinduism.

2. The lines from the Bhagavad Gita are as quoted in Sri Aurobindo, *The Message of the Gita* (Pondicherry, India: Sri Aurobindo Ashram, 1977), 204–5.

3. Judith M. Tyberg, *The Language of the Gods,* 2nd ed. (Los Angeles: East West Cultural Center, 1976), 34–35.

4. In Aurobindo, *Message of the Gita*, 205–6.

5. Ibid., 204–5.

6. Ibid., 205, 222.

7. "Guna," *Wikipedia*, accessed March 3, 2016, http://en.wikipedia.org/wiki/Gu%E1%B9%87a.

8. In Aurobindo, *Message of the Gita*, 234–35.

9. Ibid., 290–92.

10. Jayadayol Goyandka, trans., *Kalyana Kalpataru* 14, Gita Tattva no. 3 (1948): 136.

11. Swami Nidhilananda, *The Upanishads,* vol. 4 (New York: Harper & Brothers, 1959), 356–57.

12. Goyandka, *Kalyana Kalpataru*, 137.

13. "Sattvic Diet," *Wikipedia*, accessed March 3, 2016, http://en.wikipedia.org/wiki/Sattvic diet.

14. Swami Prabhupada Bhakivedanta, A C, *Bhagavad-Gita As It Is* (New York: Bhaktivedanta Book Trust, 1968), 248.

15. Rudolph Ballentine, MD, *Diet and Nutrition: A Holistic Approach,* (Honesdale, PA: Himalayan International Institute, 1982), 547–51.

16. Vijay, comp., *Sri Aurobindo and the Mother on Food* (Pondicherry, India: Sri Aurobindo Society, 1973), 58.

17. Email communication from Vijay to the author, June 5, 2013.

18. Gary Gran, "The Sattvic or Yogic Diet," *YogaChicago*, January/February 2005, accessed November 11, 2016, http://yogachicago.com/2014/03/the-sattvic-or-yogic-diet/.

19. Ibid.

Chapter 2

1. "Holism," *Wikipedia*, accessed March 3, 2016, http://en.wikipedia.org/wiki/Holism.

2. Aurobindo, *Message of the Gita*, 291–92 (see chap. 1, n. 2).

3. Ibid., 288–92.

4. Solomon Schechter, Julius H. Greenstone, Emil G. Hirsch, and Kaufmann Kohler, "Dietary Laws," *Jewish Encyclopedia*, accessed March 3, 2016, http://www.jewishencyclopedia.com/articles/5191-dietary-laws.

5. Source for animals is "Clean Animal," *Creation Wiki*, accessed March 3, 2016, http://creationwiki.org/Clean animal; for birds, "Letter of Aristeas," quoted in Rav Avraham Yitzhak Hacohen Kook, *A Vision of Vegetarianism and Peace,* ed. Rabbi David Cohen, trans. with additional notes by Jonathan Rubenstein (from his unpublished rabbinic thesis), section 13, PDF e-book.

6. Harry Rabinowicz and Rela Mintz Geffen, "Dietary Laws," *Encyclopaedia Judaica*, ed. Michael Berenbaum and Fred Skolnik, 2nd ed. vol. 5 (Detroit: Macmillan Reference USA, 2007), 650–59, *Gale Virtual Reference Library*, accessed March 3, 2016, http://go.galegroup.com/ps/i.do?id=GALE%7CCCX2587505214&v=2.1&u=gonzagaufoley&it=r&p=GVRL&sw=w&asid=6cb6737b6fae827759b913f6e05cd025. The Hirsch reference is *Horeb*, section 454.

7. Emil G. Hirsch, Henry Hyvernat Executive Committee of the Editorial Board [sic], and Louis Ginzberg, "Clean and Unclean Animals," *Jewish Encyclopedia*, accessed February 16, 2016, http://www.jewishencyclopedia.com/articles/4408-clean-and-unclean-animals. The Zarza reference is to Mekor Hayyim, "Tazria,' [sic]" beginning [of the passage].

8. Rabinowicz and Geffen, "Dietary Laws," *Encyclopedia Judaica*; the Arama reference is to *Akedat Yizhak, Sha'ar Shemini*, 60–end.

9. Arama, quoted in David Sears, *The Vision of Eden, Animal Welfare and Vegetarianism in Jewish Law and Mysticism* (Spring Valley, NY: Logo, 2011), PDF e-book, 199. Sears references Arama's Torah commentary, *Akeidas Yitzchak* ("The Binding of Isaac").

10. Ibid., [Sears], 353.

11. The source for Nachmanides and Albo is Sears, *Vision of Eden*, 215–16. For Nachmanides, Sears refers to *Commentary on the Torah, Vayikra*, ch. 11 et passim; for Albo, to *Sefer HaIkkarim* 3:15.

12. Rav Kook, *A Vision of Vegetarianism and Peace*, section 13.

13. Hirsch et al., "Clean and Unclean Animals," *Jewish Encyclopedia*. The Philo reference is "De Concupiscentia," 5–10.

14. Iamblichus, *The Life of Pythagoras or On the Pythagorean Life*, sect. 29, "Sciences and Maxims," in Kenneth Sylvan Guthrie, comp. and trans., *The Pythagorean Sourcebook and Library: An Anthology of Ancient Writings which Relate to Pythagoras and Pythagorean Philosophy*, with additional translations by Thomas Taylor and Arthur Fairbanks, Jr.; introduction and edited by David R. Fiedeler (Grand Rapids, MI: Phanes Press, 1988), 98.

15. Guthrie, *Pythagorean Sourcebook*, 19.

16. Ibid., 30.

17. Timaeus of Locri: *On the World and the Soul*, sect. 11, "Discipline," in ibid., 295.

18. Iamblichus, sect. 31, "Temperance and Self-Control, in ibid., 107.

19. Preface to "The Pythagorean Symbols or Maxims" in ibid., 159.

20. Iamblichus, sect. 24, "Dietary Suggestions," in ibid., 84.

21. Ibid.

22. Iamblichus., sect. 30, "Justice and Politics," in ibid., 103.

23. Iamblichus, sect. 31, "Temperance and Self-Control," and sect. 32, "Courage or Fortitude," in ibid., 103–112.

24. Diogenes Laertius, *The Life of Pythagoras*, sect. 12, "Diet and Sacrifices," in ibid., 145.

25. Iamblichus, sect. 3, "Journey to Egypt," in ibid., 60.

26. Porphyry, *The Life of Pythagoras*, para. 45, in ibid., 132.

27. Timaeus of Locri, sect. 11, "Discipline," in ibid., 295.

28. "The Golden Verses of Pythagoras," in ibid., 164.

29. Porphyry, para. 34, in ibid., 130.

30. Iamblichus, sect. 24, "Dietary Suggestions," in ibid., 84; Porphyry, para. 36, in ibid., 130.

31. *The Anonymous Life of Pythagoras Preserved by Photius*, sect. 1, in ibid., 137.

32. Diogenes Laertius, sect. 19, "Various Teachings," in ibid., 147.

33. "The Pythagorean Symbols or Maxims," no. 22, cited in ibid., 160.

34. Diogenes Laertius, sect. 23, "Jesting Epigrams," in ibid., 153.

35. Iamblichus, sect. 24, "Dietary Suggestions," in ibid., 84.

36. Iamblichus, sect. 35, "The Attack on Pythagoreanism," in ibid., 119.

37. Diogenes Laertius, sect. 19, "Various Teachings," in ibid., 147, 149–50.

38. Porphyry, para. 44, in ibid., 132; passages referring to the Pythagoreans from the Doxographers, trans. Arthur Fairbanks, Hippol., *Phil. 2; Dox.* 555, cited in ibid., 313.

39. Porphyry, paras 42–44, in ibid., 131–32.

40. Rudolf Steiner, "Digestion and Thinking, Digestion and Vegetarianism," lecture of October 22, 1906, in *Nutrition and Stimulants, Lectures and Extracts*, trans. Maria St. Goar (Kimberton, PA: Bio-Dynamic Farming and Gardening Association, Inc., 1991), 131.

41. Iamblichus, sect. 16, "Pythagorean Asceticism," 73; sect. 21, "The Daily Program," 82; and sect. 24, "Dietary Suggestions," 84; and Diogenes Laertius, sect. 18, "Personal Habits," 146. All in Guthrie, *Pythagorean Sourcebook*.

42. Porphyry, para. 45, in ibid., 132.

43. Porphyry, para. 34, in ibid., 130.

44. Ibid., para. 35.

45. Daisetz Teitaro Suzuki, trans., *The Lankavatara Sutra: A Mahayana Text* (London: Routledge and Kegan Paul, 1932), 212, verses 245–46. Online version, http://lirs.ru/do/lanka_eng/lanka-contents.htm#contents.

46. Ibid., 215, verses 249–50.

47. Ibid., 218, verse 254.

48. Ibid., 219–21, verses 256–59.

49. Jean Herbert, *Shinto: At the Fountainhead of Japan* (New York: Stein & Day, 1967), 79.

50. Ibid., 79–82.

51. D. C. Holton, *The National Faith of Japan* (New York: Paragon Book Reprint Corp., 1965), 233.

52. Ibid., 234.

53. Ibid., 237, 239.

54. Ibid., 239.

55. Ibid.

56. Herbert, *Shinto*, 76.

57. Holton, *The National Faith of Japan*, 240.

58. John Cook, *Diet and Your Religion* (Santa Barbara: Woodbridge Press, 1976), 93, 102.

59. Ibid., 95–98.

60. Ibid., 94.

61. Ellen G. White, *Counsels on Diet and Foods* (Hagerstown, MD.: Review and Herald, 2001), 81, 481–82. I am indebted to Cook's *Diet and Your Religion* for pointing to the Ellen White references.

62. Ibid., 92.

63. Ellen G. White, *Testimonies for the Church*, vol. 2 (Nampa, ID: Pacific Press, 1948), 63.

64. White, *Counsels on Diet and Foods*, 393–94.

65. Ibid., 468.

66. Annie Besant, *Vegetarianism in the Light of Theosophy*, Adyar Pamphlet no. 27, 3rd ed. (Adyar, India: Theosophical Publishing House, April, 1932).

67. Ibid., 10–11.

68. Ibid., 12–13.

69. Ibid., 15.

70. "Looney Law" (cited example: "Butchers cannot serve on a murder jury trial in South Carolina"), *Urban Dictionary*, accessed March 3, 2016, http://www.urbandictionary.com/define.php?term=Loony%20Law.

    "Best Ways to Avoid Jury Duty," *Baby Hatchetface Can't Lose!* accessed March 3, 2016, http://babyhatchetblog.wordpress.com/2006/09/13/best-ways-to-avoid-jury-duty/; the writer says (example #10): "Apparently if you are a butcher and are in the jury pool for a violent crimes case, the attorneys will kick you out of the box because blood and gore are desensitized parts of your everyday life."

    "Olden Day Surgeons," *Google News*, accessed March 3, 2016, http://news.google.com/newspapers?nid=2306&dat=19081128&id=vqs-nAAAAIBAJ&sjid=nAQGAAAAIBAJ&pg=3011,3259766; this is a reproduction of a newspaper story from *The Freeman*, November 28, 1908, comparing surgeons in the past to butchers because they were excluded from jury duty.

71. Besant, *Vegetarianism in the Light of Theosophy*, 23–24.

72. Ibid., 25.

73. C. W. Leadbeater, *Vegetarianism and Occultism*, pamphlet no. 33 (Adyar, India: Theosophical Publishing House, November, 1913).

74. Otoman Zar-Adusht Ha'Nish, *A Vegetarian Science of Dietetics*, 9th ed. (Los Angeles: Mazdaznan Press, 1976), 15.

75. Ibid.

76. Ibid., 24.

77. Otoman Zar-Adusht Ha'Nish, *The Power of Breath*, rev. ed. (Los Angeles: Mazdaznan Press, 1970), 208.

78. Ha'Nish, *Vegetarian Science of Dietetics*, 238–39.

79. Ha'Nish, *Power of Breath*, 185.

80. Ha'Nish, *Vegetarian Science of Dietetics*, 201.

81. Ibid., 206.

82. Ronald Kotzsch, "Who Started Macrobiotics?" *East West Journal* (May 1980): 60–67.

83. George Ohsawa, *Zen Macrobiotics* (Los Angeles: The Ohsawa Foundation, Inc., 1965), 22.

84. Ibid., 33, 57.

85. George Ohsawa, *You Are All Sanpaku* (Seacaucus, NJ: University Books, 1965), 128.

86. Ibid., 178.

87. Ohsawa, *Zen Macrobiotics*, 34.

88. Michio Kushi with Alex Jack, *The Book of Macrobiotics: The Universal Way of Health, Happiness, and Peace*, (Garden City Park, NY: Square One, 2012), 73.

89. Ibid., 72–73.

90. Ibid., 137.

91. Ibid., 138.

92. Ibid., 256–57.

93. Ibid., 257–58.

94. Ibid., 269–72.

95. Ibid., 272.

96. Ibid., 295–318.

97. Ibid., 295.

98. Rudolf Steiner, *Problems of Nutrition*, booklet (New York: Anthroposophic Press, 1973), 7.

99. Steiner, "Problems of Nutrition," lecture of January 8, 1909, in *Nutrition and Stimulants*, 146.

100. Ibid., 147–48.

101. Ibid., 148–49.

102. Ibid.

103. Ibid.

104. Steiner, "The Connection between Food and the Human Being: Raw Foods and Vegetarian Diet," lecture of July 31,1924, in *Nutrition and Stimulants*, 107.

105. Mary G. Enig, PhD, *Know Your Fats* (Silver Spring, MD: Bethesda Press, 2000), 50.

106. Email correspondence with Sally Fallon Morell, October 10, 2016. She further noted, "Zinc deficiency leads to a feeling of spaciness, which vegetarians interpret as a spiritual feeling. Sex and reproduction are impossible when zinc is low, so . . . to promote veganism or vegetarianism to young men and women before and during child-bearing age is irresponsible. . . . B_{12} deficiency can lead to irrational anger, which belies the claim that avoiding meat will make one more peaceful and eliminate war."

    Morell went on to express this opinion: "Vegan/vegetarian diets are promoted by cult gurus who want docile followers, and by the food processing industry, which makes more money on plant-based foods than animal-based foods. It engenders a spiritual pride in the followers, making them believe that they are more spiritual, pure, and holy than the rest of us, who eat a varied and nutrient-dense diet in order to have the strength and mental capacity to do the important work of making the world a better place. The only way that vegetarianism can work is in places like India, where they have good quality raw dairy products, eat lots of ghee, and have a lot of insects parts and insect feces in the grains to supply B_{12} and minerals."

107. Steiner, "Problems of Nutrition," in *Nutrition and Stimulants*, 150.

108. Steiner, "Digestion and Thinking," in *Nutrition and Stimulants*, 131–32.

109. Steiner, "Meat, Vegetarian Food, Alcohol," lecture of March 20, 1913, in *Nutrition and Stimulants*, 159.

110. Steiner, *Problems of Nutrition* (booklet), foreword.

111. Steiner, "Problems of Nutrition," in *Nutrition and Stimulants*, 151.

112. Ibid.

113. Steiner, "Digestion and Thinking," in *Nutrition and Stimulants*, 128–29.

114. Steiner, "The Effects of Spiritual Development," lecture of March 21, 1913, in *Nutrition and Stimulants*, 169–70.

115. Steiner, "Problems of Nutrition," in *Nutrition and Stimulants*, 152.

116. Steiner, "The Effects of Spiritual Development," in *Nutrition and Stimulants*, 170.

117. Steiner, "Digestion and Thinking," in *Nutrition and Stimulants*, 129.

118. Steiner, "Problems of Nutrition," in *Nutrition and Stimulants*, 152. Gerhardt Schmidt suggests that Steiner's remarks refer to raw milk.

See Gerhard Schmidt, MD, *The Dynamics of Nutrition* (Wyoming, RI: Bio-Dynamic Literature, 1980), 144.

119. Steiner, "Digestion and Thinking," in *Nutrition and Stimulants*, 131.

120. Steiner, "The Connection between Food and the Human Being," in *Nutrition and Stimulants*. See also in that book "Protein, Fats, Carbohydrates and Salts, Potatoes and Materialism, Hydrocephalus," lecture of October 22, 1923; and "Nutrition and Child Nutrition: The Digestion of Protein, Arterial Sclerosis," lecture of August 2, 1924, 66, 69, 101, 116.

121. Steiner, "Problems of Nutrition," in *Nutrition and Stimulants*, 153.

122. Dalai Lama, "Compassion for All Sentient Beings," in Kerry S. Walters and Lisa Portmess, eds., *Religious Vegetarianism, From Hesiod to the Dalai Lama* (Albany, NY: State University of New York Press, 2001), 87–91; "Sir Paul McCartney's Advice to the Dalai Lama," *The Times*, December 15, 2008, accessed March 3, 2016, http://www.thetimes.co.uk/tto/faith/article2099953.ece; "An Open Letter from Norm Phelps to the Dalai Lama – 15 Jun [sic] 2007, " *All-Creatures.org*, accessed March 3, 2016, http://www.all-creatures.org/letters/20070615-np.html.

Chapter 3

1. David Hawkins and Linus Pauling, *Orthomolecular Psychiatry: Treatment of Schizophrenia* (San Francisco: Freeman and Co., 1973), 1.

2. Ibid., 11.

3. Ibid., vi.

4. Ibid.

5. E. Cheraskin and W. M. Ringsdorf Jr., *Psychodietetics* (New York: Stein and Day, 1974), 20.

6. Abram Hoffer's foreword in Michael Lesser, MD, *The Brain Chemistry Diet* (New York: G. P. Putnam's Sons, 2002), xiv–xvi.

7. Cheraskin and Ringsdorf Jr., *Psychodietics*, 20. See also Carlton Fredericks, *Psycho-Nutrition* (New York: Grosset and Dunlap, 1976); Abram Hoffer, MD, PhD, and Morton Walker, DPM, *Putting It All Together: the New Orthomolecular Nutrition* (New Canaan, CT: Keats,

1996); and Roger J. Williams, *Nutrition against Disease* (New York: Pitman, 1971).

8. Abram Hoffer and H. Osmond, *Megavitamin Therapy* (Regina, SK: Canadian Schizophrenia Foundation, 1976), 67; Abram Hoffer, MD, PhD, and Andrew W. Saul, PhD, *Orthomolecular Medicine for Everyone* (Laguna Beach, CA: Basic Health Publications, 2008), 253–83.

9. The list includes mood disorders such as anxiety, depressions, mood swings, addictions, learning disorders such as attention-deficit/hyperactivity disorder, Down syndrome, criminal behavior, and aging-brain disorders such as senility and Alzheimer's disease. See Hoffer and Saul, *Orthomolecular Medicine for Everyone*, chaps. 5 and 14.

10. The journal is the *Journal for Orthomolecular Medicine* (formerly known as the *Journal for Orthomolecular Psychiatry*); the name of the annual international conference is Orthomolecular Medicine Today. See the *Orthomolecular Medicine* website, accessed March 4, 2016, http://www.orthomed.org/index.html.

11. American Psychiatric Association, *Megavitamin and Orthomolecular Therapy in Psychiatry* (Washington, DC: American Psychiatric Association, 1973).

12. Hoffer and Osmond, *Megavitamin Therapy*, 67; Hoffer and Walker, *Putting It All Together*, 208. For various responses, see the archives of the International Schizophrenia Foundation, accessed March 4, 2016, http://www.orthomed.org/isf/isf.html, and search "1973 task force report."

13. "Orthomolecular medicine," *Wikipedia*, accessed March 4, 2016, http://en.wikipedia.org/wiki/Orthomolecular_medicine.

14. Abram Hoffer, MD, PhD, and Andrew W. Saul, PhD, *The Vitamin Cure for Alcoholism* (Laguna Beach, CA: Basic Health Publications, 2009), 97; Hoffer and Saul, *Orthomolecular Medicine for Everyone*, 1–2, 324–25, in which on p. 2 Hoffer and Saul write, "Despite the common protestation that there are no studies showing that high-dose nutrition works, there are in fact thousands and thousands of clinical studies that do just that." In addition to the studies listed in various books, they also suggest searching the online bibliographies at www.doctoryourself.com.

15. Hoffer and Saul, *The Vitamin Cure for Alcoholism*, ix.

16. Ruth Adams and Frank Murray, *Megavitamin Therapy* (New York: Larchmont Books, 1973), 159; George Watson, *Nutrition and Your Mind* (New York: Pitman, 1971), 19, 26; Hawkins and Pauling, *Orthomolecular Psychiatry*, 1; Hoffer and Walker, *Putting It All Together*, 16–17; Williams, *Nutrition against Disease*, 11.

17. Fredericks, *Psycho-Nutrition*, 20–21; Hoffer and Walker, *Putting It All Together*, 50.

18. Fredericks, *Psycho-Nutrition*, 13–24; Hoffer and Walker, *Putting It All Together*, preface to the first edition, xi–xii, 50; Watson, *Nutrition and Your Mind*, 1–19.

19. Both Fredericks (*Psycho-Nutrition*, 13–14) and Watson (*Nutrition and Your Mind*, 1–20) have emphasized the biological causes of psychological states, denigrating psychological treatment approaches. Yet others, such as Cheraskin and Ringsdorf Jr. (*Psychodietetics*, 2) and Williams (*Nutrition against Disease*, 167–68) are more integrative, stressing the need for both treatment forms.

20. The following books emphasize the themes of right and wrong molecules and adulterated, refined, and processed foods providing wrong molecules: Adams and Murray, *Megavitamin Therapy*; Cheraskin and Ringsdorf Jr., *Psychodietetics*; Fredericks, *Psycho-Nutrition*; Hoffer and Walker, *Putting It All Together*; Williams, *Nutrition against Disease*.

21. Fredericks, *Psycho-Nutrition*, 52.

22. Hoffer and Walker, *Putting It All Together*, 123–24.

23. William Dufty, *Sugar Blues* (New York: Warner Books, 1975), 117–33.

24. Adams and Murray, *Megavitamin Therapy*, 190–225; Cheraskin and Ringsdorf Jr., *Psychodietetics*, 71–84; Fredericks, *Psycho-Nutrition*, 149–56.

25. Hoffer and Walker, *Putting It All Together*, 72–74.

26. Fredericks, *Psycho-Nutrition*, 183–84.

27. Hoffer and Walker, *Putting It All Together*, 5–6.

28. Ibid., 66.

29. Ibid., 136.

30. Ibid., 93, 125.

31. Weston A. Price, *Nutrition and Physical Degeneration*, 7th ed. (La Mesa, CA: Price-Pottenger Nutritional Foundation, 2008).

32. Ibid., 362, 366, 373, 464. Imitating native practices, Price's own recommendations were milk, green vegetables, sea foods, animal organs, high-vitamin butter, and cod liver oil. See 373.

33. Ibid., 322 ff. Price cites one researcher who associates abnormal mouth palates with 19 percent of the ordinary population, 33 percent for the insane, 55 percent for criminals, and 61 percent for "idiots." Another provides the figures of 82 percent for mental defectives, 76 percent for epileptics, and 80 percent for the insane. See 361–62, 459.

34. Ibid., 2; also see ch. 19, "Physical, Mental and Moral Deterioration," 321–47.

35. Ibid., 325.

36. Ibid., 323, 342.

37. Ibid., 304, 331, 338. Price also notes that since the majority of Down syndrome persons are born to mothers over age forty, the mother's reduced reproductive capacity is also important.

38. Ibid., 336–37.

39. Ibid., 7. The first quote paraphrases Edward Lee Thorndike of Columbia University (see p. 14).

40. Ibid., 508.

41. Ibid., 419–27.

42. Ibid., 421.

43. Ibid., 427. See also 403–4 and 409–10.

44. Ibid, 447–48. See also 348–49, 354, 356–58, 409–10, and 412–13.

45. Ibid., 358. See also 380–81.

46. The figures are based on a comparison of the US Nutrient Database with the 1975 USDA Handbook #8. The USDA has confirmed the validity of the figures but denied any association with soil depletion or environmental influences such as pollution—Kushi with Jack, *Book of Macrobiotics*, 242–43, 349 (see chap. 2, n. 88).

47. Price, *Nutrition and Physical Degeneration*, 509.

Chapter 4

1. Maoshing Ni, *The Yellow Emperor's Classic of Medicine* (Boston and London: Shambala, 1995), 4.

2. Michael Pollan, *In Defense of Food* (New York: Penguin, 2008), 3.

3. Schmidt, *Dynamics of Nutrition*, 5 (see chap. 2, n. 118).

4. Elizabeth Frazao, "America's Eating Habits: Changes and Consequences," Agricultural Information Bulletin No. (AIB-750), *USDA, Economic Research Service*, May 1999, accessed March 13, 2016, http://www.ers. usda.gov/publications/aib-agricultural-information-bulletin/aib750. aspx. Click on the link to the article "Dietary Recommendations and How They Have Changed over Time" (chap. 2 PDF), 36.

5. Ibid. ("Dietary Recommendations and How They Have Changed over Time"), 35. See also: "The Food Guide Pyramid," *Emedicinehealth*, accessed March 13, 2016, http://www.emedicinehealth.com/nutrition_and_diet/page4_em.htm; "History of USDA nutrition guides," *Wikipedia*, accessed March 13, 2016, https://en.wikipedia.org/wiki/ History_of_USDA_nutrition_guide; and "The Origin of U.S. Dietary Guidelines," *PCRM/Internet Archive Waybackachine*, accessed March 16, 2016, http://web.archive.org/web/20110224172724/http:/ www.pcrm.org/magazine/GM97Autumn/GM97Autumn2.html.

    The five food groups of 1916: 1) cereals; 2) fats and fatty foods; 3) fruits and vegetables; 4) milk and meat; 5) sugars and sugary foods. The twelve food groups of 1933: 1) dry beans, peas, and nuts; 2) butter; 3) other fats; 4) cereals and flours; 5) citrus fruits and tomatoes; 6) eggs; 7) lean meat, poultry, and fish; 8) milk; 9) potatoes and sweet potatoes; 10) sugars; 11) leafy green and yellow vegetables; 12) other vegetables and fruits. The "basic seven" of 1942: 1) beans and dried peas, eggs, fish, meat, and poultry; 2) bread, cereals, and flour; 3) butter and fortified margarine; 4) cabbage, grapefruit, oranges, salad greens, and tomatoes; 5) milk and milk products; 6) green and yellow vegetables; 7) fruit, potatoes, and other vegetables.

6. For studies relating to the disease-protective effect of fiber in complex unrefined carbohydrates, see Denis Burkitt, Kenneth Heaton, and Hugh Trowell, eds., *Dietary Fibre, Fibre-Depleted Foods, and Disease* (London: Academic Press, 1985). See also:

    *   Ancel Keys, *The Seven Countries Study* (accessed February 25, 2016; http://www.sevencountriesstudy.com/about-the-study/

investigators/ancel-keys/), which focuses on the relationship between a traditional diet (grains, vegetables, fruit, beans, and fish)
and low incidence of heart disease;

- "The China Study," *Wikipedia* (accessed February 25, 2016,
https://en.wikipedia.org/wiki/The_China_Study), which also
relates to traditional plant-based diets (rice and vegetables) and to
a lower chronic-disease incidence;

- "Lyon Diet Heart Study," *Circulation* (archives of the American
Heart Association, accessed February 25, 2016, https://circ.aha-
journals.org/content/103/13/1823.full), which relates a Mediterranean Diet (bread, pasta, olive oil, vegetables, fruit, beans,
some red meat, more poultry and fish, wine, and canola oil instead
of butter) to lower mortality and cancer rates for those recovering
from heart attacks.

7. "U.S. Senate Select Committee Report on Nutrition and Human
Needs," *Wikipedia*, accessed March 6, 2016, http://en.wikipedia.org/
wiki/U.S._Senate_Select_Committee_on_Nutrition_and_Human_
Needs.

8. "The Food Guide Pyramid," *USDA, Human Nutrition Information Service*, Home and Garden Bulletin 252, August 1992, 4.

9. "Dietary Guidelines–2010," *USDA*, accessed March 6, 2016, http://
www.cnpp.usda.gov/dietary-guidelines-2010. Click on the "Press Release" link.

10. "Click a Food Group to Explore," *USDA, ChooseMyPlate.gov*, accessed
March 6, 2016, http://www.choosemyplate.gov. Click on each menu
item and follow the links that appear to the right for relevant detail.

11. Harvard School of Public Health and the Physicians Committee for
Responsible Medicine—both long-time critics with their own food
icons and guidelines—voice criticisms. See the following:

- "New U.S. Dietary Guidelines: Progress Not Perfection," *Harvard
School of Public Health*, accessed March 7, 2016, http://www.
hsph.harvard.edu/nutritionsource/dietary-guidelines-2010/;

- "Breaking News! USDA Replaces Food Pyramid with MyPlate,"
Internet Archive Waybackmachine, accessed March 4, 2016, http://
web.archive.org/web/20131026061533/http:/www.pcrm.
org/media/online/jun2011/breaking-news-usda-replaces-
food-pyramid-with;

- "USDA's New MyPlate Icon at Odds with Federal Subsidies for Meat, Dairy," *PCRM*, accessed March 4, 2016, http://www.pcrm.org/media/news/usdas-new-myplate-icon-at-odds-with-federal;

- "Power to the Plate: Food Subsidies Should Reflect New USDA Dietary Advice," *Foodconsumer*, accessed February 26, 2016, http://www.foodconsumer.org/newsite/Nutrition/Diet/power_to_the_plate_0621110838.html.

12. See "2015-2020 Dietary Guidelines for Americans," *USDA*, accessed March 7, 2016, http://www.cnpp.usda.gov/2015-2020-dietary-guidelines-americans. For a summary and key recommendations, click on "Executive Summary."

    For the critique of the 2015-2020 Guidelines, see the following from the *Harvard School of Public Health*, all accessed March 8, 2016: "New Dietary Guidelines remove restriction on total fat and set limit for added sugars but censor conclusions of the scientific advisory committee," http://www.hsph.harvard.edu/nutritionsource/2016/01/07/new-dietary-guidelines-remove-restriction-on-total-fat-and-set-limit-for-added-sugars-but-censor-conclusions/; "2015 Guidelines will not include a focus on sustainability," http://www.hsph.harvard.edu/nutritionsource/2015/10/08/2015-dietary-guidelines-will-not-include-a-focus-on-sustainability/; "The new focus on sustainability: The Dietary Guidelines for Americans and for our planet," http://www.hsph.harvard.edu/nutritionsource/2015/06/16/the-new-focus-on-sustainability-the-dietary-guidelines-for-americans-and-for-our-planet/.

13. "Med Diet and Health," *Oldways*, accessed March 13, 2016, http://oldwayspt.org/resources/heritage-pyramids/mediterranean-diet-pyramid/med-diet-health.

14. Oldways's fourfold critique of USDA guidelines in the early 1990s (regarding fat, carbohydrate, protein, and the lack of alcohol and exercise guidelines) is no longer found at the original link on the website. In response to an inquiry, Oldways refers to the following article of founder K. Dun Gifford: "Dietary Fats, Eating Guides, and Public Policy: History, Critique, and Recommendations," *The American Journal of Medicine*, December 30, 2002, vol. 113/Supplement 9B, 89S-106S. This article largely focuses on the issue of fat in USDA guidelines, but the outline of the other critiques is also visible.

15. "Mediterranean Diet Pyramid," *Oldways*, accessed March 13, 2016, http://oldwayspt.org/resources/heritage-pyramids/mediterranean-pyramid/overview.

16. Ibid.

17. "Harvard researchers launch Healthy Eating Plate," *Harvard School of Public Health* (*HSPH*), accessed March 7, 2016, http://www.hsph. harvard.edu/news/press-releases/healthy-eating-plate/.

18. "What Should I Eat?" *HSPH*, accessed March 9, 2016, http://www. hsph.harvard.edu/nutritionsource/what-should-you-eat/.

19. "Plate power–10 tips for health eating," *HSPH*, accessed March 9, 2016, http://www.hsph.harvard.edu/nutritionsource/2013/11/06/healthy -eating-ten-nutrition-tips-for-eating-right/.

20. "Carbohydrates" and "Whole Grains," *HSPH*, both accessed March 9, 2016, http://www.hsph.harvard.edu/nutritionsource/carbohydrates/ and http://www.hsph.harvard.edu/nutritionsource/whole-grains/.

21. "Protein" and "Eggs and Heart Disease," *HSPH*, both accessed March 13, 2016, http://www.hsph.harvard.edu/nutritionsource/protein/ and http://www.hsph.harvard.edu/nutritionsource/eggs/.

22. "Fats and Cholesterol," "Ask the Expert: Healthy Fats," and "Shining the Spotlight on Trans Fats," *HSPH*, all accessed March 10, 2016, http://www.hsph.harvard.edu/nutritionsource/what-should-you -eat/fats-and-cholesterol/, http://www.hsph.harvard.edu/nutrition- source/healthy-fats/, and http://www.hsph.harvard.edu/nutrition- source/transfats/.

23. "Fiber," *HSPH*, accessed March 11, 2016, http://www.hsph.harvard. edu/nutritionsource/carbohydrates/fiber/.

24. "Vegetables and Fruits" and "Healthy Eating Plate vs. USDA's MyPlate," *HSPH*, both accessed March 11, 2016, http://www. hsph.harvard.edu/nutritionsource/what-should-you-eat/vegeta- bles-and-fruits/ and http://www.hsph.harvard.edu/nutritionsource/ healthy-eating-plate-vs-usda-myplate/.

25. "Calcium and Milk" and "Healthy Beverage Guidelines," *HSPH*, both accessed March 11, 2016, http://www.hsph.harvard.edu/nutrition- source/what-should-you-eat/calcium-and-milk/ and http://www. hsph.harvard.edu/nutritionsource/healthy-drinks-full-story/#level-3.

26. "Healthy Drinks," *HSPH*, accessed March 11, 2016, http://www.hsph. harvard.edu/nutritionsource/healthy-drinks/. See also: "Healthy Bev- erage Guidelines," *HSPH*.

27. "Salt and Sodium" and "Take Action: How to Reduce Your Intake," *HSPH*, both accessed March 11, 2016, http://www.hsph.harvard.edu/

nutritionsource/salt-and-sodium/andhttp://www.hsph.harvard.edu/nutritionsource/salt-and-sodium/take-action-on-salt/.

28. "Drinks to Consume in Moderation," "Alcohol," and "Alcohol: Balancing Risks and Benefits," *HSPH*, all accessed March 13, 2016, http://www.hsph.harvard.edu/nutritionsource/healthy-drinks/drinks-to-consume-in-moderation/, http://www.hsph.harvard.edu/nutritionsource/alcohol/ and http://www.hsph.harvard.edu/nutritionsource/alcohol-full-story/.

29. "Vitamins" and "Vitamin D and Health," *HSPH*, both accessed March 13, 2016, http://www.hsph.harvard.edu/nutritionsource/what-should-you-eat/vitamins/ and http://www.hsph.harvard.edu/nutritionsource/vitamin-d/.

30. "Healthy Eating Plate and Healthy Eating Pyramid" *HSPH*, accessed March 13, 2016, http://www.hsph.harvard.edu/nutritionsource/healthy-eating-plate/.

31. Ibid.

32. "Breaking News! USDA Replaces Food Pyramid with MyPlate," *Internet Archive Waybackmachine* (n. 11).

33. "Vegetarian Foods: Powerful for Health," *PCRM*, accessed March 13, 2016, http://www.pcrm.org/health/diets/vsk/vegetarian-starter-kit-powerful.

34. "Why the Power Plate?" *PCRM*, accessed March 13, 2016, http://www.pcrm.org/health/diets/pplate/why-power-plate.

35. "The Power Plate," *PCRM*, accessed March 13, 2016, http://pcrm.org/health/diets/pplate/power-plate. Click on "The Power Plate *All in One Guide*" on the left side of the page.

36. "Health Professionals," *PCRM*, accessed March 13, 2016, http://www.pcrm.org/health/diets/pplate/health-professionals. Click on the "Dietary Guidelines Monograph (PDF)" and see page 5 (the monograph is also found at: http://www.pcrm.org/sites/default/files/images/health/pplate/PCRMDietaryGuidelinesMonograph.pdf).

37. "The Power Plate," click on "Power Plate *All in One* Guide." See the "Whole Grains" section.

38. Ibid. See the "Vegetables" section.

39. Ibid. See the "Fruit" section.

40. Ibid. See the "Legumes" section.

41. "Health Professionals," *PCRM*. Click on the "Dietary Guidelines and Goals and Recommendations (PDF)" and see page 5 (the monograph is also found at: http://www.pcrm.org/sites/default/files/images/health/pplate/PCRMDietaryGuidelines.pdf).

42. Ibid, 7–9. See also: "The Protein Myth," *PCRM*, accessed March 13,2016,http://www.pcrm.org/health/diets/vegdiets/how-can-i-get-enough-protein-the-protein-myth.

43. "Essential Fatty Acids," *PCRM*, accessed January 31, 2016, http://www.pcrm.org/health/health-topics/essential-fatty-acids.

44. "Ask the Expert: Dietary Fiber" and "How Fiber Helps Protect Against Cancer," *PCRM*, both accessed February 28, 2016, http://www.pcrm.org/health/cancer-resources/ask/ask-the-expert-dietary-fiberandhttp://www.pcrm.org/health/cancer-resources/diet-cancer/nutrition/how-fiber-helps-protect-against-cancer.

45. "Calcium and Strong Bones," *PCRM*, accessed January 31,2016,http://www.pcrm.org/health/health-topics/calcium-and-strong-bones.

46. "Iron: the Double-Edged Sword," *PCRM*, accessed February 4, 2016, http://www.pcrm.org/health/cancer-resources/diet-cancer/nutrition/iron-the-double-edged-sword; "Power Sources," "Iron," accessed January 31, 2016, http://www.pcrm.org/health/diets/pplate/power-sources.

47. "Milk and Vitamin D" and "Power Sources," *PCRM*, both accessed February 28, 2016, http://www.pcrm.org/media/news/milk-and-vitamin-d; http://www.pcrm.org/health/diets/pplate/power-sources.

48. "Don't Vegetarians Have Trouble Getting Enough Vitamin B_{12}?" *PCRM*, accessed January 31, 2016, http://www.pcrm.org/health/diets/vegdiets/dont-vegetarians-have-trouble-getting-enough.

49. Kushi with Jack, *Book of Macrobiotics*, 126 (see chap. 2, n. 88).

50. "Healing Foods Pyramid 2010," *University of Michigan*, accessed March 7,2016, http://www.med.umich.edu/umim/food-pyramid/index.htm.

51. "Vilhjalmur Stefansson," *Wikipedia*, accessed March 7, 2016, http://en.wikipedia.org/wiki/Vilhjalmur_Stefansson.

52. Vilhjalmur Stefansson, *Not By Bread Alone* (New York: MacMillan, 1946), 41ff.

53. Ibid., 287. Fat comprised approximately 75–80 percent of the diet and meat the rest.

54. Ibid., ix, quoting Eugene Du Bois.

55. Ibid. Pemmican originating with Plains Native Americans, 189–90. In his footnote to p. 259, Stefansson reports that pemmican of North American Native Americans usually contained 50 percent fat and 50 percent lean meat, but some explorers increased fat to 60 percent. On p. 285, he speaks of standard blends containing 70–90 percent fat. Pemmican and optimal health, 279; pemmican and polar expeditions, 257.

56. Ibid., 216, 219–21, 245.

57. Ibid. Evolutionary transition, 5; incentive for a new diet, 110.

58. Ibid. Meat and fat as superior foods, 81; Far North, 25–37; "best . . . in all countries," 112; God shows preference, 113.

59. Ibid. Words *blubber* and *rich*, 117, 120; statistics from 1791 to 1940, 118–19.

60. Ibid., 123.

61. Ibid., 288.

62. Martin Katahn, PhD, *The T-Factor Diet* (New York: W.W. Norton, 2001), 38–39, 260–63.

63. Price, *Nutrition and Physical Degeneration*, 503 (see chap. 3, n. 31).

64. Ibid. Percentage summaries, 402; reversing cavities, 257, 385ff.

65. Ibid., 362, 366, 373, 464.

66. Ibid., 120–21.

67. Ibid. "Activators," 386; four groups, 253.

68. Ibid. Lions, 301–2; prospector, 250–51.

69. Ibid. Seafood and dairy as animal-fat activator sources, 491; activators no health guarantee, 263.

70. Ibid., 250.

71. Ibid., 124, 132.

72. Email correspondence with Sally Fallon Morell, October 10, 2016.

73. William T. Jarvis, PhD, "The Myth of the Healthy Savage," *Nutrition Today* (March/April 1981): 14–15, 18–22.

74. Price, *Nutrition and Physical Degeneration*: old Indian, 497; hay, 245.

75. Ibid., 358.

76. "Dietary Guidelines," *Weston A. Price Foundation,* accessed October 13, 2016, http://www.westonaprice.org/health-topics/abcs-of-nutrition/dietary-guidelines/. These guidelines largely agree with the guidelines of the Price-Pottenger Nutrition Foundation, the publisher of Weston Price's work ("PPNF Guidelines for Good Health," *Price-Pottenger Nutrition Foundation,* accessed October 17, 2016, http://ppnf.org/about/ppnf-guidelines-for-good-health/).

77. "Low-carbohydrate diet," *Wikipedia,* accessed March 15, 2016, http://en.wikipedia.org/wiki/Low-carbohydrate_diet.

78. Gary Taubes, *Good Calories, Bad Calories* (New York: Alfred A. Knopf, 2007), xi. Taubes cites Jean Brillat-Savarin's *The Physiology of Taste.*

79. Ibid., x, xiii, xv, 313–14, 348. The Stanford University School of Medicine (1943), Harvard Medical School (1948), Children's Memorial Hospital in Chicago (1950), a medical textbook written by prominent British physicians (1951), Cornell Medical School, and New York Hospital (1952) all recommended a Banting-style, low-carbohydrate (high-fat) diet, as did the well-known pediatrician Dr. Benjamin Spock, Dr. Herman Taller's book *Calories Don't Count* (1961), and Robert Atkins's *Dr. Atkins New Diet Revolution* (1973).

80. Ibid., 31–33.

81. "Low-carbohydrate diet," *Wikipedia.*

82. Ibid.

83. Robert C. Atkins, MD, *Dr. Atkins' New Diet Revolution,* rev. ed. (New York: Avon Books, 2001). Various authors represent Paleo-style diets. See Walter L. Voegtlin, *The Stone Age Diet* (New York: Vantage Press, 1975); S. Boyd Eaton, Marjorie Shostak, and Melvin Konner, *The Paleolithic Prescription* (New York: Harpercollins, 1988); Ray V. Audette, *NeanderThin* (Dallas: Paleolithic Press, 1995); Loren Cordain, PhD, *The Paleo Diet* (Hoboken, NJ: John Wiley & Sons, 2002); Mark Sisson, *The Primal Blueprint* (Malibu, CA: Primal Nutrition, 2009); and Robb Wolf, *The Paleo Solution* (Las Vegas: Victory Belt, 2010).

84. "Low-carbohydrate diet," *Wikipedia.* See also Dr. Eric C. Westman, Dr. Stephen D. Phinney, and Dr. Jeff S. Volek, *The New Atkins for a New You* (New York: Simon & Schuster, 2010), 285–90, 308; Cordain, *The Paleo Diet,* 64–69; Melvin Konner and S. Boyd Eaton, "Paleolithic Nutrition: Twenty-Five Years Later," *Nutrition in Clinical Practice* 25, no. 6 (December 2010): 594–602; Associated Press, "Carbs may be

worse for heart than fatty foods," *NBC News*, accessed March 15, 2016, http://www.nbcnews.com/id/15625548/, reported November 8, 2016.

85. Dr. Peter J. D'Adamo with Catherine Whitney, *Eat Right 4 Your Type* (New York: G. P. Putnam's Sons, 1996).

86. "What's the Most Common Blood Type?" *LiveScience*, accessed March 7, 2016, http://www.livescience.com/36559-common-blood-type-donation.html.

87. "Response to Various Critics," *Eat Right 4 Your Type*, accessed March 7, 2016, http://www.dadamo.com/science_critic.htm.

88. Rudolf Steiner, "Appetites and Anti-Appetites," lecture of April 8, 1920, extract from lecture 17, "Spiritual Science and Medicine," in *Nutrition and Stimulants*, 199–200 (see chap. 2, n. 40).

89. "Seven Countries Study," *Wikipedia*, accessed March 7, 2016, http://en.wikipedia.org/wiki/Seven_Countries_Study.

90. Taubes, *Good Calories, Bad Calories*, 4, 20, 168.

91. Ibid. George Duncan Campbell and Thomas L. Cleave wrote the book *Diabetes, Coronary Thrombosis, and the Saccharine Disease* (Bristol: John Wright, 1966).

92. For the body's preference, see Katahn, *The T-Factor Diet*, 35. For calories per gram, see Terry Shintani, MD, JD, MPH, *Eat More, Weigh Less Diet* (Kamuela, HI: Halpax, 1993), 44. These figures refer to the metabolic measure called the *caloric density*. Shintani reports that the carbohydrate figure of 4 calories per gram applies to refined carbohydrates such as flour and sugar. Whole carbohydrates contain significantly less—between 0.6 and 1 calorie per gram.

Regarding breakdown costs: Initial breakdown cost refers to the metabolic measure called the *thermic effect*. Protein metabolism costs between 20–30 percent of ingested protein calories just to break the protein down into usable forms; carbohydrate metabolism costs between 3–20 percent, depending on refinement and fiber content; fat metabolism costs about 2–3 percent. Various sources give diverse estimates. The cited estimates are a composite from the following sources:

• Katahn, *T-Factor Diet*, 34–35. Katahn indicates that fat has a 3 percent thermic effect; protein, 25 percent; and carbohydrate, normally 2–3 times as much as fat, or 6–9 percent.

- Don Amerman, "Highly Thermogenic Foods," *Livestrong.com*, accessed March 15, 2016, http://www.livestrong.com/article/512626-list-of-foods-with-high-thermic-effect/. This website gives a value of 2–3 percent for fat.

- "Burn Fat with the Thermic Effect of Food," *LeanLifters*, accessed March 15, 2016, http://leanlifters.com/thermic-effect-food-protein/. This website gives values of about 3 percent for fat, 30 percent for proteins, and 20 percent for fibrous vegetables.

- "Energy Balance, Thermic Effect of Food," *ExRx.net*, accessed March 15, 2016, http://www.exrx.net/FatLoss/EnergyBalance.html. This website gives a range of 0–3 percent for fat, 5–10 percent for carbohydrate, and 10–30 percent for protein.

- Heidi Schaefer, "How the thermic effect of foods can work to your advantage," *Examiner.com*, accessed March 15, 2016, http://www.examiner.com/article/how-the-thermic-effect-of-foods-can-work-to-your-advantage. This website notes that processed and refined flour and sugar have a thermic effect of 3 percent, along with anything from which fiber, oils, and nutrients have been removed.

93. Katahn, *The T-Factor Diet*, 19–21; 260–63.

94. Taubes, *Good Calories, Bad Calories*, 139–44, 377–78.

95. Two US government websites (*Pub Med Health* and the *National Diabetes Information Clearing House*) cite excess calories and a lack of exercise as primary causes of insulin resistance; a third (the *US Department of Health and Human Services*) mentions lack of energy balance (calories in vs. calories out) and inactivity as the primary causes of obesity; and the site for the *American Diabetes Association* also says that a high-calorie diet, whether the calories come from sugar (carbohydrate) or fat, contributes to the weight gain that can lead to diabetes. See "Metabolic Syndrome," *PubMed Health*, accessed March 7, 2016, http://www.ncbi.nlm.nih.gov/pubmedhealth/PMH0004546; "Insulin Resistance and Pre-diabetes," *National Diabetes Information Clearing House*, accessed March 7, 2016, http://diabetes.niddk.nih.gov/dm/pubs/insulinresistance/; "What Are Overweight and Obesity?" *US Department of Health & Human Services/National Institutes of Health*, accessed March 7, 2016, http://www.nhlbi.nih.gov/health/health-topics/topics/obe/; "Diabetes Myths," *American Diabetes Association*, accessed March 7, 2016, http://www.diabetes.org/diabetes-basics/diabetes-myths/.

96. Enig, *Know Your Fats*, 82 (see chap. 2, n. 105).

97. Ibid., 42, 79, 81, 178; See also Cherie Calbom, MS, "The Truth About Fats," *Sound Consumer* no. 448 (PCC Natural Markets, October 2010): 1, 4, accessed March 7, 2016, http://www.pccnaturalmarkets.com/sc/1010/sc1010-fats.html.

98. Enig, *Know Your Fats*, 43, 82.

99. Enig, *Know Your Fats*, 44, 84–85, 112; Calbom also indicates that toxins stored in animal-fat cells can lead to free radicals that are implicated in oxidizing the cholesterol found in artery plaques. For this reason, she recommends organic animal products and these in small amounts. See Calbom, *PCC Natural Markets*, "Additional research on saturated fats," accessed March 7, 2016, http://www.pccnaturalmarkets.com/sc/1010/sc1010-more-fats.html, dated October 2010.

100. Cordain, *The Paleo Diet*, 50, 218–19. Paleo-type diet proponents assert the importance of grass-fed meat for a healthy omega-3 to omega-6 fatty-acid ratio (reviewed in chapter 6).

101. Aubert in Sally Fallon, *Nourishing Traditions*, rev. 2nd ed. (Washington, DC: New Trends, 2001), 504–5. Fallon refers to Claude Aubert's book *Dis-Moi Comment Tu Cuisines* (Mens, France: Association Terre Vivante, 1987).

102. Markham Heid, "Why Full-Fat Dairy May Be Healthier than Low-Fat," *Time*, March 5, 2015, accessed March 8, 2016, http://time.com/3734033/whole-milk-dairy-fat/.

Chapter 5

1. Walters and Portmess, *Religious Vegetarianism* (see chap. 2, n. 122).

2. "Sacrifice," *Encyclopedia Britannica Online Library Edition*, accessed March 14, 2016, http://www.library.eb.com.ezproxy.spl.org:2048/eb/article-66301and article-66302. For a discussion of the myths of different cultures see Tom Standage, *An Edible History of Humanity* (New York: Walker & Company, 2009), 54–56.

3. "Human Sacrifice," *Wikipedia*, accessed March 14, 2016, http://en.wikipedia.org/wiki/Human_sacrifice.

4. Mitra Ara, *Eschatology in the Indo-Iranian Traditions: The Genesis and Transformation of a Doctrine* (New York: Peter Lang, 2008), 170.

5. As quoted in Aurobindo, *Message of the Gita*, 52 (see chap. 1, n. 2).

6. "Vedic religion," *Encyclopedia Britannica Online Library Edition*, accessed March 14, 2016, http://www.library.eb.com.ezproxy.spl.org:2048/eb/article-7618.

7. "The Rigveda (Hinduism)," *Encyclopedia Britannica Online Library Edition*, accessed March 14, 2016, http://www.library.eb.com.ezproxy.spl.org:2048/eb/article-59813.

8. "The Upanishads (Hinduism)," *Encyclopedia Britannica Online Library Edition*, accessed March 14, 2016, http://www.library.eb.com.ezproxy.spl.org:2048/eb/article-59824; "Development and Decline (Vedic religion)," accessed March 14, 2016, http://www.library.eb.com.ezproxy.spl.org:2048/eb/article-7620.

9. "Karma," *Encyclopedia Britannica Online Library Edition*, accessed March 14, 2016, http://library.eb.com.ezproxy.spl.org:2048/levels/referencecenter/article/44745#9044745.toc.

10. "Vedic religion" and "Moksha," *Encyclopedia Britannica Online Library Edition*, accessed March 14, 2016, http://library.eb.com.ezproxy.spl.org:2048/levels/referencecenter/article/53217#9053217.toc; "Ahimsa," *Encyclopedia Britannica Online Library edition*, accessed March 14, 2016, http://www.library.eb.com.ezproxy.spl.org:2048/eb/article-9004121; "Ahimsa," *Wikipedia*, accessed March 14, 2016, http://en.wikipedia.org/wiki/Ahimsa#cite_ref-43.

11. "Challenges to Brahmanism (Hinduism)," *Encyclopedia Britannica Online Library Edition*, accessed March 14, 2016, http://library.eb.com.ezproxy.spl.org:2048/levels/referencecenter/article/105952#8984.toc.

12. Ibid.

13. "Ashrama (stage)," *Wikipedia*, accessed March 14, 2016, http://en.wikipedia.org/wiki/Ashrama.

14. "The Laws of Manu," *Internet Sacred Text Archive*, accessed March 14, 2016, http://www.sacred-texts.com/hin/manu.htm; see also F. Max Müller, ed., *The Sacred Books of the East*, vol. 25, trans. George Bühler, (Oxford: Clarendon, 1886), chap. 6, 1, 33, 38–39.

15. "The Laws of Manu," chap. 6, 13–14; "Ashrama," *Encyclopedia Britannica Online Library Edition*, accessed March 14, 2016, http://www.library.eb.com.ezproxy.spl.org:2048/eb/article-9009845; "Ashrama (stage)," *Wikipedia*.

16.   "Ashramas: The Four Stages of Life (Hinduism)," *Encyclopedia Britannica Online Library Edition*, accessed March 14, 2016, http://library.eb.com.ezproxy.spl.org:2048/levels/referencecenter/article/105952#261618.toc.

17.   "Dharma and the Three Paths (Hinduism)," *Encyclopedia Britannica Online Library Edition*, accessed March 14, 2016, http://library.eb.com.ezproxy.spl.org:2048/levels/referencecenter/article/105952#261617.toc.

18.   See "The Laws of Manu": Becoming an ascetic and seeking liberation without first begetting sons and offering sacrifices caused one to "sink downwards" (chap. 6, 37). Similarly, the body is made fit for union with Brahman by studying the Vedas and making sacrifices and begetting sons (chap. 2, 28). Householders were even considered superior to the other three categories of individuals because they supported them (chap. 6, 89).

19.   "Ashramas: The Four Stages of Life (Hinduism)."

20.   "Mahabharata," *Encyclopedia Britannica Online Library Edition*, accessed March 14, 2016, http://www.library.eb.com.ezproxy.spl.org:2048/eb/article-9050089.

21.   "The Mahabharata, Book 13: Anusasana Parva," trans. Kisari Mohan Ganguli, *Mahabharataonline*, accessed March 14, 2016, http://www.mahabharataonline.com/translation/index13.php.

22.   The 30–40 percent estimate for vegetarian Hindus derives from the size of the Hindu population in India, other likely vegetarian groups (Buddhists and Jains), and the percentage totals for vegetarians in India. In 2005, Hindus made up 73.4 percent of the total population, Buddhists about 0.7 percent, and Jains 0.5 percent (therada.com references given below). In 2006, about 31 percent of India's population was vegetarian (synonymous with lacto-vegetarianism), and another 9 percent included eggs in their diets (Wikipedia reference below). Considering the small number of Buddhists and Jains (about 1.2 percent of the population combined), the percentages for lacto and lacto-ovo-vegetarians in India likely apply to Hindus, although they also include Buddhists and Jains. See "Most Hindu Nations (2005)," *Association of Religion Data Archives* (ARDA), accessed March 20, 2016, http://www.thearda.com/QuickLists/QuickList_44.asp; "Most Jainist Nations (2005)," accessed March 14, 2016, http://www.thearda.com/QuickLists/QuickList_45c.asp; "Most Buddhist Nations (2005)," accessed March 14, 2016, http://www.thearda.com/QuickLists/QuickList_38.asp (these ARDA figures come from the World Christian Database 2005);

"Vegetarianism by country," *Wikipedia*, accessed March 14, 2016, http://en.wikipedia.org/wiki/Vegetarianism_in_India#India.

23. Buddhists and Hindus were never as meticulous about applying ahimsa as Jains. See "Ahimsa," *Encyclopedia Britannica Online Library Edition*.

24. "Buddhist vegetarianism," *Wikipedia*, accessed March 14, 2016, http://en.wikipedia.org/wiki/Buddhist_vegetarianism; "The Bhikkus' Rules," *Access to Insight*, accessed March 14, 2016, http://www.accesstoinsight.org/lib/authors/ariyesako/layguide.html#fn-88, n. 88.

25. "Most Buddhist Nations (2005)," *ARDA*. The figures come from the World Christian Database 2005. Buddhists are estimated to be about 455 million. Other estimates for world Buddhists are between 350 million and over 1 billion, with a generally accepted figure of 350 million. See "Major Religions of the World Ranked by Adherents," accessed March 14, 2016, http://www.adherents.com/Religions_By_Adherents.html; "Buddhism," *Wikipedia*, accessed March 14, 2016, http://en.wikipedia.org/wiki/Buddhism.

26. "Vegetarianism and religion," *Wikipedia*, accessed March 14, 2016, http://en.wikipedia.org/wiki/vegetarianism_and_religion. Monks typically do not eat meat in China and Vietnam. In Japan and Korea, most but not all Buddhist schools eat meat. Theravadans in Sri Lanka and Southeast Asia are not vegetarians, yet both monks and the laity have the option to choose vegetarianism. In contrast to the general Mahayana position supporting vegetarianism, some Mahayana monks eat meat. In Tibetan Buddhism, vegetarianism is uncommon, yet prominent representatives such as the Dalai Lama encourage it.

27. Suzuki, *The Lankavatara Sutra*, 211 (see chap. 2, n. 45).

28. "Jain vegetarianism," *Wikipedia*, accessed March 14, 2016, http://en.wikipedia.org/wiki/Jain_vegetarianism.

29. "The Moderate Speeches—Majjhima Nikāya 55 [I 368–371], To Jivaka: Jivaka Sutta [sic]," *What the Buddha said in plain English*, accessed March 14, 2016, http://what-buddha-said.net/Canon/Sutta/MN/MN55.htm.

30. John Kahila, "Are All Buddhists Vegetarian?" *UrbanDharma.org*, accessed March 14, 2016, http://www.urbandharma.org/udharma3/vegi.html.

31. The Sutta-Nipâta [sic], "Âmagandhasutta [sic]," *Internet Sacred Text Archive*, accessed March 1, 2016, http://www.sacred-texts.com/bud/

sbe10/sbe1034.htm. In Müller, ed., *The Sacred Books of the East*, vol. 10, pt. 2, trans. V. Fausböll (Oxford: Clarendon, 1881), 40–41.

32. "Mahaparinirvana Sutra and Abstaining from Eating Meat and Fish," *Shabkar.org*, accessed March 14, 2016, http://www.shabkar.org/scripture/sutras/mahaparinirvana_sutra1.htm.

33. Venerable S. Dhammika, "Vegetarianism," *UrbanDharma.org*, accessed March 14, 2016, http://www.urbandharma.org/udharma3/vegi.html.

34. "The Bhikkus' Rules," n. 88.

35. Kahila, "Are All Buddhists Vegetarian?"

36. Samanera Kumara Liew, "Is There Something Spiritually Wholesome about Being a Vegetarian?" *UrbanDharma.org*, accessed March 14, 2016, http://www.urbandharma.org/udharma3/vegi.html.

37. Philip Kapleau, *To Cherish All Life* (Rochester, NY: The Zen Center, 1981), 33.

38. Ibid., 43.

39. Norm Phelps, *The Longest Struggle, Animal Advocacy from Pythagoras to PETA* (New York: Lantern Books, 2007), 19. The five ethical principles are nonviolence, truthfulness, not stealing, celibacy, and nonpossession or nonmaterialism.

40. "Jain vegetarianism," *Wikipedia.*

41. "Âkârâṅga Sûtra," bk. 1, lecture 1, lesson 6, *Internet Sacred Text Archive*, accessed March 1, 2016, http://www.sacred-texts.com/jai/sbe22/sbe2208.htm. In Müller, ed., *The Sacred Books of the East*, vol. 22, trans. Hermann Jacobi, Gaina [sic] Sutras, pt. 1, 11–13.

42. "Âkârâṅga Sûtra," bk. 2, lecture 15, *Internet Sacred Text Archive*, accessed March 1, 2016, http://www.sacred-texts.com/jai/sbe22/sbe2279.htm, 202. For the reference to the Akaranga Sutra verses, I am indebted to Walters and Portmess, *Religious Vegetarianism*, 43–45.

43. "Most Jainist Nations (2005)," *ARDA.*

44. "Sikhism" and "Sikh Religious Philosophy," *Sikhs.org*, both accessed March 14, 2016, http://www.sikhs.org/; http://www.sikhs.org/philos.htm.

45. "Sikhism and Jainism," *Sikhs.org*, accessed March 14, 2016, http://www.sikhs.org/relig_j.htm.

46. "Sri Guru Granth Sahib," sect. 31, Raag Malaar, part 036, *Internet Sacred Text Archive*, accessed March 14, 2016, http://www.sacred-texts.com/skh/granth/gr31.htm. For the reference to the quotation from the Sri Guru Granth Sahib, I am indebted to the article "Diet in Sikhism," *Wikipedia*, accessed March 14, 2016, http://en.wikipedia.org/wiki/Diet_in_Sikhism.

47. "Vegetarianism and religion," *Wikipedia*; "Diet in Sikhism," *Wikipedia*; and "Guru Granth Sahib," *Wikipedia*, accessed March 14, 2016, http://en.wikipedia.org/wiki/Guru_Granth_Sahib; "Jhatka," *Wikipedia*, accessed March 14, 2016, http://en.wikipedia.org/wiki/Jhatka; "Kutha meat," *Wikipedia*, accessed March 14, 2016, http://en.wikipedia.org/wiki/Kutha_meat.

48. "Most Sikh Nations (2005)," *ARDA*, accessed March 14, 2016, http://www.thearda.com/QuickLists/QuickList_49.asp. The figures come from the World Christian Database 2005.

49. Richard Alan Young, *Is God a Vegetarian?* (Chicago and La Salle, IL: Open Court, 1999), 20; Sears, *Vision of Eden*, 463 (see chap. 2, n. 9).

50. Sears, *Vision of Eden*, 463.

51. Young, *Is God a Vegetarian*, 43–44.

52. "Noahidism," *Wikipedia*, accessed March 14, 2016, http://en.wikipedia.org/wiki/Noahidism. The Talmud interprets Genesis 9:4 as a prohibition against cruelty to animals: "Do not eat flesh from an animal while it is still alive," i.e., a limb or some other part of the body removed before the animal dies. The typical translation, "Only, you shall not eat flesh with its life, that is, its blood," is, however, usually understood as a prohibition against eating blood.

53. "Shechita," *Wikipedia*, accessed March 14, 2016, http://en.wikipedia.org/wiki/Shechita.

54. Kook, *Vision of Vegetarianism and Peace* (see chap. 2, n. 5). The manuscript contains 32 sections from the lecture "Afikim Banegev" (Streams in the Desert) and 7 from "Talele Orot" (Dewdrops of Light). The PDF, however, contains only the excerpts from "Afikim Banegev." Those consulted from "Talele Orot" are found in Rabbi Abraham Isaac Kook, "On the Reasons for the Commandments," in Ezra Gellman, ed., *Essays on the Thought and Philosophy of Rabbi Kook* (Madison, NJ: Fairleigh, Dickinson University Press, 1991), 280–83.

55. Sears, *Vision of Eden*, 201.

56. Kook, "On the Reasons for the Commandments," in Gellman, *Essays*, 281.

57. Based on a review of anthropological evidence, Arnold C. Mendez Sr. concludes that cannibalism was prevalent in the pre-flood world. See his "The Wickedness of the Pre-Flood World," *Giving & Sharing*, accessed March 14, 2016, http://www.giveshare.org/evolution/wickedness-of-pre-flood-world.html.

58. "Human Sacrifice," *Wikipedia*.

59. Kook, *Vision of Vegetarianism and Peace*, sects. 1, 6 (see chap. 2, n. 5); Kook, "On the Reasons for the Commandments," in Gellman, *Essays*, 280–81.

60. Kook, *Vision of Vegetarianism and Peace*, sects. 1, 6, 14,17. See also his essay "On the Reasons for the Commandments," in Gellman, *Essays*, 281–82; and his letter to Benjamin Manashe Levin dated Jaffa, 1909, in Richard Schwartz, PhD, "The Vegetarian Teachings of Rav Kook," *The Schwartz Collection on Judaism, Vegetarianism, and Animal Rights*, accessed March 14, 2016, http://jewishveg.com/schwartz/kook-expanded.html#_ednref26.

61. Sears, *Vision of Eden*, 202.

62. Kook, *Vision of Vegetarianism and Peace*, sections 6, 8; Kook, "On the Reasons for the Commandments," in Gellman, *Essays*, 280.

63. Sears, *Vision of Eden*, 201–2.

64. "Abraham Isaac Kook," *Wikipedia*, accessed March 14, 2016, http://en.wikipedia.org/wiki/Abraham_Isaac_Kook.

65. Schwartz, "The Vegetarian Teachings of Rav Kook," *The Schwartz Collection*.

66. Ibid.

67. Kook, "On the Reasons for the Commandments," in Gellman, *Essays*, 283. Similar sentiments are expressed in: Kook, *Vision of Vegetarianism and Peace*, sect. 13.

68. Kook, *Vision of Vegetarianism and Peace*, sect. 17; Kook, "On the Reasons for the Commandments," in Gellman, *Essays*, 282. The prohibition against blood and fat is quite emphatic and repeated several times, along with the threat of banishment for nonobservance (Lev. 3:17; 7:22–27; 17:10–16).

69. Kook, *Vision of Vegetarianism and Peace*, sects 27, 31; Kook, "On the Reasons for the Commandments," in Gellman, *Essays*, 282. Other translations of the Isaiah verse speak of tasty, seasoned, savory, salty, or the finest and best fodder.

70. Kook, "On the Reasons for the Commandments," in Gellman, *Essays*, 281.

71. Rabbi J. David Bleich, quoted in Sears, *Vision of Eden*, 83.

72. Sears, *Vision of Eden*, 83, 85.

73. Rabbi Dresner quoted in Samuel H. Dresner and Seymour Siegel, *The Jewish Dietary Laws, Their Meaning in Our Time* (New York: Burning Book Press, 1966), PDF, 27–28.

74. Kook, *Vision of Vegetarianism and Peace*, 3.

75. Rabbi Dresner in Dresner and Siegel, *Jewish Dietary Laws*, 39.

76. Ibid., 20–21.

77. "Kashrut," *Wikipedia*, accessed March 14, 2016, http://en.wikipedia.org/wiki/Kashrut.

78. See Roberta Kalechofsky, "A Provegetarian Bias in Torah," in Walters and Portmess, *Religious Vegetarianism*, 99–100; see also Kalechofsky in Roberta Kalechofsky, ed. *Judaism and Animal Rights, Classical and Contemporary Responses* (Marblehead, MA: Micah, 1992), 169; Young, *Is God a Vegetarian*, 73 (referring to a statement by Rabbi Kook); and J. R. Hyland, *God's Covenant with Animals* (New York: Lantern Books, 2000), 32–33.

79. The cause of the plague has also been interpreted as faithlessness: Bruce M. Metzger and Roland E. Murphy, eds., *The New Oxford Annotated Bible* (New York: Oxford University Press, 1994), OT 182, footnote to Ex. 11:33.

80. "Vegetarianism," *Jewish Encyclopedia*, accessed March 14, 2016, http://www.jewishencyclopedia.com/articles/14657-vegetarianism.

81. Metzger and Murphy, *New Oxford Annotated Bible*, OT 882, footnote to Is. 11:6–8.

82. "Carnivore," *Wikipedia*, accessed March 14, 2016, http://en.wikipedia.org/wiki/Carnivore.

83. Sears, *Vision of Eden*, 61, 65–67.

84. Louis A. Berman, "Slaughter as a Mode of Worship," in Kalechofsky, ed., *Judaism and Animal Rights*, 85–86.

85. Psalms: 40:6–8, 50:8–13, 51:16, and Proverbs 21:3; prophets: 1 Samuel 15:22, Isaiah 1:11; Jeremiah 6:20, 7:22; Hosea 6:6; Micah 6:6–8; Amos 5:22–25. Commentators: Berman in Kalechofsky, ed., *Judaism and Animal Rights*, 88; Phelps, *The Longest Struggle*, 45; Hyland, *God's Covenant*, 3–14, 34–35; and Keith Akers, *The Lost Religion of Jesus* (New York: Lantern Books, 2000), 105–9. With the exception of Amos, all passages specifically criticize "burnt offerings" (Heb. *'olah*), the offerings discussed in Leviticus 1 that were offerings of praise and thanksgiving (in contrast to all other offerings, including meat offerings for consumption). Thus, these passages appear to criticize praise and thanksgiving that is not genuine. Amos criticizes various kinds of offerings, including burnt offerings.

86. Young, *Is God a Vegetarian*, 69–71.

87. Berman, in Kalechofsky, ed., *Judaism and Animal Rights*, 150–52.

88. Sears, *Vision of Eden*, 196–200.

89. Dresner in *Jewish Dietary Laws*, PDF, 38.

90. *The Jewish Vegetarian Society*, accessed March 14, 2016, http://www.jvs.org.uk/home/.

91. Rabbi Joseph Rosenfeld, "The Ultimate Ideal," accessed March 14, 2016, http://jvs.org.uk//wp-content/uploads/2012/02/The-Jewish-Vegetarian-issue-1.pdf, PDF, 11.

92. The premise of Will Tuttle's book *The World Peace Diet* (New York: Lantern Books, 2005) is that abusing, killing, and eating animals is at the root of all human and social ills. Consequently, a vegetarian diet is the key to harmony and peace. He writes in the preface (p. xiii):
    "Finding our lives beset with stress and a range of daunting problems of our own making, we rightly yearn to understand the source of our frustrating inability to live in harmony on this earth. When we look deeply enough, we discover a disturbing force that is fundamental in generating our dilemmas and crises, a force that is not actually hidden at all, but is staring up at us every day from our plates! It has been lying undiscovered all along in the most obvious of places: It is our food."

93. *Jewish Vegetarians of North America* (JVNA), accessed March 14, 2016, http://jewishveg.com/.

94. "Genesis 9:3—Permission to Eat Meat?" *JVNA*, accessed March 14, 2016, http://jewishveg.com/whats-jewish-about-being-veg/genesis-93-%E2%80%93-permission-eat-meat.

95. "Isn't Kosher Meat Humane?" *JVNA*, accessed March 14, 2016, http://jewishveg.com/faq-isnt-kosher-meat-humane.

96. Ibid.

97. "A Jewish Vegetarian Response to Efforts to Ban Shechita," *The Jewish Vegetarian Society*, accessed March 14, 2016, http://www.jvs.org.uk/jewish-vegetarian-response-efforts-ban-shechita/.

98. "Amirim," *Wikipedia*, accessed March 14, 2016, http://en.wikipedia.org/wiki/Amirim; Elliott Goldstein, "Place in Focus: Amirim," *Jewish Agency for Israel*, accessed March 14, 2016, https://web.archive.org/web/20070126104141/http://www.partner.org.il/kavimut/places-amirim-0107.html.

99. "About us," *The Shamayim V'Aretz Institute*, accessed March 14, 2016, http://www.shamayimvaretz.org/about.html.

100. The phrase "the healing medicine" is used in the communion ritual of the Christian Community, a movement for religious renewal founded in Germany in the early part of the twentieth century under the inspiration of Rudolf Steiner.

101. Matthew 21:12–13; Mark 11:15–19; Luke 19:45–48; and John 2:13–16.

102. On Jesus as a vegetarian, see Akers, *The Lost Religion of Jesus*, 125–34; Young, *Is God a Vegetarian*, 1–13, 127–38; Phelps, *The Longest Struggle*, 50–51; and Andrew Linzey, "Vegetarianism as a Biblical Ideal," in Walters and Portmess, *Religious Vegetarianism*, 133–34.

103. "Mark 7," *Bible Hub*, accessed March 15, 2016, http://biblehub.com/interlinear/mark/7.htm.

104. "Did Christ Declare All Foods Clean? Misunderstandings regarding Mark 7:19," *Bible Things in Bible Ways*, accessed March 15, 2016, http://biblethingsinbibleways.wordpress.com/2013/05/12/did-christ-declare-all-foods-clean-misunderstandings-regarding-mark-719/.

105. "Christian Vegetarianism," *Wikipedia*, accessed March 15, 2016, http://en.wikipedia.org/wiki/Christian_vegetarianism#cite_ref-19. It is argued that Peter was himself a vegetarian on the basis of his own

statement in the *Clementine Homilies*. The *Homilies*, however, are associated with the Ebionite sect, which did not believe among other things in the divinity of Jesus and was considered heretical.

106. Metzger and Murphy, *New Oxford Annotated Bible*, NT 183, note to verse 20.

107. Ibid., NT 303, note to verses 4:3–5.

108. Alexander Basnar, "Gilt das Blutverbot Immer Noch?" *Hausgemeinde*, accessed March 18, 2016, https://hausgemeinde.files.wordpress.com/2016/03/gilt-das-blutverbot-immer-noch.pdf, PDF, 7.

109. Augustine, "Contra Faustum," book 32, para. 13, *New Advent*, accessed March 15, 2016, http://www.newadvent.org/fathers/140632.htm.

110. Cyril of Jerusalem, Catechetical Lecture Four, "On the Ten Points of Doctrine," Concerning Meats, para. 28, *New Advent*, accessed March 15, 2016, http://www.newadvent.org/fathers/310104.htm.

111. For references to Gangrene, Orleans, Constance, Leo VI, Calixtus II, and Calvin, see P. J. Verdam, LLD, *Mosaic Law in Practice and Study throughout the Ages* (Kampen, Germany: J. H. Kok, 1959), 19. For the Verdam references, I am indebted to Alexander Basnar (see n. 108) and, via Basnar, to Dr. Thomas Schiffmacher, "The Biblical Prohibition from Eating Blood," *Contra Mundum*, accessed March 15, 2016, http://www.contra-mundum.org/schirrmacher.html. For references to Gregory III and Trullo, see David Grumett and Rachel Muers, *Eating and Believing: Interdisciplinary Perspectives on Vegetarianism and Theology* (London: Continuum), Kindle ed., 33, 39. For Gregory III, also see "Seven Laws of Noah," *Wikipedia*, accessed March 15, 2016, http://en.wikipedia.org/wiki/Seven_Laws_of_Noah, note 51 (Bishop Karl Josef von Hefele's commentary on canon II of the Council of Gangra [sic]). For references to Pulleyn and Stephen of Tournay, see Dr. Karl Böckenhoff, *Speisesatzungern Mosaisher Art in Mittelaltlichen Kirchenrechtsquellen des Morgen- und Abendlandes* (Münster: Aschendorffschen Verlag, 1907), PDF, 120–23 (for this reference, I am also indebted to Schiffmeyer).

112. "The Bible and Morality, Biblical Roots of Christian Conduct," *Pontifical Biblical Commission*, Cultural background, accessed March 15, 2016, http://www.vatican.va/roman_curia/congregations/cfaith/pcb_documents/rc_con_cfaith_doc_20080511_bibbia-e-morale_en.html, 13.

113. Böckenhoff, *Speisesatzungern*, 37–40; Schiffmacher, "Biblical Prohibition," *Contra Mundum*, 2.

114. "Question Number 786," *Orthodox Answers*, accessed March 16, 2016, http://orthodox-church.info/answer/786/.

115. Basnar, "Gilt das Blutverbot Immer Noch?" *Hausgemeinde*, 4 and 7; Böckenhoff, *Speisesatzungern*, 37–40.

116. "Christian Vegetarianism," *Wikipedia*.

117. "St. Francis of Paola," *Catholic Online*, accessed March 17, 2016, http://www.catholic.org/saints/saint.php?saint_id=645.

118. "Christian Vegetarianism," *Wikipedia*.

119. Lt. Colonel Maxwell Ryan, "The Gospel of Vegetarianism," *The Salvationist*, accessed March 2, 2016, http://salvationist.ca/2010/10/the-gospel-of-vegetarianism/.

120. "Scriptures, The Doctrine and Covenants, Section 89," *The Church of Jesus Christ of Latter-Day Saints*, accessed March 15, 2016, https://www.lds.org/scriptures/dc-testament/dc/89.4?lang=eng, verses 12–13. I am indebted for the reference to John Cook's *Diet and Your Religion* (see chap. 2, n. 58).

121. "Doctrine and Covenants Student Manual, Section 89, The Word of Wisdom," *The Church of Jesus Christ of Latter-Day Saints*, accessed March 15, 2016, http://www.lds.org/manual/doctrine-and-covenants-student-manual/section-81-89/section-89-the-word-of-wisdom?lang=eng.

122. *LDS Veg Homepage*, accessed March 15, 2016, http://www.ldsveg.org/.

123. *Christian Vegetarian Association (CVA)*, accessed March 15, 2016, http://christianveg.org/default.htm; *Christian Vegetarian Association UK (CVAUK)*, accessed March 15, 2016, http://www.christianvegetarians.com/.

124. "Honoring God's Creation—Replies" (see the remarks to the headings "God gives Noah permission to eat meat" and "Didn't Jesus eat meat?"), *CVA*, accessed March 17, 2016, http://christianveg.org/hgc-replies.htm.

125. Young, *Is God a Vegetarian*, 59.

126. "Vegetarianism's Benefits: From Christian Vegetarian Association" (see the sections "Heart Disease" and "Obesity and Diabetes"), *CVA*, accessed March 17, 2016, http://christianveg.org/vegbenefits.htm.

127. "CVAUK Mission," *CVAUK*, accessed March 17, 2016, http://www.christianvegetarians.com/home.html; "Christianity and Vegetarianism," *CVAUK*, accessed March 17, 2016, http://www.vegan-shoes.com/CVAUK-Leaflet.pdf.

128. "Honoring God's Creation—Replies" (see the remarks to the heading "Eat whatever is sold in the meat market"), *CVA*, accessed March 15, 2016, http://www.all-creatures.org/cva/hgc-replies.htm.

129. *The Noble Qu'ran*, accessed March 15, 2016, http://quran.com/. Verse 56.21 regarding "meat of fowl" refers to an afterlife recompense banquet. For the references, I am indebted to the website *Diet in Islam*, accessed March 15, 2016, http://www.inter-islam.org/Lifestyle/diet.htm.

130. Kook, *Vision of Vegetarianism and Peace*, section 14.

131. Steiner, "The Effects of Nicotine; Vegetarian and Meat Diets; Absinth," lecture of January 13, 1923, in *Nutrition and Stimulants*, 47–48 (see chap. 2, n. 40).

132. "Bacon/Pork Products," *Eat Right for Your Blood Type*, accessed March 15, 2016, http://www.dadamo.com/typebase4/depictor5.pl?43.

133. "Dhabihah," *Wikipedia*, accessed March 15, 2016, http://en.wikipedia.org/wiki/Dhabihah.

134. Ibid.; see also Dr. Abdul Majid Katme, "An Assessment of the Muslim Method of Slaughter," *Guideways*, accessed March 15, 2016, http://www.guidedways.com/articles/halalslaughtermethod.php#dhabh.

135. Andy Coughlin, "Animals Feel the Pain of Religious Slaughter," *New Scientist*, accessed March 15, 2016, http://www.newscientist.com/article/dn17972-animals-feel-the-pain-of-religious-slaughter.html?full=true&print=true.

136. "Dhabihah," *Wikipedia*.

137. Steven Rosen, *Diet for Transcendence: Vegetarianism and the World Religions* (Badger, CA: Torchlight, 1997). See the chapter on Islam.

138. Rosen cites M. R. Bawa Muhaiyaddeen, *Asma' ul-Husna: The 99 Beautiful Names of Allah* (Philadelphia: Fellowship Press, 1979), 183.

139. *Islamic Concern*, accessed March 15, 2016, http://www.islamiccon-cern.com/.

140. "Facts about the Source of Some Halal Meat," *Islamic Concern*, accessed March 15, 2016, http://www.islamicconcern.com/halalmeat_sum-mary.asp.

141. "Kashrut," *Wikipedia*, accessed March 15, 2016, http://en.wikipedia.org/wiki/Kashrut.

142. "The Bhagavadgita (Hinduism)," *Encyclopedia Britannica Online Library Edition*, accessed March 15, 2016, http://www.library.eb.com.ezproxy.spl.org:2048/eb/article-59830.

143. Aurobindo, *Message of the Gita*, 22 (see chap. 1, n. 2).

144. Ibid., 4, footnote 1. Sri Aurobindo rejects the understanding of the Bhagavad Gita teaching as "an allegory of the inner life" instead of an actual physical battle.

145. Ibid., 278.

146. Ibid., 12.

147. "Dharma and the Three Paths (Hinduism)," *Encyclopedia Britannica Online Library Edition*, accessed March 15, 2016, http://library.eb.com.ez-proxy.spl.org:2048/levels/referencecenter/article/105952#261617.toc.

148. Vijay, comp., *Sri Aurobindo and the Mother on Food*, 10–11 (see chap. 1, n. 16).

149. Further applicable comments:

- No healthy primitive societies, past or present, or contemporary indigenous groups exclude animal products from their diet. See Douglas Dupler, Rebecca J. Frey, PhD, and Helen Davidson, "Vegetarianism," in *Gale Encyclopedia of Alternative and Complimentary Medicine, 4th Edition* (Farmington Hills, MI: Gale, 2014), 2496–2503.

- Quotation from the rule of St. Benedict (whose rule did forbid meat for monks): "Except the sick who are very weak, let all abstain entirely from the flesh of four-footed animals." See Andrew Linzey, "Vegetarianism as a Biblical Ideal," in Walters and Portmess, *Religious Vegetarianism*, 137; Linzey refers to chaps. 39 and 46 of the *Rule of St. Benedict*.

- The Roman priest (and antipope) Novatian's suggestion that God allowed meat because of the increased need for strength to meet the rigors of life outside of paradise. See Novatian, "On the Jewish Meats," chapter 2, *New Advent*, accessed March 2, 2016, www.newadvent.org/fathers/0512.htm:

  > And since now it was no more a paradise to be tended, but a whole world to be cultivated, the more robust food of flesh is offered to men, that for the advantage of culture something more might be added to the vigour of the human body.

  I am indebted to Richard Alan Young (*Is God a Vegetarian?*, 131) for the Novatian reference.

150. Fallon, *Nourishing Traditions*, 504–5 (see chap. 4, n. 101). Fallon quotes Claude Aubert's book *Dis-Moi Comment Tu Cuisines* (Mens, France: Association Terre Vivante, 1987) regarding research on the growth rate of rats using different combinations of corn, beans, and fish.

151. Rudolph Ballentine speaks of spiritual masters reportedly living for years without food, and Gabriel Cousens of the twentieth-century Catholic nun Therese Neumann living on the Christian communion host; see Ballentine, *Diet and Nutrition*, 574 (see chap. 1, n. 15). See also Gabriel Cousens, MD, *Spiritual Nutrition* (Berkeley, CA: North Atlantic Books, 2005), 132. A current example of someone reportedly living without food is the German stigmatic Judith von Halle; see Robert Powell, *Cultivating Inner Radiance and the Body of Immortality* (Great Barrington, MA: Lindisfarne, 2012), 11.

152. Email correspondence with Sally Fallon Morell, October 10, 2016.

153. Ibid.

154. On attention to children's instincts, see Rudolf Steiner, "Nutrition and Child Nutrition, Digestion of Protein, Arterial Sclerosis," lecture of August 2, 1924, and "Healthy Instinct for Food," extract from The Education of the Child (1907), both in *Nutrition and Stimulants*, 121 and 182 (see chap. 2, n. 40). On nutrition and health education after puberty, see Steiner, "Teaching Children about Nutrition," lecture of September 5, 1919, extract from lecture 14, "Practical Advice for Teachers," in *Nutrition and Stimulants*, 186–187.

155. Peter Singer, *Animal Liberation* (New York: Harper Perennial, 1975), 2009.

156. Richard H. Schwartz, Ph.D., *Judaism and Vegetarianism* (New York: Lantern Books, 2001), 125.

Chapter 6

1. John N. Cole, *Amaranth from the Past for the Future* (Emmaus, PA: Rodale Press, 1979), 62–63; Maguelonne Toussaint-Samat, *A History of Food*, trans. Anthea Bell (Malden, MA: Blackwell, 1994), 128.

2. Standage, *Edible History*, 11 (see chap. 5, n. 2).

3. Tamara Andrews, *Nectar and Ambrosia* (Santa Barbara, CA: ABC-CLIO, 2000), 74.

4. Anthony Christie, *Chinese Mythology* (Middlesex: Paul Hamlyn, 1968), 93.

5. Andrews, *Nectar and Ambrosia*, 149 (millet) and 193 (quinoa).

6. Cole, *Amaranth*, 21.

7. Ballentine, *Diet and Nutrition*, 49–50, 65 (see chap. 1, n. 15).

8. Andrews, *Nectar and Ambrosia*, 202.

9. Ibid., 71.

10. Cole, *Amaranth*, 49–50.

11. Andrews, *Nectar and Ambrosia*, 214. For the myths about quinoa and spelt, see the Arrowhead Mills brochures *The Life Story of Quinoa* and *The Life Story of Spelt* (Hereford, TX: Arrowhead Mills, 1993); also see Andrews, *Nectar and Ambrosia*, 74, and Cole, *Amaranth*, 57.

12. Lorenz Schaller, "Healing Foods: Cereal Grains of Peace," *Sharing News: A Wholistic Journal*,1987; and "About Cereal Grains," *The Cerealist*, no. 1(1989): 8. Both publications are by the Kusa Seed Society, Ojai, CA, copyright Lorenz Schaller.

13. Andrews, *Nectar and Ambrosia*, 214.

14. Cole, *Amaranth*, 31, 61.

15. Erich Neumann, *The Great Mother: An Analysis of the Archetype* (Princeton, NJ: Princeton University Press, 1970), 285.

16. Standage, *Edible History*, ix.

17. Toussaint-Samat, *A History of Food*, 156–57.

18. Dawn E. Bastian and Judy K. Mitchell, *Handbook of Native American Mythology* (Santa Barbara, CA: ABC-CLIO, 2004), 70.

19. Toussaint-Samat, *A History of Food*, 125.

20. Sir James George Frazer, OM, *The Golden Bough*, pt. 4, vol. 2, Adonis, Attis, Osiris (New York: St. Martin's Press, 1976), 7; Andrews, *Nectar and Ambrosia*, 245.

21. Standage, *Edible History*, 13.

22. Ibid., 15.

23. Ara, *Eschatology in the Indo-Iranian Traditions* (see chap. 5, n. 4). See especially the chapter "Old Europe: Theoretical Perspectives" and p. 109 regarding the germination of seeds.

24. Andrews, *Nectar and Ambrosia*, 244.

25. Frazer, *Golden Bough*, pt. 4, vol. 2, 16, 112–14, 159.

26. Andrews, *Nectar and Ambrosia*, 20.

27. Joseph Campbell, *The Mythic Image* (Princeton, NJ: Princeton University Press, 1974), 426.

28. Frazer, *Golden Bough*, pt. 4, vol. I, 6ff., 227ff., 263ff., 298; pt. 4, vol. 2, 3ff., 113, 126, 159; pt. 5, vol. 1, *Spirits of the Corn and of the Wild*, especially 35, 214. On Tammuz also being known as Tiamant, see Neumann, *Great Mother*, 183.

29. Frazer, *Golden Bough*, pt. 4, vol. 2, 114.

30. Ibid., 114; pt. 5, vol. 1, 90–91.

31. Commentaries to books 2 and 4 of Patanjali's *Yogasutras* use agriculture and rice farming to explain karma and rebirth to ordinary people. See Karl Potter, "The Karma Theory and Its Implications in Some Indian Philosophical Systems," in Wendy Doniger O'Flaherty, ed., *Karma and Rebirth in Classical Indian Traditions* (Berkeley: University of California Press, 1980), 245, 248.

32. "Paleolithic Diet," *Wikipedia*, accessed March 15, 2016, http://en.wikipedia.org/wiki/Paleolithic_diet. Walter Voegtlin's book *The Stone Age Diet* (see chap. 4, n. 83) appeared, as did Singer's *Animal Liberation*, in 1975 (see chap. 5, n. 155).

33. Peter Singer, "All Animal Rights Are Equal," from *Animal Rights and Human Obligations*, Tom Regan and Peter Singer, eds., 2nd ed. (Englewood Cliffs, NJ: Prentice Hall, 1989), online file accessed March 15, 2016, http://www2.webster.edu/~corbetre/philosophy/animals/singer-text.html. The article originally appeared in *Philosophic Exchange* 1, no. 5 (Summer 1974).

34. "Paleolithic Diet," *Wikipedia.*

35. "Origins of Agriculture," in Solomon H. Katz, ed., *Encyclopedia of Food and Culture*, vol. 1 (New York: Charles Scribner's Sons, 2003), 52.

36. Ibid., 50–51.

37. "Methods of Paleo Nutrition," in Katz, *Encyclopedia of Food and Culture*, vol. 3, 37.

38. "Prehistoric Societies, Stone Age Nutrition," in Katz, *Encyclopedia of Food and Culture*, vol. 3, 130.

39. Ibid., 132–33.

40. "Paleolithic Diet," *Wikipedia.*

41. "Prehistoric Societies, Stone Age Nutrition," in Katz, *Encyclopedia of Food and Culture*, vol. 3, 133–34.

42. "Methods of Paleo Nutrition," in Katz, *Encyclopedia of Food and Culture*, vol. 3, 36.

43. "Paleolithic Diet," *Wikipedia.*

44. The percentages for typical consumption patterns add up to 100 by including 3 percent for alcohol consumption. See "Prehistoric Societies, Stone Age Nutrition," in Katz, *Encyclopedia of Food and Culture*, vol. 3, 134.

45. Ibid., 134–36.

46. A. Ströhle, M. Wolters, and A. Hahn, "Human Nutrition in the Context of Evolutionary Medicine," *Wiener Klinische Wochenschrift* 121, nos. 5–6 (March 2009): 173–87, abstract, *PubMed*, accessed March 15, 2016, http://www.ncbi.nlm.nih.gov/pubmed/19412746.

47. Loren Cordain acknowledges the criticism about a Paleo-style diet's high cost, yet he asserts that, at least in the West, such a diet can contribute to lowered health costs. See Cordain, "Paleolithic Diet," *Wikipedia.*

48. Melvin Konner and S. Boyd Eaton, "Paleolithic Nutrition: Twenty-Five Years Later," *Nutrition in Clinical Practice* 25, no. 6 (December 2010): 594–602. Eaton and Konner (along with Marjorie Shostak) coauthored one of the first books on Paleo diets, *The Paleolithic Prescription* (see chap. 4, n. 83).

49. Paleo authors who discourage the use of grains and other complex carbohydrates include Loren Cordain, *The Paleo Diet*; Mark Sisson, *The Primal Blueprint*; and Robb Wolf, *The Paleo Solution* (see chap. 4, n. 83 for all three books). Gary Taubes also concludes that grains and other starchy complex carbohydrates are too problematic and best excluded: Taubes, *Good Calories, Bad Calories*, 454–56 (see chap. 4, n. 78).

50. Fallon, *Nourishing Traditions*, 56 (see chap. 4, n. 101).

51. Gluten is difficult to digest, and intolerance to it is linked to many diseases: ibid. "U.S. wheat flour the most indigestible": Julia Ross, *The Mood Cure* (New York: Viking, 2002), 126. Wheat gluten content has increased 500 times and coeliac disease rates quadrupled: Dr. Alison Adams, "What Happened to Wheat?" *One Radio Network*, accessed March 15, 2016, http://oneradionetwork.com/latest/what-happened-to-wheat-article/.

52. "Phytic Acid," *Wikipedia*, accessed March 15, 2016, http://en.wikipedia.org/wiki/Phytic_acid. Other carbohydrate foods such as sesame seeds, nuts, and legumes have more phytic acid than have grains.

53. "Niacin," in Katz, *Encyclopedia of Food and Culture*, vol. 2, 553.

54. Ibid.

55. Andrew Weil, MD, "Are Phytates Bad or Good?" (Q and A Library), *DrWeil.com*, accessed March 15, 2016, http://www.drweil.com/drw/u/QAA400758/Are-Phytates-Bad-or-Good.html.

56. Ballentine, *Diet and Nutrition*, 71–73.

57. "Excess Phytates in the Diet: Overview," *Diagnose Me.com*, accessed March 19, 2016, http://www.diagnose-me.com/symptoms-of/excess-phytates-in-diet.html; "Method of treatment of Parkinson's disease using phytic acid," *United States Patent and Trademark Office*, accessed March 19, 2016, http://patft.uspto.gov/netacgi/nph-Parser?Sect2=PTO1&Sect2=HITOFF&p=1&u=/netahtml/PTO/search-bool.html&r=1&f=G&l=50&d=PALL&RefSrch=yes&Query=PN/5206226; "Phytates Revisited—What are Phytates?" *Paleo Plan*, accessed March 19, 2016, http://www.paleoplan.com/2015/06-03/phytates-revisited-what-are-phytates/.

58. "Lectin," *Wikipedia*, accessed March 15, 2016, http://en.wikipedia. org/wiki/Lectin; "The Lectin Connection," *Eat Right for Your Type*, accessed March 20, 2016, http://www.dadamo.com/txt/index.pl?1007; Carolyn Pierini, CLS (ACSP), CNC, "Lectins, Their Damaging Role in Intestinal Health, Rheumatoid Arthritis, and Weight Loss," *Vitamin Research Products*, accessed March 15, 2016, http://www.vrp.com/digestive-health/lectins-their-damaging-role-in-intestinal-health-rheumatoid-arthritis-and-weight-loss; Mark Sisson, "The Lowdown on Lectins," *Mark's Daily Apple*, accessed March 15, 2016, http://www. marksdailyapple.com/lectins/#axzz2SgJIcUbo.

59. Ballentine, *Diet and Nutrition*, 69–70.

60. Ibid. See also Toussaint-Samat, *A History of Food*, 140–41, 144–45.

61. Toussaint-Samat, *A History of Food*, 71–73.

62. Ibid., 76–78.

63. "Low-carbohydrate diet," *Wikipedia*, accessed March 15, 2016, http:// en.wikipedia.org/wiki/Low-carbohydrate_diet. The author says this:

> While diet devoid of essential fatty acids (EFAs) and essential amino acids (EAAs) will result in eventual death, a diet completely without carbohydrates can be maintained indefinitely because triglycerides (which make up fat stored in the body and dietary fat) include a (glycerol) molecule which the body can easily convert to glucose.

Wikipedia adds that when carbohydrates are absent, the body uses fatty acids and ketones for energy, as well as the glucose supplied by protein conversion (*gluconeogenesis*). In this way, normal levels of glucose are maintained without carbohydrates.

64. Taubes, *Good Calories, Bad Calories*, 454–56.

Chapter 7

1. "The Ornish Diet (The Science of Appetite)," *Time 2007 Special*, accessed March 15, 2016, http://content.time.com/time/specials/2007/ article/0,28804,1626795_1626678_1626544,00.html; "The Weight Watchers Diet," *Time 2007 Special*, accessed March 15, 2016, http:// content.time.com/time/specials/2007/article/0,28804,1626795 _1626678_1626534,00.html; "The Atkins Diet," *Time 2007 Special*, accessed March 15, 2016, http://content.time.com/time/specials/2007/article/0,28804,1626795_1626678_1626539,00.html.

These three are named the "Big Three" and represent the three main diet types: low fat, low calorie, and low carbohydrate.

2. Robert C. Atkins, MD, *Atkins for Life* (New York: St. Martin's Press, 2003), 23–24, 45–46.

3. Ibid., 63; Westman, Phinney, and Volek, *The New Atkins*, 39–45, 70–71, 260–71 (see chap. 4, n. 84).

4. Westman, Phinney, and Volek, *The New Atkins*, xv.

5. Ibid., 45, 49. See also Atkins, *Atkins for Life*, 51–53, 62–63.

6. "Low-carbohydrate diet," *Wikipedia* (see chap. 6, n. 63).

7. Taubes, *Good Calories, Bad Calories*, 319 (see chap. 4, n. 78); Westman, Phinney, and Volek, *The New Atkins*, 287.

8. On fasting, see Taubes, *Good Calories, Bad Calories*, 319. On protection against cellular injury, see "Low-carbohydrate diet," *Wikipedia*.

9. Westman, Phinney, and Volek, *The New Atkins*, 285–86; "Ketogenic diet," *Wikipedia*, accessed March 15, 2016, http://en.wikipedia.org/wiki/Ketogenic_diet.

10. Westman, Phinney, and Volek, *The New Atkins*, 40–41.

11. Sora Song, "Health: Atkins Trims the Fat," *Time*, February 2, 2004, accessed March 15, 2016, http://content.time.com/time/magazine/article/0,9171,993244,00.html.

12. Associated Press, "Carbs may be worse for heart than fatty foods," *NBC News*, November 8, 2006, accessed March 15, 2016, http://www.nbc-news.com/id/15625548/; Westman, Phinney, and Volek, *The New Atkins*, 286–290; "Low-carbohydrate diet," *Wikipedia*.

13. Westman, Phinney, and Volek, *The New Atkins*, 308; "Low-carbohydrate diet," *Wikipedia*.

14. "Atkins Diet," *Wikipedia*, accessed March 15, 2016, http://en.wikipedia.org/wiki/Atkins_diet.

15. Nancy Hellmich, "Researchers chew the fat on merits of the Atkins diet," *USA Today*, accessed March 15, 2016, http://www.usatoday.com/news/health/2002-08-06-atkins_x.htm.

16. On low energy, see Cordain, *Paleo Diet*, 65 (see chap. 4, n. 83). On impaired functioning, see Dean Ornish, MD, "Was Dr. Atkins Right?" *Journal of the American Dietetic Association* 104, no. 4 (April 2004):

540; and Katahn, *T-Factor Diet*, 242–43 (see chap. 4, n. 62). Both authors refer to R. R. Wing, J. A. Vazquez, and C. M. Ryan, "Cognitive Effects of Ketogenic Weight-Reducing Diets," *International Journal of Obesity and Related Metabolic Disorders* 19, no. 11 (1995): 811–16.

17. Different sources give diverse estimates for macronutrient thermic effects. The cited estimates are a composite (see chap. 4, n. 92).

18. Shintani, *Eat More, Weigh Less Diet*, 56 (see chap. 4, n. 92). The figures are 40 percent fat, 45 percent carbohydrate, and 15 percent protein, compared with 10 percent fat, 75 percent carbohydrate, and 15 percent protein. Katahn (in *T-Factor Diet*, 35) also refers to this phenomenon.

19. Sri Aurobindo indicates that the gunas reflect characteristic qualities as well as effects on the body and that the character of tamas is inertia. Rudoph Ballentine adds that tamas creates heaviness and lethargy, promoting sluggishness, decreased alertness, and even sleep. Aurobindo, *Message of the Gita*, 26, 234, 296 (see chap. 1, n. 2); Ballentine, *Diet and Nutrition*, 547–50 (see chap. 1, n. 15).

20. Ballentine, *Diet and Nutrition*, 548–50. As indicated in chapter 1, fish and wild game are associated with the rajas guna, and carbohydrates such as grains and fruit (and fresh raw milk) with sattva. Sri Aurobindo relates sattva to intelligence, conserving energy, and clarity; and rajas to force and action (Aurobindo, *Message of the Gita*, 26, 295–96).

21. "Most whole natural foods (with the exception of meat, which contains no carbohydrate) contain a balance of the three major nutrients as well as appropriate amounts of vitamins and minerals." Ballentine, *Diet and Nutrition*, 47–48.

22. "Low-carbohydrate diet," *Wikipedia*. Essential fatty acids, or EFAs, cannot be manufactured by the body and must be obtained by diet. The same is true for proteins (essential amino acids, or EAAs), but not carbohydrates (there are no essential carbohydrates).

23. Westman, Phinney, and Volek, *The New Atkins*, 72; Taubes, *Good Calories, Bad Calories*, 324.

24. Atkins, *Atkins for Life*, 63.

25. Various authors represent Paleo-style diets: Walter L. Voegtlin's *Stone Age Diet*; S. Boyd Eaton, Marjorie Shostak, and Melvin Konner's *Paleolithic Prescription*; Ray V. Audette's *NeanderThin*; Loren Cordain's *Paleo Diet*; Mark Sisson's *Primal Blueprint*; and Robb Wolf's *Paleo Solution*. See chap. 4, n. 83 for full publishing details.

26. Cordain, *Paleo Diet*, 218; Jennifer McLagan, *Fat* (Berkeley, CA: Ten Speed, 2008), 9.

27. Cordain, *Paleo Diet*, 11–14.

28. Don Amerman, "Highly Thermogenic Foods" (see chap. 4, n. 92).

29. Cordain, *Paleo Diet*, 68.

30. Cordain, *Paleo Diet*, 40, 101; "The Dangers of a High-Protein Diet," *Raw Food Explained.com, Lesson 85*, accessed March 15, 2016, http://www.rawfoodexplained.com/the-dangers-of-a-high-protein-diet.

31. Cordain, *Paleo Diet*, 34 and 211.

32. Steiner, "Problems of Nutrition," in *Nutrition and Stimulants*, 148–49 (see chap. 2, n. 40).

33. Ballentine, *Diet and Nutrition*, 547–51.

34. Dean Ornish, MD, *Eat More, Weigh Less* (NY: Harper Collins, 2001), 34–35.

35. Ibid., 8; "Dean Ornish," *Wikipedia*, accessed March 15, 2016, https://en.wikipedia.org/wiki/Dean_Ornish.

36. Dean Ornish, MD, "The Case for Low Fat," *Time*, September 2, 2002, accessed March 15, 2016, http://content.time.com/time/magazine/article/0,9171,1003161,00.html.

37. Ornish, *Eat More, Weigh Less*, xiii.

38. Terry Shintani, MD, JD, MPH, *The Hawaii Diet* (New York: Pocket Books, 1999), 32.

39. Ibid., xiii.

40. Katahn, *T-Factor Diet*, 48. Twenty to forty grams of fat equals 180–360 calories (9 calories/gram x 20–40 grams). Using Dr. Terry Shintani's figure of a 2,500 calorie diet for an average sedentary man and active woman, 180–360 calories equals about 7–14 percent of daily calories, and 30–60 grams (270–540 calories) about 11–22 percent.

41. Ibid.,11–12, 263–265.

42. Shintani, *Eat More, Weigh Less Diet*, 44.

43. Katahn, *T-Factor Diet*, 37.

44. Ibid., 39.

45. Ibid., 35.

46. Ibid. On converting carbs increases thermic effect, see pp. 35, 260–63; on the body would rather speed up metabolic rate, see 36.

47. Ornish, *Eat More, Weigh Less*, v.

48. "Adolf Hitler and Vegetarianism," *Wikipedia*, accessed March 15, 2016, http://en.wikipedia.org/wiki/Adolf_Hitler_and_vegetarianism.

49. Health Magazine, *The Diet Advisor* (Alexandria, VA: Time Life Books, 2000), 19.

50. Low-carbohydrate and low-fat diets also include exercise, yet attention is more directed to the metabolic principles leading to weight loss. Dean Ornish notes that excessive exercise isn't necessary with his diet; just 20–60 minutes of walking is sufficient. Terry Shintani recommends 30 minutes of exercise 4 times a week. See Ornish, *Eat More, Weigh Less*, 46; Shintani, *Eat More, Weigh Less Diet*, 122.

51. Health Magazine, *The Diet Advisor*, 172, 175.

52. Health Magazine, *The Diet Advisor*: low-carb diets lead to overeating, 17; low-carb diets stress the kidneys, 29; fat is one of life's pleasure, 73; too little fat and lack of exercise elevates blood triglycerides, 31.

53. Ornish, *Eat More, Weigh Less*, xiii.

Chapter 8

1. Neumann, *Great Mother*, 285 (see chap. 6, n. 15).

2. Ibid., 285.

3. Ibid., 60.

4. Ballentine, *Diet and Nutrition*, 69–73 (see chap. 1, n. 15); Toussaint-Samat, *A History of Food*, 140–41, 144–45, 177 (see chap. 6, n. 1). Toussaint-Samat also mentions the alternative of mixing protein-rich millet with refined flour and adds that cereals were made more digestible by roasting them.

5. On Indian practices and parboiling, see Ballentine, *Diet and Nutrition*, 76–78; on cracks being repaired, see Margaret Visser, *Much Depends on Dinner* (New York: Grove Press, 1986), 185.

6. Visser, *Much Depends on* Dinner, 210–20.

7. Steiner, "Milling and Baking," in *Nutrition and Stimulants*, 211–14 (see chap. 2, n. 40). These indications were compiled by Fr. Schyre from

remarks made by Rudolf Steiner on various occasions. Schyre published them in *Mitteilungen des Landwirtschaftlichen Versuchsringes der Anthroposophischen Gesellschaft* (*Newsletter of the Anthroposophical Society's Agricultural Experiments*), no. 14, 2nd year, March 1928.

8. Melissa Diane Smith, *Going against the Grain* (Chicago: Contemporary Books, 2002), 9, 57.

9. Fallon, *Nourishing Traditions*, xi (see chap. 4, n. 101).

10. "Sprouting," *Wikipedia*, accessed March 15, 2016, http://en.wikipedia.org/wiki/Sprouting; Fallon, *Nourishing Traditions*, 112. Critics point to fantastic claims about vitamin and mineral increases through sprouting and emphasize that nutrient percentages per gram of weight actually remain about the same. They also note that nutrient levels hardly change for sprouted and unsprouted whole grain bread. Yet there are important benefits to sprouted flour, such as changing starch molecules into more digestible vegetable sugars, creating enzymes that aid digestion, and neutralizing antinutrients, all of which improve tolerance to wheat bread among those who had been previously intolerant. See "Sprouted Bread," *Wikipedia*, accessed March 15, 2016, http://en.wikipedia.org/wiki/Sprouted_bread; "About Sprouted Flour and Related Info," *Summers Sprouted Flour Co.*, accessed March 15, 2016, http://www.creatingheaven.net/eeproducts/eesfc/about_sprouted.html.

11. Fallon, *Nourishing Traditions*, xii. For paragraph references see pages xi, 25, 47, 452–53, 476, 489, 499.

12. Betty Fussell, *The Story of Corn* (New York: Alfred A. Knopf, 1992), 176.

13. Bob Lignon, "Growing with Grains" (interview with Lorenz Schaller), *Macrobiotics Today* (Nov/Dec 1991): 7–8.

14. Fallon, *Nourishing Traditions*, 112, 463.

15. Price, *Nutrition and Physical Degeneration*, 245 (see chap. 3, n. 31).

16. J. Jayaraj and R. K. Murali Baskaran, "Control of moths in stored grain," *The Hindu*, February 7, 2013.

17. Fallon, *Nourishing Traditions*, 495.

18. Rudolph Ballentine, MD, *Transition to Vegetarianism* (Honesdale, PA: Himalayan Institute Press, 1999), 139, 229, 231. In addition to using turmeric, cumin, and coriander, Ballentine lists the following to make beans less gassy: the spices ginger, black mustard seeds, cardamom,

cloves, and black pepper; and the herbs bay leaves, thyme, sage, and marjoram (onions and garlic also help to stimulate digestion; see p. 100).

19. Ibid., 100.

20. Fallon, *Nourishing Traditions*, 80–81, 185.

21. "Sattvic Diet," *Wikipedia* (see chap. 1, n. 13); and a conversation with Atmavadan Reddy during a visit to a Sri Aurobindo dairy operation in January, 2014. Gerhardt Schmidt suggests that Rudolf Steiner's remarks about milk (see chapter 2) also refer to raw milk: Schmidt, *Dynamics of Nutrition*, 144 (see chap. 2, n. 118).

22. Ballentine, *Diet and Nutrition*, 129–32; Ballentine, *Transition to Vegetarianism*, 207–8.

23. Fallon, *Nourishing Traditions*, 545.

24. Ballentine, *Transition to Vegetarianism*, 225.

25. Stephen Uprichard, "Lorenz Schaller New Age Seed Man," *Macrobiotics Today* (November 1986): 9. Schaller notes that grains were traditionally cut and left on the fields for proper sun curing. He laments that today crops are bred with an industrial bias that favors immature harvesting: see Bob Lignon, "Growing with Grains" (interview with Lorenz Schaller), *Macrobiotics Today* (November/December 1991): 7–8.

26. Ballentine, *Transition to Vegetarianism*, 119–20.

27. Ballentine, *Diet and Nutrition*, 564–67.

28. Ibid., 574; Cousens, *Spiritual Nutrition*, 132, 204–10 (see chap. 5, n. 151).

29. The apostle Paul's Letter to the Hebrews 9:27. In addition to the Letter to the Hebrews, the *New Catholic Encyclopedia* refers to Luke 16:19–31 and 23:43, and 2 Corinthians 5:10. See *New Catholic Encyclopedia*, 2nd ed. vol. 9, Mab-Mor, "Metempsychosis" (Washington, DC: Catholic University of America, 2003), 556.

30. Anonymous, *Meditations on the Tarot, a Journey into Christian Hermeticism* (New York: Tarcher/Putnam, 2002), 93. Originally published in French in 1980 and in English in 1985.

31. Ibid., 361. The anonymous author writes that belief in reincarnation would deflect attention from the process of purgation, illumination, and union that accompanies every death, with potentially disastrous results.

32. Ibid., 256.

33. Ibid., 576.

34. Ibid., 580.

35. Ibid., 472.

36. Ibid., 571–72.

37. Rudolf Steiner, *An Outline of Esoteric Science*, trans. Catherine E. Cree-ger (Great Barrington, MA: Anthroposophic Press, 1997), 30–58 (the chapter is entitled "The Makeup of the Human Being"). See also "The Essential Nature of the Human Being," chap. 1 of Steiner's *Theosophy* (Hudson, NY: Anthroposophic Press, 1994).

38. "The *I am* is the divine name": Metzger and Murphy, *New Oxford Annotated Bible*, 140 NT, footnote to John 8:58 (see chap. 5, n. 79). The footnote cites Exodus 3:14, where Moses is commissioned by God to bring the Israelites out of Egypt. When Moses asks who he shall say sent him, God replies: "Thus you shall say to the Israelites, '*I am* has sent me to you.'" In John 8:58, Jesus identifies himself with this same name ("Very truly I tell you, before Abraham was, *I am*"). In response, his listeners pick up stones to throw, but he escapes unharmed (the passage indicates the blasphemy of invoking the divine name and using it to refer to oneself).

39. Anonymous, *Meditations on the Tarot*, 208.

40. Metzger and Murphy, "Apocalyptic Literature," *New Oxford Annotated Bible*, 363 NT.

41. Laurence A. Moran, "ABO Blood Types," *Sandwalk, Strolling with a Skeptical Biochemist*, accessed March 15, 2016, http://sandwalk.blogspot.com/2007/02/abo-blood-types.html; Kevin Richardson, "The Scientific Argument against Blood Type Diets," *Naturally Intense Personal Training Blog*, accessed March 15, 2016, http://www.naturallyintense.net/blog/diet/the-scientific-argument-against-blood-type-diets/; "Blood Type Diet," *Wikipedia*, accessed March 15, 2016, http://en.wikipedia.org/wiki/Blood_type_diet.

42. "Blood Type Diet," *Wikipedia*; "The Scientific Argument against Blood Type Diets," *Naturally Intense Personal Training Blog*; Barry Eade, "Which Human Blood Group Evolved First?" *Focus Science and Technology*, accessed March 15, 2016, http://sciencefocus.com/qa/which-human-blood-group-evolved-first. About type A appearing, disappearing, and then reappearing, see Dr. Peter D'Adamo's review of a recent study in the journal of *Molecular Biology and Evolution*:

"Response to Various Critics," *Eat Right 4 Your Type,* accessed March 15, 2016, http://www.dadamo.com/science_critic.htm.

43. Stefansson, *Not By Bread Alone,* 1–13 (see chap. 4, n. 52); Rob Dunn, "Human Ancestors Were Nearly All Vegetarians," *Scientific American* (July 23, 2012), accessed March 15, 2016, http://blogs.scientificamerican.com/guest-blog/2012/07/23/human-ancestors-were-nearly-all-vegetarians/; D'Adamo with Whitney, *Eat Right 4 Your Type* (see chap. 4, n. 85).

44. Moran, "ABO Blood Types," *Sandwalk.* The quote is found at the end of the article in Moran's first comment posted Wednesday, February 21, 2007.

45. Rudolf Steiner, lecture of December 29, 1911, published as *The World of the Senses and the World of the Spirit,* Collected Works 134 (North Vancouver, BC: Steiner Book Centre, 1979).

46. "Berachos 17," Adages of Chachamim, verse (g), accessed February 17, 2016, http://www.dafyomi.co.il/berachos/points/br-ps-017.htm. For this reference, I am indebted to Rabbi David Sears, *The Vision of Eden,* 352 (see chap. 2, n. 9).

47. Ballentine, *Transition to Vegetarianism,* 184.

48. Ibid., xiv. Ballentine's *Transition to Vegetarianism* is highly recommended for its wealth of tips and valuable information.

49. Cousens, *Spiritual Nutrition,* 236–37 (see chap. 5, n. 151).

50. Aurobindo, *Message of the Gita,* 234–35 (see chap. 1, n. 2).

Afterword

1. See Fallon, *Nourishing Traditions,* 452–454 (see chap. 4, n. 101).

Appendix A

1. For Adonis, Attis, and Osiris, see Frazer, *Golden Bough,* pt. 4, vol. 1, 6f., 227f., 263f., 298 and pt. 4, vol. 2, 3f., 113, 126, 159; for Spirits of the Corn and of the Wild, see pt. 5, vol. 1, especially 35 and 214 (see chap. 6, n. 20).

2. Ibid., pt. 4, vol. 2, 126f and pt. 5, vol. 1, 214.

3. Ibid., pt. 5, vol. 1, 176–77.

4. Andrews, *Nectar and Ambrosia*, 74 (see chap. 6, n. 3); Campbell, *Historical Atlas of World Mythology*, vol. 1, part 2 (New York: Harper & Row, 1988), 207; Fussell, *Story of Corn*, 53 (see chap. 8, n. 12); Visser, *Much Depends on Dinner*, 35 (see chap. 8, n. 5).

5. Andrews, *Nectar and Ambrosia*, 200, 215.

6. Campbell, *Historical Atlas of World Mythology*, vol. 2, pt. 1 (also1988), 36–37.

7. Ibid., vol. 2, pt. 2 (1989), 131.

8. Ibid., vol. 2, pt. 3 (1989), 72–73.

9. Ibid, vol. 2, pt. 3, 305.

10. Campbell, *The Mythic Image*, 158 (see chap. 6, n. 27).

11. Ibid, 420.

12. Christie, *Chinese Mythology*, 93 (see chap. 6, n. 4).

13. Louis Herbert Gray, AM, PhD, ed., *The Mythology of All Races*, vol. 8 (New York: Cooper Square, 1964), 232.

14. Visser, *Much Depends on Dinner*, 166.

15. Neumann, *Great Mother*, 151–152 (see chap. 6, n. 15).

16. Ibid., 183; Campbell, *Historical Atlas of World Mythology*, vol. 2, pt. 1, 37.

17. Neumann, *Great* Mother, 186.

18. Ibid., 189–191.

19. Ibid., 279.

20. Campbell, *Historical Atlas of World Mythology*, vol. 2, pt. 1, 37.

21. Ibid., 75.

22. Campbell, *The Mythic Image*, 420, 422.

23. Andrews, *Nectar and Ambrosia*, 20.

24. Campbell, *The Mythic Image*, 158.

25. Gray, *Mythology of All Races*, vol. 3, 46–47.

26. Ibid., vol. 4, 239–243.

27. Ibid., vol. 10, 201.

28. Visser, *Much Depends on Dinner*, 170.

29. Cole, *Amaranth*, 18–20 (see chap. 6, n. 1).

30. Frazer, *Golden Bough*, pt. 5, vol. 2, 48.

31. Ibid., 82–83.

32. Ibid., 86–89.

33. Ibid., 93–94.

34. Ibid.,109.

35. Ibid., 167.

36. Neumann, *Great Mother*, 192.

37. Campbell, *Historical Atlas of World Mythology*, vol. 2, pt. 1, 72–73, 76.

38. Fussell, *Story of Corn*, 41.

39. Toussaint-Samat, *History of Food*, 169 (see chap. 6, n. 1).

40. Fussell, *Story of Corn*, 291–92, 298.

41. Frazer, *Golden Bough*, pt. 4, vol. 1, 272–273.

42. Ibid., pt. 4, vol. 2, 12–13, 16.

43. Ibid., 114.

44. Ibid., pt. 5, vol. 1, 54, 90f.

45. Ibid., pt. 5, vol. 2, 167.

46. Ibid., pt. 4, vol. 1, 159.

47. Ibid., pt. 5, vol. 2, 167–168.

48. Ibid., pt. 6, 420f.

49. "James George Frazier," *Wikipedia*, accessed March 15, 2016, http:// en.wikipedia.org/wiki/James_George_Frazer; "Dying-and-rising god," *Wikipedia*, accessed March 15, 2016, https://en.wikipedia.org/wiki/ Dying-and-rising_god; Mary Beard, "Frazier, Leach, and Virgil: the Popularity (and Unpopularity) of the Golden Bough," *Comparative Studies in Society and History* 34:2 (April 1992): 203–24; "Sir James George Frazer," *Encyclopedia Britannica On-Line*, accessed March 15, 2016, www. britannica.com/EBchecked/topic/217662/Sir-James-George-Frazer.

50. Fussell, *The Story of Corn*, 30, 33, and 39.

51. Campbell, *Historical Atlas of World Mythology*, vol. 2, pt. 1, 73.

52. Ibid., 36.

53. At least the Avestan tradition attributes the demand for sacrificial killing to the influence of the evil spirit. See Ara, *Eschatology in the Indo-Iranian Traditions*, 170 (see chap. 5, n. 4).

Appendix B

1. "History of Alcoholic Beverages," *Wikipedia*, accessed March 3, 2016, https://en.wikipedia.org/wiki/History_of_alcoholic_beverages; "Religion and Alcohol," *Wikipedia*, accessed March 3, 2016, https://en.wikipedia.org/wiki/Religion_and_alcohol.

2. Ibid; see also "Christian Views on Alcohol," *Wikipedia*, accessed March 3, 2016, https://en.wikipedia.org/wiki/Christian_views_on_alcohol.

3. Steiner, "Vegetarian and Meat Diets, Milk, Alcohol," lecture of December 17, 1908, in *Nutrition and Stimulants* (see chap. 2, n. 40).

4. Ibid., "Problems of Nutrition," lecture of January 8, 1909.

5. Ibid., "Meat, Vegetarian Food, Alcohol," lecture of March 20, 1913.

6. Ibid., "The Process of Nutrition," lecture of September 16, 1922.

7. Ibid., "The Effect of Alcohol," lecture of January 8, 1923.

8. Ibid., "Alcohol," lecture of February 16, 1924.

9. Steiner, "Foundations of Esotericism: Lecture XXX," lecture of November 4, 1905, *Rudolf Steiner Archive and e.Lib*, accessed February 14, 2016, http://wn.rsarchive.org/Lectures/GA093a/English/RSP1982/19051104p01.html. Also found in excerpt form as "Different Forms of Nourishment in Human Evolution" in Steiner, *Nutrition and Stimulants*, 208-10.

Appendix C

1. Cousens, *Spiritual Nutrition*, 191, 355 (see chap. 5, n. 151).

2. Edmond Bordeaux Szekely, trans. and ed., *The Essene Gospel of Peace* (online text), accessed February 15, 2016, http://www.essene.com/GospelOfPeace/peace1.html.

3. Cousens, *Spiritual Nutrition*, 289–297.

4. "Edmond Bordeaux Szekely," *Wikipedia*, accessed March 15, 2016, https://en.wikipedia.org/wiki/Edmund_Bordeaux_Szekely.

5. Cousens, *Spiritual Nutrition*, 304.

6. Steiner, "The Connection between Food & the Human Being: Raw Foods and Vegetarian Diet," lecture of July 31, 1924, *Nutrition and Stimulants* (see chap. 2, n. 40).

7. Steiner, "The Effect of Cooking; the Tomato," lecture of June 16, 1924, *Nutrition and Stimulants*.

8. "Edmund Bordeaux Szekely," *Wikipedia*; "Raw Foodism," *Wikipedia*, accessed March 15, 2016, https://en.wikipedia.org/wiki/Raw_foodism; "Edmund Bordeaux Szekely," *Poetry Chaikhana: Sacred Poetry from around the World*, accessed March 15, 2016, http://www.poetry-chaikhana.com/Poets/S/SzekelyEdmon/index.html; Trimm, James "Topic: Essene Gospel of Peace," *Nazarene Space*, accessed March 15, 2016, http://nazarenespace.com/main/search/search?q=szekely.

9. See *Poetry Chaikhana*.

10. "Raw Foodism," *Wikipedia*.

11. Fallon, *Nourishing Traditions*, 47, 178 (see chap. 4, n. 101). Fallon refers to the following authors with their works: Edward Howell, MD, *Enzymes for Health and Longevity* (Woodstock Valley, CT: Omangod Press, 1980); Edward Howell, MD, *Enzyme Nutrition* (Wayne, NJ: Avery Publishing Group, 1985); Henry G. Bieler, MD, *Food is Your Best Medicine* (Ballentine Books, 1965).

12. Fallon, *Nourishing Traditions*, xi, 47.

13. Ibid., 178. Regarding raw vegetables, Fallon cites Bieler, *Food Is Your Best Medicine*.

14. Ibid., 47.

15. "Chakra," *Wikipedia*, accessed February 15, 2016, https://en.wikipedia.org/wiki/Chakra.

BIBLIOGRAPHY

Adams, Ruth, and Frank Murray. *Megavitamin Therapy*. New York: Larchmont Books, 1973.

Akers, Keith. *The Lost Religion of Jesus*. New York: Lantern Books, 2000.

American Psychiatric Association. *Megavitamin and Orthomolecular Therapy in Psychiatry*. Washington, DC: American Psychiatric Association, 1973.

Andrews, Tamara. *Nectar and Ambrosia*. Santa Barbara, CA: ABC-CLIO, 2000.

Anonymous. *Meditations on the Tarot: A Journey into Christian Hermeticism*. New York: Tarcher/Putnam, 2002.

Ara, Mitra. *Eschatology in the Indo-Iranian Traditions: The Genesis and Transformation of a Doctrine*. New York: Peter Lang, 2008.

Arrowhead Mills. *The Life Story of Quinoa* and *The Life Story of Spelt* (brochures). Hereford TX: Arrowhead Mills, 1993.

Atkins, Robert C., MD. *Atkins for Life*. New York: St. Martin's Press, 2003.

_____. *Dr. Atkins' New Diet Revolution*. Rev. ed. New York: Avon Books, 2001.

Aurobindo, Sri. *The Message of the Gita*. Pondicherry, India: Sri Aurobindo Ashram, 1977.

Ballentine, Rudolph, MD. *Diet and Nutrition: A Holistic Approach*. Honesdale, PA: Himalayan International Institute, 1982.

_____. *Transition to Vegetarianism*. Honesdale, PA: Himalayan Institute Press, 1999.

Bastian, Dawn E., and Judy K. Mitchell. *Handbook of Native American Mythology*. Santa Barbara, CA: ABC-CLIO, 2004.

Bawa Muhaiyaddeen, Asma' ul-Husna. *The 99 Beautiful Names of Allah*. Philadelphia, PA: Fellowship Press, 1979.

Beard, Mary. "Frazier, Leach, and Virgil: the Popularity (and Unpopularity) of the Golden Bough." *Comparative Studies in Society and History* 34, no. 2 (April 1992): 203–24.

Besant, Annie. *Vegetarianism in the Light of Theosophy.* Adyar Pamphlet 27. 3rd ed. Adyar, India: Theosophical Publishing House, April, 1932.

Bhakivedanta A. C., Swami Prabhupada. *Bhagavad Gita As It Is.* New York: Bhaktivedanta Book Trust, 1968.

Böckenhoff, Karl. *Speisesatzungern Mosaisher Art in Mittelaltlichen Kirchen-rechtsquellen des Morgen- und Abendlandes.* Münster: Aschendorffschen Verlag, 1907. PDF.

Burkitt, Denis, Kenneth Heaton, and Hugh Trowell, eds. *Dietary Fibre, Fibre-Depleted Foods, and Disease.* London: Academic Press, 1985.

Calbom, Cherie, MS. "The Truth about Fats." *Sound Consumer* (PCC Natural Markets), no. 448 (October 2010): 1, 4.

Campbell, Joseph. *Historical Atlas of World Mythology.* Vols. 1 and 2. New York: Harper & Row, 1988 and 1989.

_____. *The Mythic Image.* Princeton, NJ: Princeton University Press, 1974.

Cheraskin, E., and W. M. Ringsdorf Jr. *Psychodietetics.* New York: Stein and Day, 1974.

Christie, Anthony. *Chinese Mythology.* Middlesex: Paul Hamlyn, 1968.

Cole, John. *Amaranth from the Past for the Future.* Emmaeus, PA: Rodale Press, 1979.

Cook, John. *Diet and Your Religion.* Santa Barbara, CA: Woodbridge Press, 1976.

Cordain, Loren, PhD. *The Paleo Diet.* Hoboken, NJ: John Wiley & Sons, 2002.

Cousens, Gabriel, MD. *Spiritual Nutrition.* Berkeley, CA: North Atlantic Books, 2005.

D'Adamo, Dr. Peter J., with Catherine Whitney. *Eat Right 4 Your Type.* New York: G. P. Putnam's Sons, 1996.

Dresner, Samuel H. *The Jewish Dietary Laws: Their Meaning in Our Time.* New York: Burning Book Press, 1966. PDF.

Dufty, William. *Sugar Blues.* New York: Warner Books, 1975.

Easton, Stuart. *Man and World in the Light of Anthroposophy*. Spring Valley, NY: Anthroposophical Press, 1975.

Encyclopedia of Food and Culture. Edited by Solomon H. Katz. Vols. 1–3. New York: Charles Scribner's Sons. 2003.

Enig, Mary G., PhD. *Know Your Fats*. Silver Spring, MD: Bethesda Press, 2000.

Fallon, Sally. *Nourishing Traditions*. Rev. 2nd ed. Washington, DC: New Trends, 2001.

Frazer, Sir James George, OM. *The Golden Bough*. (Multiple volumes.) New York: St. Martin's Press, 1976.

Fredericks, Carlton. *Psycho-Nutrition*. New York: Grosset and Dunlap, 1976.

Fussell, Betty. *The Story of Corn*. New York: Alfred A. Knopf, 1992.

Gaina Sutras, The Sacred Books of the East. Edited by F. Max Müller. Vol. 22, pt. 1. Translated by Hermann Jacobi. Oxford: Clarendon Press, 1884.

Gale Encyclopedia of Alternative and Complimentary Medicine, The. 4th ed. 4 vols. Farmington Hills, MI: Gale, 2014. See especially Douglas Dupler, Rebecca J. Frey, PhD, and Helen Davidson: "Vegetarianism," 2496–2503.

Gellman, Ezra, ed. *Essays on the Thought of Rabbi Kook*. See Abraham Isaac Kook, "On the Reasons for the Commandments." Dickinson University Press, 1991.

Gray, Louis Herbert, AM, PhD, ed. *The Mythology of All Races*. (Multiple volumes.) New York: Cooper Square, 1964.

Grumett, David, and Rachel Muers, eds. *Interdisciplinary Perspectives on Vegetarianism and Theology*. London: T & T Clark, 2008.

Ha'Nish, Otoman Zar-Adusht. *A Vegetarian Science of Dietetics*. 9th edition. Los Angeles: Mazdaznan Press, 1976.

_____. *The Power of Breath*. Rev. ed. Los Angeles: Mazdaznan Press, 1970.

Hawkins, David, and Linus Pauling. *Orthomolecular Psychiatry: Treatment of Schizophrenia*. San Francisco: Freeman and Co., 1973.

Health Magazine. *The Diet Advisor*. Alexandria, VA: Time Life Books, 2000.

Herbert, Jean. *Shinto: At the Fountainhead of Japan*. New York: Stein and Day, 1967.

Hoffer, Abram, and H. Osmond. *Megavitamin Therapy*. Regina, SK: Canadian Schizophrenia Foundation, 1976.

Hoffer, Abram, MD, PhD and Andrew W. Saul, PhD. *Orthomolecular Medicine for Everyone*. Laguna Beach, CA: Basic Health Publications, 2008.

_____. *The Vitamin Cure for Alcoholism*. Laguna Beach, CA: Basic Health Publications, 2009.

Hoffer, Abram, MD, PhD and Morton Walker, DPM. *Putting It All Together: The New Orthomolecular Nutrition*. New Canaan, CT: Keats, 1996.

Holton, D. C. *The National Faith of Japan*. New York: Paragon Book Reprint Corp., 1965.

Hyland, J. R. *God's Covenant with Animals*. New York: Lantern Books, 2000.

Jack, Alex. "The Taste of America." *East West Journal* (April 1979): 48.

Kalechofsky, Roberta, ed. *Judaism and Animal Rights, Classical and Contemporary Responses*. Marblehead, MA: Micah, 1992.

Kapleau, Philip. *To Cherish All Life*. Rochester. NY: The Zen Center, 1981.

Katahn, Martin, PhD. *The T-Factor Diet*. New York: W. W. Norton, 2001.

Keen, Sam. "Eating Our Way to Enlightenment." *Psychology Today* (October 1978): 62–87.

Konner, Melvin, and S. Boyd Eaton. "Paleolithic Nutrition: Twenty-Five Years Later." *Nutrition in Clinical Practice* 25, no. 6 (December 2010): 594–602.

Kook, Rav Avraham Yitzhak Hacohen. *A Vision of Vegetarianism and Peace*. Edited by David Cohen. Translated, with additional notes, by Jonathan Rubenstein (from his unpublished rabbinic thesis). PDF.

Kotzsch, Ronald. "Who Started Macrobiotics?" *East West Journal* (May 1980): 60–67.

Kushi, Michio. "U.F.O.'s Without Sensationalism." *East West Journal* (February 1979): 60.

_____, with Alex Jack. *The Book of Macrobiotics: The Universal Way of Health, Happiness, and Peace*. Garden City Park, NY: Square One, 2012.

Laws of Manu, The: The Sacred Books of the East. Edited by F. Max Müller. Vol. 25. Translated by George Bühler. Oxford: Clarendon Press, 1886.

Leadbeater, C. W. *Vegetarianism and Occultism*. Adyar Pamphlet 33. Adyar, India: Theosophical Publishing House, November, 1913.

Lesser, Michael, MD. *The Brain Chemistry Diet*. New York: G. P. Putnam's Sons, 2002.

Lignon, Bob. "Growing with Grains" (interview with Lorenz Schaller). *Macrobiotics Today* (Nov/Dec 1991): 7–8.

McLagan, Jennifer. *Fat*. Berkeley, CA: Ten Speed Press, 2008.

Neumann, Erich. *The Great Mother: An Analysis of the Archetype*. Princeton, NJ: Princeton University Press, 1970.

New Catholic Encyclopedia. 2nd edition. Vol. 9 (Mab–Mor). "Metempsychosis," 556. The Catholic University of America, 2003.

New Oxford Annotated Bible, The. Edited by Bruce M. Metzger and Roland E. Murphy. New York: Oxford University Press, 1994.

Ni, Maoshing. *The Yellow Emperor's Classic of Medicine*. Boston and London: Shambala, 1995.

Nidhilananda, Swami. *The Upanishads*. Vol. 4. New York: Harper & Brothers, 1959.

O'Flaherty, Wendy Doniger, ed. *Karma and Rebirth in Classical Indian Traditions*. See Karl Potter. "The Karma Theory and Its Implications in Some Indian Philosophical Systems." Berkeley: University of California Press, 1980.

Ohsawa, George. *You Are All Sanpaku*, Seacaucus, NJ: University Books, 1965.

_____. *Zen Macrobiotics*. Los Angeles: Ohsawa Foundation, 1965.

Ornish, Dean, MD. *Eat More, Weigh Less*. New York: Harper Collins, 2001.

_____. "Was Dr. Atkins Right?" *Journal of the American Dietetic Association* 104, no. 4 (April 2004): 540.

Phelps, Norm. *The Great Compassion: Buddhism and Animal Rights*. New York: Lantern Books, 2004.

_____. *The Longest Struggle: Animal Advocacy from Pythagoras to PETA*. New York: Lantern Books, 2007.

Phillips, David. *From Soil to Psyche*. Santa Barbara, CA: Woodbridge Press, 1977.

Pollan, Michael. *In Defense of Food*. New York: Penguin, 2008.

Powell, Robert. *Cultivating Inner Radiance and the Body of Immortality*. Great Barrington, MA: Lindisfarne, 2012.

Price, Weston A., DDS. *Nutrition and Physical Degeneration*. La Mesa, CA: Price-Pottenger Nutrition Foundation, 2008.

Pythagorean Sourcebook and Library: An Anthology of Ancient Writings which Relate to Pythagoras and Pythagorean Philosophy. Kenneth Sylvan Guthrie, comp. and trans. Additional translations by Thomas Taylor and Arthur Fairbanks, Jr. Introduction and edited by David R. Fiedeler. Grand Rapids, MI: Phanes Press, 1988.

Rosen, Steven. *Diet for Transcendence: Vegetarianism and the World Religions*. Badger, CA: Torchlight, 1997.

Ross, Julia. *The Mood Cure*. New York: Viking, 2002.

Schaller, Lorenz. "About Cereal Grains." *The Cerealist* (Ojai, CA: Kusa Seed Society), no. 1 (1989): 8.

_____. "Healing Foods: Cereal Grains of Peace." Reprinted from *Sharing News: A Wholistic Journal*. Ojai, CA, 1987.

Schmidt, Gerhard, MD. *The Dynamics of Nutrition*. Wyoming, RI: Bio-Dynamic Literature, 1980.

Schwartz, Richard H., PhD. *Judaism and Vegetarianism*. New York: Lantern Books, 2001.

Sears, David. *The Vision of Eden: Animal Welfare and Vegetarianism in Jewish Law and Mysticism*. Spring Valley, NY: Logo, 2011. PDF e-book.

Shintani, Terry, MD, JD, MPH. *Eat More, Weigh Less Diet*. Kamuela, HI: Halpax, 1993.

_____. *The Hawaii Diet*. New York: Pocket Books, 1999.

Singer, Peter. *Animal Liberation*. New York: Harper Perennial, 2009.

Sisson, Mark. *The Primal Blueprint*. Malibu, CA: Primal Nutrition, 2009.

Smith, Melissa Diane. *Going Against the Grain*. Chicago: Contemporary Books, 2002.

Standage, Tom. *An Edible History of Humanity*. New York: Walker & Company, 2009.

Stefansson, Vilhjalmur. *Not By Bread Alone*. New York: MacMillan, 1946.

Steiner, Rudolf. *Nutrition and Stimulants: Lectures and Extracts*. Translated by Maria St. Goar. Kimberton, PA: Bio-Dynamic Farming and Gardening Assoc., 1991.

_____. *Outline of Esoteric Science, An.* Translated by Catherine E. Creeger. Steiner Books/Anthroposophic Press, 1997.

_____. *Problems of Nutrition* (booklet). New York: Anthroposophic Press, 1973.

_____. *Theosophy.* Translated by Catherine E. Creeger. Anthroposophic Press, 1994.

_____. *World of the Senses, The, and the World of the Spirit.* Hanover lecture of December 29, 1911. See Collected Works. Vol. 134. North Vancouver, BC: Steiner Book Centre, 1979.

Sutta-Nipâta [sic], *The Sacred Books of the East.* Edited by F. Max Müller. Vol. 10, pt. 2. Translated by V. Fausböll. Oxford: Clarendon Press, 1881.

Suzuki, Daisetz Teitaro, trans. *The Lankavatara Sutra: A Mahayana Text.* London: Routledge and Kegan Paul, 1932.

Taubes, Gary. *Good Calories, Bad Calories.* New York: Alfred A. Knopf, 2007.

Toussaint-Samat, Maguelonne. *A History of Food.* Translated by Anthea Bell. Malden, MA: Blackwell, 1994.

Tuttle, Will, PhD, *The World Peace Diet,* New York: Lantern Books, 2005.

Tyberg, Judith M. *The Language of the Gods.* 2nd ed. Los Angeles: East West Cultural Centre, 1976.

Uprichard, Stephen. "Lorenz Schaller New Age Seed Man." *Macrobiotics Today* (November 1986): 9.

US Department of Agriculture, Human Nutrition Information Service. *The Food Guide Pyramid.* Home and Garden Bulletin 252. August 1992.

Verdam, P. J., LLD. *Mosaic Law in Practice and Study throughout the Ages.* Kampen, Netherlands: J. H. Kok, 1959.

Visser, Margaret. *Much Depends on Dinner.* New York: Grove Press, 1986.

Vijay, comp. *Sri Aurobindo and the Mother on Food.* Pondicherry, India: Sri Aurobindo Society, 1973.

Walters, Kerry S., and Lisa Portmess, eds. *Religious Vegetarianism: From Hesiod to the Dalai Lama.* Albany, NY: State University of New York Press, 2001.

Watson, George. *Nutrition and Your Mind.* New York: Pitman, 1971.

Westman, Dr. Eric C., Dr. Stephen D. Phinney, and Dr. Jeff S. Volek. *The New Atkins for a New You.* New York: Simon & Schuster, 2010.

White, Ellen G. *Counsels on Diet and Foods.* Hagerstown, Md.: Review and Herald, 2001.

_____. *The Ministry of Healing.* Nampa, ID: Pacific Press, 1942.

_____. *Testimonies for the Church.* Vols. 2–3. Nampa, ID: Pacific Press, 1948.

Williams, Roger J. *Nutrition against Disease.* New York: Pitman, 1971.

Wolf, Robb. *The Paleo Solution.* Las Vegas: Victory Belt, 2010.

Young, Richard Alan. *Is God a Vegetarian?* Chicago and La Salle, IL: Open Court, 1999.

INDEX

A

Abrahamic traditions, 113, 130–31, 160,
    169–70
abstention
    from alcohol, 249–51
    Gentiles and, 150
    from meat, 14, 20, 122, 151–52
    by spiritual masters, 297(n)
Academy for Nutrition and Dietetics,
    85
Acts, Book of, 150
Adam and Eve, 132–33
Adonis (god), 185, 243
African natives, 97–98, 182
aggressiveness, 38, 45, 105–6, 145,
    207
agricultural revolution
    blood type and, 229–30
    carbohydrates and, 199, 217, 233,
        235–36
    dairy products and, 222
    grain in, 182–83, 218–23, 233
    health decline during, 189–90, 217
agriculture, 40, 184–85
AHA. *See* American Heart Association
ahimsa (nonviolence), xviii, 117,
    119–20, 123–24, 127, 172
Akaranga Sutra, 127–28
Albo, Joseph, 17, 143–45
alcohol
    Buddhism and, 25, 77
    in food guides, 83
    in Paleo-style diets, 195

qualities of, 11–12, 36
spiritual teachings on, 47, 249–54
alcoholism, 196–97
Alfassa, Mirra, 172–73
allergies, 196
Alzheimer's disease, 203
Amaghanda Sutra, 124, 149
amaranth, 181–82, 246
ambiguity/ambivalence, 116, 169–70,
    174, 237
American Dietetic Association, 85, 109,
    204
American Heart Association, 107,
    204
American Psychiatric Association,
    55
amino acids, 87
Amirim village, 146–47
amylase enzyme, 193
Angra Mainyu (evil spirit), 115, 186
animal-based foods. *See also* dairy; meats
    and meat-eating
    aggression and, 38, 45, 105–6, 145, 207
    effects of avoiding, 20
    human development and, 112–14
    in traditional diets, 97–98
    vitamin B12 in, 87–89
    yang quality of, 36
animal-fat activators, 94–95, 98–99
Animal Liberation (Singer), xix, 176,
    189
animal-rights movement, 237

grain (*continued*)
    transformation of, 218–23
    whole, 80–81, 101, 111
grain effigies, 148, 185
grain-fed animals, 110–11, 191, 195–96,
        220
Gran, Gary, 13–14
Grandin, Temple, 139
grass-fed animals, 101, 110–11, 191,
        195–96, 206, 220
Great Mother (archetype), 182, 245
Greek mythology, 184–85
Gregory III (pope), 154
grihastha (householder), 117
gunas (primal qualities), xv–xvi, 7–14,
        48, 234, 305(n)
Guru Granth Sahib scriptures, 129
gut bacteria, 198

H

Hades (god), 184
halal standards (meat acceptable to
        Muslims), 168–69
Ha'Nish, Otoman Zar-Adusht, 33–34,
        48
Harvard School of Public Health
        (HSPH), 75, 79–84
harvesting, 221
Hawaii Diet, 208
Healing Foods Pyramid, 88–89, 89(f)
health
    agricultural revolution and, 189–90,
        217
    alcohol and, 249
    animals food and, 157–58
    carbohydrates and, 217,
        236
    grains and, 181
    meat and, 11, 32, 67–68, 297(n)
    Paleo-style diets and, 193–94
    vegetarianism and, 85, 232–33
health foods, xviii
healthy eating patterns, 74
Healthy Eating Plate, 79–83

Healthy Eating Pyramid, 83–84
Healthy Foods Pyramid, 79, 83–84
heart disease
    cholesterol and, 107–8, 110
    Ornish diet and, 208
    phytates protecting against, 197
    risk of, 83, 110, 194, 204
heavy metals, 197
herbs, 181
Hermeticism, 258–59
hermit (life stage), 117, 122. *See also*
        ascetics and asceticism
Hinayana Buddhism. *See* Theravada
        Buddhism
Hinduism. *See also* Brahmanism; Vedic
        culture
    animal sacrifice in, 114–16
    life stages or castes in, xv–xvi,
        117–18, 174–75
    meat-eating in, 118–20
    vegetarianism and, 113, 123, 169,
        286(n)
Hippocrates, 201
Hirsch, Raphael, 16–17
Hitler, Adolph, 46, 211
Hoffer, Abram, 54, 58–59
holistic viewpoint
    in Bhagavad Gita, 9–10, 14–16, 27,
        111–12
    of food groupings, 67–68
    macrobiotics and, 38, 42
    sattvic diet and, 51, 170
honey, 23, 127
Hopi people, 245
host (communion), 148
hot foods, as *rajasic,* 10–11
householder (life stage), 117, 122,
        174–75
HSPH. *See* Harvard School of Public
        Health
Huichol people, 244, 246
Huitzilopochtli (god), 246
human beings
    adaption to new foods by, 189,
        223